www.harco...yn...

Bringing you products from all Harcourt Health Sciences companies including Baillière Tindall, Churchill Livingstone, Mosby and W.B. Saunders

- **Browse** for latest informa... ...ooks, journals and electronic products

- **Search** for information on over 20 000 published titles with full product information including tables of contents and sample chapters

- **Keep up to date** with our extensive publishing programme in your field by registering with **eAlert** or requesting postal updates

- **Secure online ordering** with prompt delivery, as well as full contact details to order by phone, fax or post

- **News** of special features and promotions

If you are based in the following countries, please visit the country-specific site to receive full details of product availability and local ordering information

USA: www.harcourthealth.com

Canada: www.harcourtcanada.com

Australia: www.harcourt.com.au

Book No. **05194475**

30121 0 05194475

Managing and Implementing Decisions in Health Care

For Baillière Tindall:

Senior Commissioning Editor: Jacqueline Curthoys
Project Development Manager: Karen Gilmour
Project Manager: Jane Dingwall
Design Direction: George Ajayi

Six Steps to **Effective Management**

Managing and Implementing Decisions in Health Care

Edited by

Ann P Young BA MBA RGN RNT FRSH

Subject Leader, Strategic and International Management,
East London Business School,
University of East London, Dagenham, Essex

Mary Cooke RN CM RNT BSc(Hons) PGCE MSc(Econs)

Senior Research Fellow, University College Northampton;
Teacher and Assessor, Cambridge University, Cambridge

Foreword by

Pippa Gough MSc RN RM HV PGCEA

Fellow, King's Fund, London

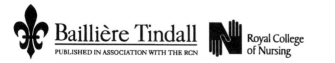

Baillière Tindall
PUBLISHED IN ASSOCIATION WITH THE RCN

Royal College of Nursing

EDINBURGH   LONDON   NEW YORK   PHILADELPHIA   SYDNEY   TORONTO   2002

Baillière Tindall
An imprint of Harcourt Publishers Limited

© Harcourt Publishers Limited 2002

✠ is a registered trademark of Harcourt Publishers Limited

The right of Ann Young and Mary Cooke to be identified as editors of this work has been asserted by them in accordance with the Copyright, Designs and Patents Act 1988

First published 2002

ISBN 0 7020 2516 X

British Library Cataloguing in Publication Data
A catalogue record for this book is available from the British Library

Library of Congress Cataloging in Publication Data
A catalog record for this book is available from the Library of Congress

Note
Medical knowledge is constantly changing. As new information becomes available, changes in treatment, procedures, equipment and the use of drugs become necessary. The editors, contributors and the publishers have taken care to ensure that the information given in this text is accurate and up to date. However, readers are strongly advised to confirm that the information, especially with regard to drug usage, complies with the latest legislation and standards of practice.

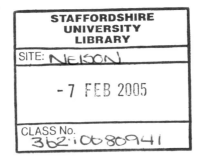

The publisher's policy is to use **paper manufactured from sustainable forests**

Printed in China

05194475

Six Steps to Effective Management series

Series editor: *Ann Young*

Managing the Business of Health Care
Edited by Julie Hyde and Frances Cooper

Managing and Implementing Decisions in Health Care
Edited by Ann Young and Mary Cooke

Managing and Leading Innovation in Health Care
Edited by Elizabeth Howkins and Cynthia Thornton

Managing Communication in Health Care
Edited by Mark Darley

Managing Diversity and Inequality in Health Care
Edited by Carol Baxter

Managing and Supporting People in Health Care
Edited by Margaret Buttigieg and Surrinder Kaur

About the series

The Six Steps to Effective Management series comes at a time when the speed and extent of change within health care have rarely been greater, and the challenges facing nurses and everyone working within the health care sector are extensive. The series identifies and discusses those challenges and suggests ways of managing them. It aims to be unique in that it links theory with practice through the application of evidence where available and includes case studies which build on sound and relevant theoretical material.

All nurses are required by the clinical governance agenda to have a grasp of management principles. The *Six Steps to Effective Management* series is both practical enough to appeal to the practitioner and theoretical enough to be useful to those undertaking courses at undergraduate or diploma level. The books are relevant to all nurses.

The series comprises six volumes that are carefully constructed to contain a mix of theoretical and practical approaches, research and case studies, including a variety of perspectives from different sectors of health care. Each volume is relevant, realistic and practical to encourage reflection and critical thinking to prepare readers for flexible and adaptable styles of management.

For more information on this series please contact: Harcourt Health Sciences Health Professions Marketing Department on +44 20 7424 4200.

Contents

Contributors   xii

Application Contributors   xiii

Foreword   xv

Preface   xvii

Section One   THE CONTEXT OF DECISION MAKING   1

Chapter One   **The political context of decision making**   3
Ann P Young

Application 1.1   *Ann P Young*
Facing the wider issues of recruitment difficulties   22
Application 1.2   *Ann P Young*
Department of Health publications   25

Chapter Two   **The influence of professional and statutory bodies on decision making**   27
Abigail Masterson and Ailsa Cameron

Application 2.1   *Abigail Masterson and Ailsa Cameron*
Case study: the development of specialist and advanced practice roles   39
Application 2.2   *Leslie Gelling and Mary Cooke*
The role of RCN interest groups in local decisions   46

Chapter Three   **Organisational culture and decision making**   50
Margaret Todd

Application 3.1   *Ann P Young*
Reflections of organisational culture in managerial job descriptions   65
Application 3.2   *Ann P Young*
Interview with the manager of a unit for those with behavioural disorders   72

Section Two   DECISION MAKING IN PRACTICE   77

Chapter Four   **The characteristics of decision making in health care**   79
David Sandland

Application 4.1   *Jane Hubert and Jennifer Gosling*
A day in the life of . . .   100
Application 4.2   *Mary Cooke*
Evaluating decisions: a case study from a
rural practice   108

Chapter Five   The practitioner as manager   **113**
Elizabeth A Smith and Ann P Young

Application 5.1   *Samantha Lawrence and Mary Cooke*
Managing staff and residents in a nursing
home: conflicts in decision making   125

Chapter Six   Affecting decisions through networks
and group processes   **128**
Debbie Lee

Application 6.1   *Ann P Young*
Networking by middle managers in health care   144
Application 6.2   *Ann P Young*
Team roles and decision making   148

Section Three   USER PARTICIPATION IN DECISION
MAKING   **151**

Chapter Seven   Patient empowerment and the power
of patients   **155**
Mary Cooke

Application 7.1   *Mary Cooke*
Empowerment of patients   173
Application 7.2   *Mary Cooke*
Empowerment of users   177
Application 7.3   *Mary Cooke*
Complaints and complainants   180

Chapter Eight   Consumer groups and community voices   **182**
Mary Cooke

Application 8.1   *Mary Cooke*
Grassroots organisations and user support groups   200

Chapter Nine   Patients' rights and responsibilities   **203**
Trevor Ride

Application 9.1   *Mary Cooke*
Patients' rights and responsibilities and The NHS Plan   223

Contents

Six Steps to **Effective Management**

Section Four   THE IMPLEMENTATION OF STRATEGY AT LOCAL LEVEL   231

Chapter Ten   **The practitioner and strategic decision making** 233
Mary Cooke

Application 10.1   *Josephine Nwaelene*
User involvement in strategic information
planning in a chemical pathology unit: extracts from a
management project   247
Application 10.2   *Lenore Anderson*
Reengineering: a case study   251

Chapter Eleven   **Autonomy and initiative in
implementing strategic decisions**   256
Ann P Young

Application 11.1   *Ann P Young*
Managerial perceptions of initiative   272
Application 11.2   *Ann P Young*
Assertiveness and leadership skills   276

Chapter Twelve   **Using clinical research to underpin
decision making in health care: a case study approach**   280
Christopher Loughlan

Application 12.1   *Christopher Loughlan*
Findings and methodology   291

Section Five   MANAGING RISK AND CRISIS   293

Chapter Thirteen   **Managing risk and crisis: legal and
ethical implications**   295
Beverley Hunt

Application 13.1   *Beverley Hunt*
Guidelines and protocols: issues of legal liability   314
Application 13.2   *Lenore Anderson*
The importance of documentation in
assessing risk   319

Chapter Fourteen   **Assessing and managing risk**   323
Lenore Anderson

Application 14.1   *Lenore Anderson*
Implementing risk management strategies   344
Application 14.2   *Mike Flynn*
Managing children's services: a risky business   347

Contents

Chapter 15   **Crisis management: creating order out of chaos**   351
Trevor Dolan and Nigel Northcott

Application 15.1   *Mary Cooke*
Interview with a clinical manager in A&E   365

Index   369

Contents

xi

Contributors

Lenore Anderson BSc(Hons) CertEd DipNurs(Lond) RN SCM
Senior Nurse, Central Nursing, Addenbrooke's NHS Trust, Cambridge

Ailsa Cameron BA(Hons) MSc
Research Fellow, School for Policy Studies, University of Bristol, Bristol

Mary Cooke RN CM RNT BSc(Hons) PGCE MSc(Econs)
Senior Research Fellow, University College Northampton; Teacher and
Assessor, Cambridge University, Cambridge

Trevor Dolan RGN RSCN BA(Hons)
Director, Alternative Strategies, Organisation Consulting Associates and
Senior Lecturer, Health Management, Oxford Brookes University, Oxford

Beverley Hunt RGN BEd(Hons) MA
Medical Law and Ethics and Fellow in Education and Leadership
Development, King's Fund, London

Debbie Lee RGN CIM DipN MBA
Chief Executive, LMTG Associates Ltd, Harrogate

Christopher Loughlan BSc CertEd DipEd MEd PhD
Research and Development and Teaching Manager, Addenbrooke's
NHS Trust, Cambridge

Abigail Masterson MN BSc RGN PGCEA
Director, Abi Masterson Consulting Ltd, Southampton

Nigel Northcott PhD RGN MA(Ed) DipN
Independent Nurse/Management/Education Consultant

Trevor Ride MA BA(Hons) RN DipNurs DipHSM
Consultant in Nursing and Health Policy, Office of Nursing Policy
Associates, Cheshunt, Hertfordshire

David Sandland BSc MSc DMS PhD
Associate Lecturer, University of East London, East London Business
School, Dagenham, Essex

Elizabeth A Smith
St Mary's Convent and Nursing Home Chiswick, London

Margaret Todd RNLD RMN RGN DipN(Lond) BA(Hons) MBA
Senior Lecturer, University of Hertfordshire, Department of Health
and Social Care, Hatfield, Hertfordshire

Ann P Young BA MBA RGN RNT FRSH
Subject Leader, Strategic and International Management, East
London Business School, University of East London, Dagenham, Essex

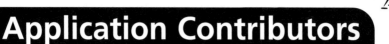

Application Contributors

Lenore Anderson BSc(Hons) CertEd DipNurs(Lond) RN SCM
Senior Nurse, Central Nursing, Addenbrooke's NHS Trust, Cambridge

Ailsa Cameron BA(Oxon) MSc(Lond)
Research Fellow, School for Policy Studies, University of Bristol, Bristol

Mary Cooke RN CM RNT BSc(Hons) PGCE MSc(Econs)
Senior Research Fellow, University College Northampton; Teacher and
Assessor, Cambridge University, Cambridge

Michael J Flynn RSCN RGN MBA
General Manager – Child Health, The Medway NHS Trust, Medway
Maritime Hospital, Gillingham, Kent

Sue Fraser-Betts RGN SCM BSc
Matron, BUPA Hartswood Hospital, Eagleway, Brentwood, Essex

Leslie Gelling BSc(Hons) MA RGN
Nurse Researcher, Academic Neurosurgery Unit, University of
Cambridge, Cambridge

Jennifer Gosling BA(Hons) MSc
Practice Manager, Iveagh House Surgery, London

Diane Horsington RGN BSc
Deputy General Manager, Emergency Patient Service/Medicine,
Medway Maritime Hospital, Gillingham, Kent

Jane Hubert RGN DMS
Service Manager – Surgery, The Royal Free Hospital NHS Trust,
London

Beverley Hunt RGN BEd(Hons) MA
Medical Law and Ethics and Fellow in Education and Leadership
Development, King's Fund, London

Samantha Lawrence BSc(Hons) DipN(Lond) RGN MCI Mgmt (NVQ5)
ENB 941 998 D32/33
Formerly matron/manager

Christopher Loughlan BSc CertEd DipEd MEd PhD
Research and Development and Teaching Manager, Addenbrooke's
NHS Trust, Cambridge

Abigail Masterson MN BSc RGN PGCEA
Director, Abi Masterson Consulting Ltd, Southampton

Six Steps to **Effective Management**

Josephine Chibuzor Nwaelene BSc(Hons) MBA
Biomedical Scientist, The Royal London Hospital, London

Ann P Young BA MBA RGN RNT FRSH
Subject Leader, Strategic and International Management, East
London Business School, University of East London, Dagenham, Essex

Application Contributors

Foreword

Modernising the health services requires fundamental and radical change at all levels of service. New organisational structures are demanding different accountabilities and altered management relationships. Change of this scope and nature requires a capturing of the hearts and minds of the people providing the care and a recognition of their potential to inform and shape strategic and operational decisions. If health care professionals, with special reference to nurses, are not enabled to 'get on board' in this way then the modernisation agenda will fail.

To be able to rise to this challenge and participate in re-shaping and improving services, nurses and other professionals need to be equipped to manage complexity, uncertainty, ambiguity and intractability of problems which exist in a concentration such as is not found elsewhere in the service industries. The NHS is characterised by 'wicked' problems which complicate the decision-making process and make absolute or perfect solutions intangible. No single approach or strategy will fit all the situations that arise. Practitioners and managers must be skilled in selecting the right tools for the particular circumstances that face them. They also need to recognise that the world of health care is at best chaotic and messy and that a muddling through, or incremental, approach to decision making is probably the best that it gets.

Currently, the complexity of decision making has been compounded by the pace of modernising reform which has created an environment which demands more patient-focused services; has more complex lines of accountability and responsibility – the consequence of flatter organisations and the increasing emphasis on interorganisational partnership working; needs new roles which have a greater emphasis on strong interpersonal relationships and political sophistication; and sustains pressure to innovate continuously to improve service delivery and quality. These reforms are of course to be applauded; but there also needs to be a recognition of the toll this can take on sometimes struggling, over-stretched health care workers.

In response, leadership development and management training now needs to understand how people change, adapt and apply learning about decision making in the workplace. Practitioners must be able to transfer their learning back into organisations in ways that develop organisational memory and deliver change. Support is needed to enable people to put new ideas into practice. It is not enough simply to have knowledge without it being applied and the learning drawn from experience of applying knowledge. This may sometimes mean dealing with failure as well as success; but failure may provide some of the most powerful learning.

This book aims to smooth some of the pain of application by explicating some of the theoretical aspects of managing in the NHS and also by providing real life examples of how nurses and others have adapted their skills learned in the clinical areas and around management tables, to new ways of managing in the new NHS. As such it is a timely and ambitious book which breaks new ground by bringing together in one place insights into the complexity of decision making in today's changing health services and highlighting the way in which health care professionals can participate actively in this process. As such it makes compelling and essential reading.

Pippa Gough

Preface

There are two common misconceptions about decision making. The first is that this is a rational and scientific process and the second that a decision is made at a specific point in time. In fact, making decisions is an incredibly complex and ongoing activity involving an interaction between the individual and the whole organisation in which that person operates. These beliefs underpin the contributions to this book on managing and implementing decisions in health care.

This volume forms part of a series that addresses issues in health care that have become increasingly critical as the rate of change continually accelerates. In such circumstances, old patterns of behaviour may become inappropriate while members of the professional health care team may be hurried into making decisions without due consideration of broader and longer term consequences. The approach taken in this series is to avoid telling practitioners and managers what they should be doing. Prescriptions will usually only work once diagnosis has been made. With many variations possible, a much more constructive approach is to enable analysis of a range of situations and then to select action from a number of possibilities. The book is structured to facilitate this approach with a number of chapters that provide relevant theoretical material followed by 'applications' to illustrate how professionals and managers have made and implemented decisions in practice. Such an approach, it is hoped, will encourage critical thinking and reflection and aid application to practice in flexible and appropriate ways.

The volume is divided into five sections and starts by exploring the context in which health care decision making takes place. Section One emphasises the political, professional and cultural features of decision making. One of the particular problems facing health care in the UK, particularly the NHS, is the high public profile it holds. Political involvement in response to public opinion is inevitable, making the implementation of strategic long-term decisions difficult. The power of health care professionals in this process has also been critical and although this influence has largely been medical, nursing and other paraprofessions are waking up to the possibility of influencing decisions at operational and local levels in important ways. Moving from the national to the local context of decision making, the part played by organisational culture is introduced, a theme revisited throughout the book.

Section Two is about practice. Its focus is very much on how decisions are made on a day-to-day basis. Starting with a comprehensive analysis of the nature and types of decision making, Section Two asks the reader to apply these frameworks to the realities faced by practitioners and managers in a range of settings, acute and primary care, urban and rural, NHS and private sector. The inevitable involvement of the practitioner in a management role is explored and the central importance of making and implementing decisions through team processes and networks is underlined.

Having taken a broad sweep across the context and content of decision making in Sections One and Two, the book turns to more specific issues in the remaining Sections Three, Four and Five. Particularly problematic areas of decision making are selected for this purpose: user participation; practitioner involvement in strategic implementation; and the management of risk and crisis.

Section Three explores the issues around user participation, including the relationships between patients, users, consumers and the communities being served. Although empowerment has become a rather overused word in recent literature, the issue of patient and community empowerment has not yet been fully tackled. The realities arising out of some theoretical possibilities are presented. Some progress has been made, as demonstrated by the applications, but more remains to be done. The balance between rights and responsibilities also needs further work and the part played by patients' charters is explored.

The nature of change in health care has largely followed a top-down approach with strategic decisions being imposed on middle managers and practitioners as a result of political and/or business-orientated actions. Section Four looks at the interface of organisational demands and individual autonomy at the point of strategic implementation. Although broad frameworks might be set, the ability of practitioners and managers to make a difference is emphasised. Calling on professional support, building small successes that have the potential to escalate and arguing on the basis of research findings are just some of the tools that can be used to influence decisions about implementation. The key importance of individual skills in self-assertion and leadership is emphasised and is particularly important to professional groups that are largely female and/or non-white.

Section Five, on managing risk and crisis, provides possible approaches but no easy answers. The legal basis of risk and crisis management is presented and some ways of dealing with and developing relevant documentation are put forward. Various practical tools are also suggested. Although a number of crisis points exist in health care, the book concludes by focusing on acute care as the problems of accident and emergency departments and insufficient hospital beds are still a long way from being resolved. However, some of the lessons learned here are applicable to any crisis situation at both practical and ethical levels.

It is not necessary to read this book from cover to cover. Although, as explained above, the material is organised into a logical sequence, it is both possible and likely that the reader will dip into sections in order to meet a particular need. Sound information is provided in the longer theory-based chapters while it is hoped that the mix of experiences described and exercises suggested in the applications will enable readers to relate to and interact with the material in ways that will help them address real situations in their own working lives.

Ann Young and Mary Cooke

Section **One**

THE CONTEXT OF DECISION MAKING

OVERVIEW

How decisions are made is very dependent on the context in which the decision makers find themselves. Decision making is therefore likely to follow different pathways depending on the political, structural and organisational frameworks found.

The aim of Section One of this book is to highlight a number of these contextual issues that underpin decision making in health care. The main emphasis is on UK health care but some points of comparison with the rest of Europe are made and the literature used draws on US material as well as that from Europe. It has to be admitted, though, that the contexts explored are advanced Western democracies rather than newly developing countries where the influences on decision making may be rather different.

Section One consists of three largely theoretical chapters with supporting material applying the concepts presented in a number of different ways. Chapter One, the political context of decision making, identifies a number of broad-ranging influences on the decision-making process, whether in the public or private health care sector. Two applications serve to illustrate the political face of health care decision making. The first takes the sensitive issue of staffing difficulties at practitioner level. The second invites the reader to use the Internet to visit the Department of Health. A series of activities bring home the uncertainties and lack of overall control in individual organisations faced with a massive amount of policy material from government.

Chapter Two moves from the very wide-ranging perspective of Chapter One to a closer focus on one professional group, nursing, although much that is presented is typical of other paramedical groups in health care. The relationship between the UK government as represented by the Department of Health and the civil service, the statutory and professional bodies for nursing and the major employee of nurses, the NHS, is explored.

The third chapter of Section One, while also taking a broad contextual approach to decision making, focuses on the organisation and examines the pervasive effect of workplace culture on how decisions are made. Culture is seen as being inexorably linked, not only to the way people work but how they think and view their world. However, Todd makes the important point that it is unlikely, particularly in a professional organisation, that only one culture exists. She highlights the important effects of subcultures, particularly in the management of change. A consideration of this leads the reader on to Section Two where the practicalities of managing decisions are the main theme.

Chapter **One**

The political context of decision making

Ann P Young

- ● Decision making in a democratic context
- ● The role of the state and Parliamentary political parties in decision making
- ● Decision making and stakeholder power
- ● Changing political frameworks: learning from history?
- ● Conclusion

O VERVIEW

Much that is written about decision making assumes that this is a rational activity, thought through on a logical basis and following a clear sequence of events. The reality, as any manager knows well, is very different. Decisions may only be argued as rational after the event. Acceptable reasons are found to justify or persuade others to accept decisions already made for very different reasons.

This chapter will particularly explore the effect of the political context on decision making in health care. It will take the word 'politics' to include both the national political processes of Parliamentary parties as well as the effects of power relations at organizational level. In highlighting some of the influences that underpin decisions in the health sector, it is suggested that the questions raised should be kept in mind when reading the other chapters of this volume.

The chapter concludes by reflecting on future patterns of decision making.

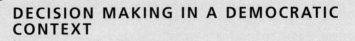

DECISION MAKING IN A DEMOCRATIC CONTEXT

The context of decision making

Managers can make decisions:

- autocratically with or without consultation
- democratically where subordinates have an equal say in the decision
- by consensus where all parties discuss until they agree a decision.

Within the organisational setting, managers usually reach some kind of balance between these different decision-making techniques, depending on organisational culture, personal style and the particular needs pertaining at the time. However, there is a pressure in large bureaucratic organisations, typical of many NHS organisations and the larger private health care companies, to impose decisions on subordinates. For two reasons, this may seem inappropriate or unacceptable. First, as citizens of a democracy, particularly when working in the public sector, employees value concepts such as equality and choice. Second, the professionals who usually make up a large proportion of the health care workforce value their own autonomy and expect some degree of consultation and involvement in the decision-making process. Some of these issues are now discussed in more detail.

Decision making in a democracy

'The creed of democracy and equality must always be given vigorous and vociferous support' said Dahl (1961, p. 95) when exploring democracy and power in an American city. The word 'democracy' carries such a positive aura that even those governments that require a considerable stretch of the imagination to be called 'democratic' attach the name to themselves; for example, 'the people's democratic socialist republic', where a single party system claims to rule in the interests of the people as a whole. The Western pattern emphasises a different aspect of democracy.

Democracy (rule by the people) in the modern state has to be by representation through election to a policy-making body (Wollheim 1975). Occasionally specific issues may be taken to the electorate for a direct decision by means of a referendum but its timing and content will be decided by government. Such an event is rare in the UK. Decisions are usually made on the basis of majorities but a key characteristic is 'the granting of the right of political expression to minorities' (Burnham 1941, p. 162).

However, for a number of reasons, decision making fails to match democratic expectations.

Sources of influence in the political arena

Firstly, how can a democratic system work amid inequality? Sources of influence are likely to include:

- social standing
- access to cash, credit and wealth
- access to legal powers of office
- popularity and
- control over information.

Dahl (1961) suggested that virtually no-one, certainly no group, is entirely lacking in access to some of these resources although they are unequally distributed. However, a resource is only a potential source of influence. Some individuals can choose not to use resources or to use them in different ways at different times for both 'objective' reasons, relating to location, wealth, education and occupation, and 'subjective' reasons at a more personal and individual level. Some of these points can be applied to health care. With this sitting mainly in the public sector in the UK, it might be reasonable to expect democratic decision making at macro level. However, commissioning authorities are largely appointed rather than elected and seem distant to the electorate.

Although more information is now being made available, for example with the publication of local patient charter results, it is fragmented and patchy and needs to be made more cohesive at organisational level. If information on needs, costing, the development of standards and public/patient views could be brought together and shared more widely between stakeholders, the quality of decision making might be enhanced (Young 1996a).

The political processes of decision making

A second reason for democratic decision making to be flawed is the way in which political processes can very successfully prevent access of some individuals and groups in spite of their potential influence through the resources mentioned above. Bachrach & Baratz's work (1970) on this made a major contribution to decision making in identifying the 'mobilisation of bias' to keep certain

The political context of decision making

policy conflicts out of the agenda. The process can thus act as a filter to allow certain items through while blocking others. They suggested that political systems and subsystems operate systematically and consistently to the benefit of certain persons and groups at the expense of others.

Decision making involves rituals and game rules, biased in favour of those maintaining the status quo who may be a minority or elite group. Advocates of change must win at all stages of the political process, while the defenders of existing policy must win at only one stage of the process. This 'one stage' is, not surprisingly, at the point of implementation, although for an unwanted issue to get this far is almost a failure of power on the part of the powerful! For change, certain stages must be achieved.

- Stage 1: an issue must be recognised.
- Stage 2: it must then be made visible.
- Stage 3: it must get access to the relevant decision-making arena.
- Stage 4: finally, it must succeed at the implementation stage.

Although some aspects of a power struggle may be apparent at the latter three stages, at stage 1, a power struggle appears to be absent as not even the less powerful may recognise it as a struggle.

These realities of decision making are important to health services. Identifying which groups are influential within the process may not change it but may facilitate the more effective use of political resources and increase the amount of influence exerted (see below re stakeholders). In order to change the process, more structural changes are necessary from an unhealthy concentration of power in a centralised elite to one involving local groups to a greater degree than is currently the case. However, decentralisation can take two distinct forms. Managerial decentralisation, seen in the NHS to some extent, works on a business model to improve efficiency and quality to local users. Not yet seen is political decentralisation of health care with local decision making enhancing local democracy although a number of techniques are being tried to gather these 'local voices'. However, gathering local views may be insufficient, as Popay & Williams (1994) identified.

> On the policy front, it is likely that many NHS managers and professionals will not have the skills necessary to listen to what local people have to say as residents or as patients. (p. 93)

Professional attitudes about the role of experts may be part of the problem, preventing a democratic approach (see below).

Matching policy aims and actual outcomes

A third influence on decision making are the outcomes required. 'Policy should be judged by its actual impact rather than its intentions' (Lowe 1993, p. 46). This seems to be a wise statement, bearing in mind that intentions are often unclear and conflicting. A welfare state has broad aims of universal access, equality and social justice. These have to be achieved within economic efficiency and individual freedom, creating a practical implementation problem. One way for the state to deal with this is to leave wide the gap between policy and implementation. This can also happen at organisational level between strategic decisions and operational action. Discretion is built into the system but, as a result, the clarity of outcomes is often fudged.

In health care, evidence of success or failure is often clouded in rhetoric and dressed up in scientific guise, for example with published quantitative measures. However, the selection of these measures is subject to bias.

> Who chooses what measures is a question that should be asked. The government has been largely instrumental in leading this process, with managers and professionals following behind, and the measures chosen relied initially on what was most readily available, not necessarily on what was most useful and reliable. (Young 1996a, p. 350)

Young also pointed out that a reliance on quantitative data omitted a range of key issues that are qualitative in nature and these are particularly important to health care professionals.

THE ROLE OF THE STATE AND PARLIAMENTARY POLITICAL PARTIES IN DECISION MAKING

The role of the state

The state has a long history, around 5000 years, but not surprisingly has changed its nature over this time. On the whole, there is agreement that it plays an economic role and is therefore the body which has a monopoly over taxation and money supply (Needle 1994).

The modern state usually possesses a set of clearly differentiated political institutions:

The political context of decision making

- an executive
- a legislature
- a judiciary
- armed forces and police (not discussed in this chapter).

These do not necessarily constitute a united body and tensions exist between and within them. For health care organisations, the relationship between statute, statutory instrument, NHS executive guidelines and legal interpretations in the courts can lead to some confusion over what the state is requiring of its health care managers. For example, to fulfil a contract set through the commissioning process (NHS Act 1990) within an imposed price tariff that is not based on true costs (NHS Executive) as well as ensuring the safety of patients in conditions of resource shortages (the civil law on negligence) is a tall order.

The legislature, i.e. Parliament, is often seen as the site of state regulation. However, there are a number of ways in which the state controls its citizenry that avoid the necessity of taking new statutes through the full Parliamentary process. For example, delegated legislation through statutory instruments and rules can be drawn up by some nominated body (so enabled by statute) and will become law once approved by the Secretary of State. Most Acts of Parliament require clarification as they contain insufficient detail. Codes of practice are often developed which, although not legally enforceable, can be sufficiently powerful to seriously embarrass those not following them, for example in the field of employment. In these two circumstances, the question needs to be asked: who has been given (or taken) the power to supplement formal legislative process and how did they acquire this? The extent to which the state legislature can actually exert control is also debatable. Burnham (1941) suggested that sovereignty had been slipping away from Parliament since World War I, and the issues around the European Community are but the most recent examples of this. Certainly, the development of the European Community has already had a number of effects at organisational level. Although the UK opted out of the Social Chapter of the Maastricht Treaty, regulations from Brussels have already taken precedence over national rulings, particularly in the area of Health & Safety at work and employment issues. The current debate over entry into economic monetary union has major implications for the role of government over the economy.

Separate from legislation, the state executive aims to regulate through bureaucratic processes. The power of the civil service may have been reduced as large chunks have been hived off into semi-privatised agencies but the government still relies on its civil servants to shift through large volumes of information and suggest possible decisions. The advice given usually remains invisible. For example, in the area of health care, not all reports that have been commissioned have been published and one has to wonder what happens if recommendations are not in line with a government decision already made. Government itself has its executive arm in the offices of Prime Minister and Cabinet. Again, decisions made here lack visibility and potentially lose some accountability to the citizenry.

The third branch of state control is the judiciary. Although the UK citizen has the right to trial by jury, most criminal justice is enacted at magistrate level, usually without a jury. Civil law totally relies for its interpretation on judges. England is unusual in the development of civil law through the courts rather than the legislature. Civil law is therefore often known as judge-made law (Pannett 1992) and the aims of the state judiciary may not always be congruent with either its executive or legislature. For example, the release of information may be required by a court hearing a case whereas the executive might deem some information as too sensitive for public consumption. The government might call on the Official Secrets Act only to be overruled by the judges.

The control of the judiciary, although officially by the Head of State, is usually identified as being in the hands of an elite upper class who may also wield considerable power over the legislature and the executive. As described by Jessop (in Waters 1994, p. 229):

> The state is not an independent and sovereign political subject but is an instrument of coercion and administration which can be used for various purposes by whatever interests manage to appropriate it.

The interests of certain political parties are discussed next.

Political parties and decision making

Assumptions have been made that different political parties are 'disposed to think and behave in certain ways, prefer certain kinds of conduct and disposed to make certain choices' (Oakeshott 1975, p. 23). Historically, the UK has supported a laissez-faire approach to government. Oakeshott labels this as being conservative:

> To be conservative is to prefer the familiar to the unknown, to prefer the tried to the untried, fact to mystery, the actual to the possible, the limited to the unbounded, the near to the distant, the

The political context of decision making

sufficient to the superabundant, the convenient to the perfect, present laughter to utopian bliss. (p. 24)

Conservatism prefers 'to enforce a rule it has got rather than invent a new one' (p. 46) and to encourage citizens to make their own choices without much government imposition of others' beliefs and activities. It therefore supports an individualistic citizen.

By contrast, socialism is hostile to laissez-faire and economic competition, believing instead in collective and cooperative action as a means of improving the conditions of the poor (Cole 1975). Although socialism developed in a number of different ways, the version most often found in Western labour and socialist parties is Fabian socialism. This non-revolutionary approach relies on justice and human brotherhood, rather than class power, with the expectation that extended suffrage and responsible government will extract concessions from the ruling class and claim an increasing share of political authority (Cole 1975, p. 93).

Conservative and socialist thinking present two political extremes but in reality neither the UK Conservative nor Labour party is typical of these beliefs although some elements are recognisable. Instead, Hayek (1975) proposed that the underlying political order in the UK (as elsewhere in the Anglo-Saxon world) was liberal. Key concepts within this type of political order are:

- individual liberty under the law
- self-generating or spontaneous order in social affairs
- the greater utilisation of its citizens' knowledge and skill than is possible under central direction
- protection of a recognisable individual private domain
- enforcement of universal rules of just conduct.

The liberal concept therefore is inseparable from the institution of private property and the market as well as having strong links with a common-law conception of justice (i.e. the duty of care owed to each other and the role of individual consent rather than state coercion). Hayek went on to explain that where the market does not produce some services adequately, government has the discretion to dispose of some of its resources in services to its citizens.

The liberal underpinning to a number of political parties in the West and elsewhere is apparent. Using the example of health care policy, Saltman & Von Otter (1995) were unable to link the current changes towards more marketised health care systems in Europe to any particular political party and in the UK, Ham (1997b) identified increasing convergence between the main political parties over the future of health care.

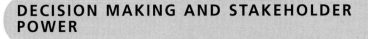
DECISION MAKING AND STAKEHOLDER POWER

Although important, the broad context discussed above must be set within the more local arena of the health care organisation. Here, a number of influences affect the decision-making process and one way of analysing, and using, these is through stakeholder power.

Stakeholder analysis

Stakeholders are groups or individuals who have a stake in or an expectation of the organisation's performance (Johnson & Scholes 1999). They can be external or internal to the organisation, will share attitudes and expectations with others, probably belong to more than one stakeholder group and will surface as a result of events. The concept of stakeholders can, therefore, be a useful one in relation to decision making if their existence is then linked to the amount of power that they have.

Common sources of organisational power have been identified as follows:

- hierarchy and status
- influencing and negotiating skills
- control of strategic resources
- possession of knowledge and associated skills useful to the organisation
- internal and external networks
- involvement in strategic implementation, for example through the exercise of managerial discretion in how strategy will be translated into operations.

For stakeholder analysis to be carried out, the relative power of the stakeholders needs to be assessed. For example, status can be measured by position in the hierarchy, salary relative to others and average grade of staff managed. The size of the budget managed, particularly if it is discretionary, will be an indicator. Symbols of power are very pervasive in organisations and very important as indicators. For example, the size of office, the allocation of a car parking space and the existence of a personal assistant are just a few commonly found.

Johnson & Scholes went on to demonstrate how stakeholder mapping could be done. They suggested two possible matrices:

The political context of decision making

11

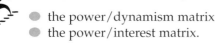

● the power/dynamism matrix
● the power/interest matrix.

In the first the level of power of stakeholders is mapped against how predictable their behaviour is likely to be, those on the low-power/high-predictability quadrant creating the fewest problems while those with high power and behaving unpredictably present the greatest danger or opportunities. The second matrix maps power against level of interest in the change proposed. Low-power/low-interest stakeholders require minimal effort while high-power stakeholders with a high level of interest are inevitably the key players of any potential change.

This exercise can be applied to health care organisations to suggest the effect of employees, managers, the chief executive, external customers, patients, relatives, the general public, and any others that are relevant, on the particular organisational changes being examined. However, the rest of this section concentrates on the power of professionals as key stakeholders in health care.

The professional as stakeholder

Health care professionals are finding that power seems to have shifted and there is a need for them to act in a consciously political way in relation to decision making rather than relying on their position as professional expert.

In the past, health care was dominated by the medical profession through their role as 'gatekeepers'. Also playing a part are the professions allied to medicine (PAMs) which include nursing, physiotherapy, radiography and midwifery and those more closely linked to administration, e.g. accountancy and personnel. Such a list demonstrates the difficulty of categorisation as well as hinting at the changing nature of professional influence in health care. In addition, the relationship of the professional to the decision-making process is varied. Professionals work in a number of different organisations, from public to private sector or as the bosses of their own small businesses. A large number of health carers still work for the NHS but increasingly a spell in a private hospital or clinic is being seen as a sensible career option while some, either through choice or forced redundancy, are taking the self-employed route through agency work, consultancy or setting up their own specialist clinic or nursing home.

It is therefore important to view professional power as a fluid state of affairs. There are differences of power between and within professions with changing coalitions and 'horizontal fissures' (Armstrong 1984) of differential privilege and status. For example, cardiac surgeons carry more power than public health physicians and intensive care nurses more prestige than nurses caring for the elderly infirm. In addition, in the health care arena, Abbott (1988) emphasised the interdependence of professional development. For example, nurses have been eager to extend their role into work traditionally undertaken by doctors who, in turn, have been willing to allow this in order to maintain control over less determinate areas of knowledge.

The changing context in which health care organisations operate has had an important effect on professional relationships. It is suggested that the current transitions in health care may affect clinical managers' power bases as follows.

1. Power under challenge and probably reducing:

● existing power as traditional working patterns change
● formal authority from position in the hierarchy
● control of knowledge and information as this becomes more transparent.

2. Power changing but some potential opportunities still existing:

● control of scarce resources, for example finance
● use of organisational structures, rules and regulations
● involvement with interpersonal alliances and networks.

3. Power can grow if manager can get involved:

● control of boundaries/interfaces
● control of technology.

Two aspects of resources are particularly relevant to health care professionals at this time.

Financial control

Finance looms large in any debate on organisational control. Clinical professionals have become involved with budgetary planning and control where previously this was not included in their role and their awareness of the financial function has increased rapidly. Decisions on the physical resources are the easiest to juggle with in the short term but, for most professionals, the debate is now firmly on making efficiency savings from the human resource and this has had particular implications for professional power (see below).

The political context of decision making

The control of knowledge

It is important for the continuation of any profession that it can maintain a discrete body of knowledge that is not readily accessible to those outside the profession. The control of this knowledge is therefore an important power mechanism. However, a number of far-reaching changes have seriously undermined this position.

- The increasing transparency of expert knowledge as the media and advances in information technology have enabled a wide audience to access previously hidden knowledge.
- A shifting in the specific knowledge base of most health care professionals with rapid changes in job content and government support of the use of health care assistants with National Vocational Qualifications (NVQs), who sit outside the professional framework.

Evidence on the amount of power exerted by different groups of professionals is difficult to come by. Although there are suggestions that professional power is declining or certainly facing serious challenges, other evidence points to continuing professional domination. It is likely that the medical profession has had to lose some ground in the face of external regulation over individual salaries or payments as well as through central budgets and non-financial measures of quality audit and managed care.

The techniques used by professionals to reduce the impact of change seem to follow two routes. First is the invasion of management posts by doctors and nurses who, although to some extent being management trained, do not identify themselves with a managerialist culture. Second is a refusal by doctors either to become involved in or even to recognise the validity of managerial authority. Harrison & Pollitt (1994) suggest that three approaches are available to health care politicians and executives:

- to challenge the professionals
- to incorporate them or
- to change the environment.

Even so, success is likely to be restricted and governments need to acknowledge the limits to external professional regulation, particularly of the doctors. Users also resist changes in decision-making processes. Spiers (1995) suggested a basic unwillingness for involvement when people enter the system as patients as they collude with doctors to maintain the status quo. Such attitudes underlie some of the difficulties of implementing change in health care.

CHANGING POLITICAL FRAMEWORKS: LEARNING FROM HISTORY?

The hope is that the introduction of change, even if unwanted or painful, will in some way be beneficial. There is also the argument that history will be of value in understanding the present and thereby learning from it. 'History does not precisely repeat itself' (Thane 1982, p. 2) and this idea has been applied to organisations as the concept of organisational learning. This section, within the frameworks already discussed, will explore how change appears to have impacted on health care at operational level.

The visibility of change

One visible aspect of the change process is restructuring at both sector and organisational levels. There is an expectation, certainly in the UK, that it is a necessary concomitant of change. The introduction of planned markets into health care, probably one of the most marked changes to health care in recent times, required a dismantling of previous structures and the development of reconfigured ones in order to manage the purchaser/provider split. The nature of restructuring at organisational level is a reflection on how the process of reform is managed. General trends in both private and public organisations are to reduce bureaucracy, remove layers and encourage multiskilling and flexibility of the workforce but variations are found in how it is done. Ham (1997a) saw a 'big bang' approach as being typical of the UK. An incremental approach is more likely in The Netherlands where politically there is more emphasis on consensus and coalition which will lead to a gradual evolution of organisational structures while the bottom-up process in Sweden has led to a number of natural experiments in design (Ham 1997a).

Usually, such restructuring at organisational level is not imposed in detail by central policy makers. However, the Norwegian government believed strongly that organisational design would have a significant impact on the content of decisions made and it appeared to reserve the right of government to design the organisational apparatus within which its political goals were to be achieved (Pettigrew et al 1992).

The UK history of laissez-faire would make such an approach difficult in this country. Instead, policy ambiguities have allowed quite marked discretion to local purchasers and professional providers. Hunter (1998), in reviewing Rivett's history of the NHS, *From Cradle to Grave*, commented on the reasonable success of policy at the level of high politics but highlighted the weaknesses at micro-management level. He compared this to the US 'non-system' of health care which was more successful at this level in spite of it standing for all that the UK sought to eradicate. The US achieved 'reform without reform' with a decentralised and highly pluralistic pattern of care (Ham 1997a), while in the UK, the approach of the NHS to the medical profession and the effectiveness of intervention has proved 'somewhat feeble and wimpish' (Hunter 1998).

Enough research has been done to demonstrate the potential importance of restructuring on the implementation of change in both public and private organisations. However, Beer et al (1990) demonstrated that the top-down imposition of formal structures does not always lead to desired outcomes, for example in the implementation of total quality management (TQM). Also important are the level of agreement on objectives, continuities with the past and relationships between different power groups.

The imposition of new accountability measures

One of the drivers of the decision-making process is accountability. The nature of this accountability may vary between the public and private sectors but changes imposed by government over the last 15 years have brought these two sectors closer.

In spite of rhetoric to the contrary, the underlying reason for the introduction of both general management and planned markets into public health care was doubtless to drive down costs and exert stronger financial control over the seemingly bottomless pit of health care expenditure. The introduction of general management in the mid-1980s made little impact on controlling costs through business plans and devolved budgets. Professionals in the clinical areas saw it as unacceptable that accountants should have a major influence on decisions that affect clinical care and were also concerned that a short-term view would take precedence over long-term benefits that initially seemed more expensive (Young 1996b).

It is, however, difficult to get away from an expenditure-based accountability system in the public sector. As pointed out in the Local Government Training Board's Discussion Paper (1988):

> The budget in the public domain is an act of political choice. Government taxes rather than sells. The budget sets out the choice as to the desirable level of taxation and expenditure and the

The context of decision making

choices made on the allocation of that expenditure. The budget will normally be kept to. It will not be changed merely because demand for a service is greater than is provided for. (p. 3)

While this was written about the macro-level of resource allocation, much of what is stated still applies at organisational level with financial accountability taking place within a context that is political and power contested. However, the situation may have changed from that described in 1988 with the introduction of managed markets in the public sphere.

The argument has been proposed that accountability to the user can best be achieved through the use of a market model. The user is viewed as a consumer and, within this consumerist model, government-set accountability measures have been highly influential. The Patient's Charter (DoH 1995), now in its second edition, raised the profile of quality to the public with its list of rights and expectations. Although the rights already existed, the list of expectations that 'the NHS is aiming to achieve' (p. 4) and the publication of local providers' success in meeting Charter targets has had a marked effect on NHS trusts.

The concept of the market is basically an economic one. According to neo-classical economic theory, in a true marketplace, quantity, demand and price are inextricably linked (Begg et al 1991). Therefore, the ability of the provider to alter price in response to demand and the existence of competitors to force cost efficiencies are essential prerequisites for a system that meets consumer needs. In the NHS, these prerequisites do not exist. However, the private sector has also had to control costs. Their advantage is operating in a freer market than that found in the public sector, with an ability to select their patients. No emergency admissions and the power to turn away patients at preadmission assessment if it seems likely that their overall health profile would lead to complications (better dealt with in an NHS hospital!) enable effective control over length of stay and therefore costs. This highlights the practical difficulties of the public sector attempting to work with a market model, however diluted.

It is therefore difficult to conclude that the introduction of some form of market has improved financial accountability. An increased emphasis on quality is potentially positive when the consumer rather than the purchaser is put in the centre of the frame but the lack of influence by some groups of users reinforces the ethical argument against a market-based accountability on the basis of inbuilt inequalities (Young 1996a).

Oakley (1994) has summarised the situation as follows.

The political context of decision making

17

While both government rhetoric and welfare practice enforce the view that individualised and marketised welfare is ensuring significant gains in terms of choice and cost containment, the evidence points in the opposite direction. Changes in health, education and welfare provision have introduced more choice for a few, at the expense of a lower quality of service for many. This is one of the hidden costs of a quasi-market system. Part of the economic efficiency of the old welfare state lay in the equitable distribution of a wide range of social costs and benefits. (p. 15)

Strategy or muddle at organisational level

As well as plenty of opinion, there are a number of recent studies on perceptions of change at the level of public sector and health care organisations. A number of issues are worth commenting on. First is the assumption that strategy develops in a way that is logical, clear and unambiguous. Most strategy is incremental.

> When well managed major organisations make significant changes in strategy, the approaches they use frequently bear little resemblance to the rational-analytical systems so often touted in the planning literature. . . . The processes used to arrive at the total strategy are typically fragmented, evolutionary and largely intuitive. (Quinn 1991, p. 96)

For health care, the strategic identification of objectives can be problematic. Using the example of the introduction of marketing to the NHS, Beenstock & Mabbott (1996) identified that the industrial and commercial realms have fairly single-minded business objectives compared to the public sector, but 'the NHS would always be anything but single-minded because it has a multiplicity of stakeholders with diverse objectives'. The survey they carried out indicated the view that the strategic status of marketing was an aspiration rather than a reality.

Second, the implementation of strategy in the top-down manner normally expected in organisations is bound to meet difficulties as it does not match the incremental practices with which people are comfortable. Grafting on new activities is unlikely to work (Whittington et al 1994). The change has to spread through the organisation and that process is complex and slow. Research in the NHS and the private sector showed that these implications were only slowly being recognised and grasped by management. In the meantime, managers, particularly in the NHS, are likely to face continuing 'manager bashing' as a result of their failure to demonstrate a reasonable congruence between a policy and its implementation (Hunter 1996). Although managers are in an agency relationship with government, there is a mismatch here between expectation and reality.

Structural changes in organisations also hamper the idealised view of strategic implementation. As Whittington et al (1994) found, 'The tension between the need for decentralised accountability and strategic coherence' seemed inherent in the market-driven change examined. However, some decentralisation offered the professionals 'new areas of opportunity and discretion, new ways of playing political games or exercising their skills' (p. 843).

Strategic implementation takes place within a certain organisational culture. There are a number of definitions of this but most would agree it includes power relations and history. A clear example of the effect of organisational culture on change was given by Parker & Dent (1996). Their study of the introduction of resource management in a UK health district highlighted the difficulties of a managerially initiated change making little headway with the clinicians. Getting doctors to even recognise legal-rational authority was a problem, let alone respond to it. These professionals could not be forced to do anything. Managerial attempts to create a unified culture were clearly unrealistic.

The conclusions of Lowndes (1997) from research into local authorities are probably typical of much change in health care as well. There appeared to be no one 'new management', nor one process of managerial change.

> While external triggers to management change are important, the susceptibility of individual authorities to change, and the direction of that change, is related to internal power relations and to local sensibilities and circumstances. Management change is a non-linear process, involving continuities between old and new approaches, movements forward and backward, and change at different levels. (p. 93)

As one interviewee put it: 'We are learning to accommodate mess' (p. 85).

CONCLUSION

In writing a chapter on the political context of decision making, the author is immediately faced with the problem of a change of political context. Governments change at regular intervals; in the UK the maximum time between general elections is 5 years and is often less. One such election took place in May 1997, resulting in a shift from a Conservative to a Labour government. It was with a consciousness of this that this chapter's approach focused on broad rather than specific issues. However, it does look as if changes that were in progress prior to New Labour's election and changes that they have introduced since have not initiated any cataclysmic differences, but are more fine tuning. Although the rhetoric has altered, the purchaser/provider split remains, restructuring continues to be a fact of life and doctors still have a powerful voice.

However, some trends are discernible, as follows.

● Different approaches to commissioning are being tried with primary care groups. Some even have formal nurse representation.
● New ways of collecting consumer/patient input are in place.
● Attempts are being made to return to a more holistic approach to care that had been fragmented by the separation of care into acute and community-based trusts and commissioning authorities. This restructuring has been under way for some time through mergers and the development of new authorities.

As seems to be inevitable with the political context being so important, the use of rhetoric to convey messages can either communicate the facts or cloud the issue. One thing is for sure: change will continue but quite in which direction and to what extent will remain unclear. One can always be wise after the event!

References

Abbott A 1988 The system of professions. Chicago University Press, Chicago

Armstrong P 1984 Competition between the organizational professions and the evolution of management control strategies. In: Thompson K (ed) Work, employment and unemployment. Open University Press, Buckingham

Bachrach P, Baratz M 1970 Power and poverty; theory and practice. Oxford University Press, New York

Beenstock J, Mabbott I 1996 This little trust went to market. Health Service Journal January 4: 23

Beer M, Eisenstat R, Spector B 1990 The critical path to corporate renewal. Harvard Business School Press, Harvard

Begg D, Fischer S, Dornbusch R 1991 Economics, 2nd edn. McGraw Hill, London

Burnham J 1941 The managerial revolution. Greenwood Press, Connecticut

Cole G 1975 What is socialism? In: De Crespigny A, Cronin J (eds) Ideologies of politics. Oxford University Press, Oxford, pp. 79–105

Dahl P 1961 Who governs? Democracy and power in an American city. Yale University Press, New Haven

Department of Health 1995 The Patient's Charter and you. HMSO, London

Ham C (ed) 1997a Health care reform: learning from international experience. Open University Press, Buckingham

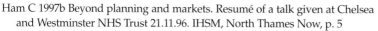

Ham C 1997b Beyond planning and markets. Resumé of a talk given at Chelsea and Westminster NHS Trust 21.11.96. IHSM, North Thames Now, p. 5

Harrison S, Pollitt C 1994 Controlling health professionals: the future of work and organization in the NHS. Open University Press, Buckingham

Hayek F 1975 The principles of a liberal social order. In: De Crespigny A, Cronin J (eds) Ideologies of politics. Oxford University Press, Oxford, pp. 55–75

Hunter D 1996 Give merit where it's due. Health Service Journal March 21: 21

Hunter D 1998 Our flexible friend: a review of *From Cradle to Grave* by G. Rivett. Health Service Journal January 8: 36–37

Johnson G, Scholes K 1999 Exploring corporate strategy, 5th edn. Prentice Hall, London

Local Government Training Board 1988 Management in the public domain: a discussion paper. LGTB, Luton

Lowe R 1993 The welfare state in Britain since 1945. Macmillan, Basingstoke

Lowndes V 1997 'We are learning to accommodate mess': four propositions about management change in local governance. Public Policy and Administration 12(2): 80–94

Needle D 1994 Business in context: an introduction to business and its environment, 2nd edn. Chapman and Hall, London

Oakeshott M 1975 On being conservative. In: De Crespigny A, Cronin J (eds) Ideologies of politics. Oxford University Press, Oxford, pp. 23–51

Oakley A 1994 Introduction. In: Oakley A, Williams AS (eds) The politics of the welfare state. UCL Press, London

Pannett A 1992 Law of torts, 6th edn. Pitman, London

Parker M, Dent M 1996 Managers, doctors and culture: changing an English health district. Administration and Society 28(3): 335–361

Pettigrew A, Ferlie E, McKee L 1992 Shaping strategic change: making change in large organizations – the case of the NHS. Sage, London

Popay J, Williams G 1994 Local voices in the NHS: needs, effectiveness and sufficiency. In: Oakley A, Williams AS (eds) The politics of the welfare state. UCL Press, London, pp. 75–97.

Quinn J 1991 Strategies for change. In: Mintzberg H, Quinn J (eds) The strategy process, 2nd edn. Prentice Hall, London

Saltman R, Von Otter C (eds) 1995 Implementing planned markets in health care. Open University Press, Buckingham

Spiers J 1995 The empowered patient. IHSM Network 2(1): 4–5

Thane P 1982 The foundations of the welfare state. Longman, London

Waters M 1994 Modern sociological theory. Sage, London

Whittington R, Macnulty T, Whipp R 1994 Market driven change in professional services; problems and processes. Journal of Management Studies 31(6): 829–845

Wollheim R 1975 Democracy. In: De Crespigny A, Cronin J (eds) Ideologies of politics. Oxford University Press, Oxford, pp. 109–130

Young AP 1996a Who sets the business agenda? Journal of Nursing Management 4: 347–352

Young AP 1996b Marketing: a flawed concept when applied to health care? British Journal of Nursing 5(15): 937–940

The political context of decision making

Application **1:1**

Ann P Young

Facing the wider issues of recruitment difficulties

One of the challenges facing health care today is the difficulty of recruiting and retaining certain groups of staff, most notably the lower paid professional groups such as nurses. This has led to bed closures with delays to operations and life-threatening situations with shortages of intensive care facilities. Below are presented two responses, the first from a political perspective which focuses on levels of pay and a lack of family-friendly policies, the second a managerial response from an NHS trust which, although including the very measures that UNISON deplores, is taking action on a number of other strategies.

NEWS....October 2000 LOW PAY HINDERS RECRUITMENT, PAY REVIEW BODY TOLD (excerpts from an article reproduced on www.unison.org.uk/news/focus/pages/news11.html)

'Trusts face an uphill struggle to meet the target of recruiting 20,000 new nurses when 68% of existing staff would not recommend nursing as a career.' That was the stark message that UNISON nurses took to the Nurses and Midwives Pay Review Body, when the union gave its oral evidence. UNISON national secretary for health Paul Marks pointed out that 'the best advertisement for a job is recommendation and yet UNISON's survey shows that the vast majority of nurses would not recommend it as a career. This is hardly surprising when you consider that nearly a third of nurses have to take a second job just to make ends meet.'

'UNISON is very concerned that trusts rely too heavily on short term solutions – 61% use bank and agency staff to combat staff shortages and 16% recruit from abroad – instead of looking at wider issues such as introducing family-friendly policies to encourage and help nurses to stay on the wards.' UNISON told the review body that more needs to be done for the low paid.

. . .Gail Adams, chair of UNISON's national nursing sector committee, said, 'Trusts do not always see what is under their noses,

The context of decision making

but look to the Philippines, Australia and New Zealand to fill staff shortages. They are not developing and using the skills they already have, but – unless something is done – we will lose those resources as more and more nursing health care assistants leave.'

UNISON is recommending a significant overall increase in pay and a boost to the lowest paid by deleting the bottom three points of the HCA grades. ...In addition, the union is proposing consolidation of discretionary points for the more senior grades, so that they become part of the existing salary structure.

—NHS TRUST NURSING AND MIDWIFERY ADVISORY COMMITTEE Minutes of meeting held at 11.00 am on Wednesday 19th July 2000 (Part of the minutes of this meeting is reproduced below with permission from Addenbrooke's NHS Trust)

RECRUITMENT ISSUES

Recruitment Manager attended for this item.

Overseas trip to the Philippines

Staff will be representing the Trust on this recruitment initiative at the end of July. Due to closed beds and expansion of the critical care unit the number of nurses that are being sought has risen to 86. Overseas interviews check list has been prepared. These nurses will require support during their adaptation period. CVs are available for managers to view and the calibre of nurses remains good. The start dates for these nurses will be October (first group of 40) and the second group in November. Accommodation issues are being considered.

Telephone interviewing candidates

A check list pro-forma has been produced for telephone interviewing candidates but this is an area where extreme caution is required. UKCC declarations and requirements for references need to be carefully specified.

Job fairs

Recruitment is pleased to coordinate attendance at various events but the success of each one needs to be evaluated. A diary of recruitment events is available; events that have recently been attended include:

Facing the wider issues of recruitment difficulties

23

Six Steps to **Effective Management**

> *College of Health Studies open days* – these are attended regularly and a large number of Trust representatives attend. In future it will not be necessary for so many to attend but written information to be made available for people to take away with contact names and numbers.
>
> *East of England Show* – this was an enjoyable event but not very productive in terms of recruitment. It has highlighted the need to have interesting demonstrations available to catch people's attention.
>
> *Trust open day* – this is a very good event for recruitment for all staff groups.
>
> Future events include Guild Hall and RCN job fair in October.
>
> ## Advertising agents
>
> This is currently out to tender via Procurement. Four agencies have been interviewed and further information is being collected.
>
> ## Websites
>
> Jobs in Health is the site that is currently used and this contract is up for review in May 2001. Jobs on County is another site that is being used which is free of charge. The Trust website is currently being revamped by the PR Department.
>   There will be a recruitment study day looking at recruitment issues including target areas, overseas, New Deal, employing disabled people, return to practice, etc. This will be targeted at service centre managers and those involved in recruitment.
>
> ## Interviewing process
>
> There are many ad hoc enquiries for nursing vacancies and delays are occurring in shortlisting these people for interview. In future all applications will be sent to managers with a covering letter to gain information on whether or not the candidates are suitable for interview.

COMMENT

The conflict between the need to make short-term decisions versus the desirability of taking a longer term perspective will be a continuing thread of this volume. The situation above also highlights the complex nature of many health care problems where the political, financial and professional agendas collide.

The context of decision making

Application **1:2**

Ann P Young

Department of Health publications

Decision making in UK health care, and most particularly in the NHS, has to take place within governmental control. This is probably appreciated by all those working in managerial posts. However, the scale of this control may not be realised by individuals.

A visit to the Department of Health website at http:/www.doh. gov.uk/ will demonstrate both the scale and breadth of this control. It is suggested to the reader that such a visit is made even if you do not have access to the web at work or home; local colleges and libraries all have this facility.

A number of activities should be undertaken. First go to the home page (www.doh.gov.uk/dhhome.htm).

1. Click on 'What's new'. These pages will give you, in date sequence (most recent first), a list of bulletins, reviews, guidance notes, statistics, reports and consultation documents. Count how many have been issued over the last month. At the time of writing, these were being produced at the rate of five or six every week. Although not all will be relevant to every manager, there are still a large number that do need some kind of managerial response. Identify those that might apply to you over the last 3 months. Then return to the home page.

2. Now click on 'Publications'. The page will give you several options.

   'COIN' (DH Circulars on the Internet) will enable you to search by subject in alphabetical order. Click on the chosen letter (e.g. M for management), click again on the particular management subcategory you want to view and a list of relevant circulars will be displayed.

   If you want to explore a wider range of publications, return to the publications page and select 'POINT' (Publications on the Internet). This will provide a search tool. Type in a category, being as precise as possible. For example, if you type in 'nursing' and 'management', you will get a list of over 30 documents. Try refining your search, for example, 'nursing' and 'management' and 'security'. You can then select a particular document to view.

3. If you require a broader search tool, then return to the home page and select 'Search'. This will draw on a wider database.

Discussion questions

- What are the advantages of using the Internet access rather than paper copy?
- Apart from possible difficulties of access, can you think of any disadvantages, organisational and/or personal? How might these be overcome?

The context of decision making

Chapter Two

The influence of professional and statutory bodies on decision making

Abigail Masterson and Ailsa Cameron

- Introduction
- The key stakeholders
- Nursing: the drive for professional status
- The relationship between nurses and health care
- Political decision making and nursing
- Professional advancement
- Conclusion

OVERVIEW

In this chapter we aim to illustrate the impact of professional and statutory bodies on decision making in health care. We describe the respective roles of the Royal College of Nursing (RCN), the National Boards and the United Kingdom Central Council for Nursing, Midwifery and Health Visiting (UKCC). We then explore the interaction between these organisations and the institutions of health care and the impact of those organisations on the decision-making processes that govern the way that nursing services are provided and affect the career pathways and opportunities available to individual practitioners. This exploration, we believe, can enable nurses to gain a greater understanding of the processes by which decisions are made and implemented at the macro policy level and the consequences of that decision making on individual practitioners. Through such study nurses individually and collectively may become more able to influence the decision making process itself and not merely react to an agenda that is controlled and set by others.

INTRODUCTION

In order to understand the influence the professional and statutory bodies have on decision making it is necessary to describe the policy process itself. In a democracy such as the United Kingdom the policy process is a continuous activity that involves constant negotiation and bartering between groups in society in an attempt to develop and implement government policy. This process involves a range of actors such as government ministers and civil servants but also includes groups with particular expertise and knowledge who seek to influence how and which decisions are made (Cameron 1999). These groups are often referred to as interest groups and in relation to the health policy process include professional organisations such as the RCN, the Royal College of Midwives and the British Medical Association, regulatory bodies like the UKCC and the National Boards and trade unions such as UNISON.

The political theorist David Easton described the political process as a series of systems, in which different groups make demands of the political system; these demands are fed into the decision-making process and are converted into outcomes or policies. The decision-making system is consequently dynamic and open to influence from the wider environment (Ham 1992). In considering the influence of professional and statutory bodies on decision making in health care, it is useful therefore to conceptualise organisations such as the UKCC and the RCN as interest groups making demands on the political process.

THE KEY STAKEHOLDERS

In order to understand how the statutory and professional bodies relate to each other and to government and health care providers it is necessary to briefly review the organisations involved.

Statutory bodies

Self-regulation is commonly accepted as one of the key attributes of a profession (Davies 1995). In the latter part of the 19th century there was much discussion and discord with regard to the desirability of setting up a professional register to ensure a nationally recognised standard of training and the restriction of the use of the

The context of decision making

term 'nurse'. This fight for professional self-regulation was led by the newly formed College of Nursing (later to become the RCN). Three Nurses Registration Acts in 1919 resulted in the establishment of General Nursing Councils (GNCs) in Scotland, England and Wales. The majority of the Councils' members were elected by the nurses themselves and the GNCs laid down rules regarding curriculum content and length of training and maintained the register of qualified staff. Following this the 1979 Nurses, Midwives and Health Visitor's Act established the UKCC and the four National Boards (Scotland, Northern Ireland, England and Wales) to regulate the nursing, midwifery and health-visiting professions.

The UKCC aimed to establish and improve standards of professional conduct and the development of the professions in the interests of the public. 'Professional self-regulation is a privilege and responsibility conferred on a profession by the public through the state' (UKCC 1997, p. 10). The purpose of statutory regulation is to protect the public from the harm that could be caused by the activities of an unregulated professional. The accountability of the regulator is to the public first and secondly to the professions that establish and fund it (JM Consulting 1999). Professional self-regulation generally, despite the government's commitment to strengthening it (DoH 1997, 1999, NHSE 1999), appears to be coming under increasing attack. This may well be the consequence of recent inquiries into medical malpractice such as the 'Bristol' case and certainly in relation to nursing, midwifery and health visiting, the government has suggested that a more open, responsive and accountable system of professional self-regulation is needed (DoH 1999).

Currently the roles of the statutory regulatory bodies for nursing, midwifery and health visiting are changing again with the establishment of a new council – the Nursing and Midwifery Council – to replace the existing five bodies. The new council has UK-wide powers and national offices and will meet on a rotating basis in England, Scotland, Wales and Northern Ireland. The main functions of the new council are to:

- develop and set standards for practice, education and conduct and to monitor their effectiveness
- maintain a register of professionals deemed fit to practise
- ensure that courses of nursing and midwifery education lead to suitable outcomes for admission to the Register and to meet European obligations
- operate investigative, disciplinary and remedial procedures in relation to professional conduct and performance

The influence of professional and statutory bodies

29

● provide guidance to and influence all concerned with safe practice by these professions.

Royal College of Nursing

The RCN was established in 1916 and is a registered charity. All members must be qualified nurses or nursing students. The RCN has possessed a Royal Charter since 1928 and one of its objectives is to promote the science and art of nursing. The RCN aims to promote the interests of nurses and patients on a wide range of health issues through working with the government, Members of Parliament, other unions, professional bodies and voluntary organisations. It acts as the voice of British nursing abroad and is represented on many European, Commonwealth and international bodies such as the International Council of Nurses.

Congress, the main debating forum of the RCN, plays a major part in initiating policy, which is then taken forward by its Council. There are teams of professional advisers, educators and researchers responsible for responding to members' professional needs, promoting professional awareness and formulating and publishing specialist professional opinion. The RCN is the only trade union/professional organisation that is concerned purely with nursing. It is the world's largest professional union of nurses, with more than 300 000 members. The RCN is run by nurses and claims to be the fastest growing trade union in the UK.

As Hart (1994) notes, the RCN was a prime mover in the movement for the professionalisation of nursing in the early part of the 20th century and this is still reflected in how the organisation projects itself today. The RCN ties itself so tightly to the professional voice of nursing that it is often confused with nursing's statutory bodies. The RCN offers a wide range of postregistration educational opportunities for its members from conferences and short courses through to Masters degrees. It offers a wide variety of special interest groups that members can belong to, has substantial research and practice development programmes and has the largest nursing library in Europe. It also provides significant industrial relations support and indemnity insurance.

The National Health Service

The National Health Service (NHS) was formally established on 5 July 1948 but its final shape was the result of a move towards increased state involvement in health care which began in the late 19th century. The two world wars highlighted the marked disparity in health service provision across the UK and the feasibility of centralising the organisation and management of health care. Advances in medical science and effective utilisation of the policy process ensured that medicine had a significant influence on the final shape of the service. Consequently, the model of health and health care that has had the greatest influence on the NHS is the 'medical model'. Indeed, health has usually been seen as synonymous with the elimination of medically defined disease and as a result acute and curative services such as surgery have been a priority for funding although this is currently under review.

The NHS employs over 332 000 nurses, midwives and health visitors (DoH 1999). Nurses, midwives and health visitors are the largest of the health professions and the biggest staff group in the NHS. There are four chief nursing officers (CNO), one for each of the countries that make up the UK. They are the most senior nursing advisers to government ministers and act as a conduit between government policy and nurses, midwives and health visitors in practice in their respective countries. In England, there are three assistant CNOs and approximately 30 nursing officers covering everything from public health, community services for older people to critical care.

The CNO has input into every policy that is generated by the Department of Health and some policy from other departments such as Employment and Education. These posts are civil service posts and so postholders must support government policy regardless of their own political views.

Since its inception the NHS has constantly been scrutinised on grounds of cost and efficiency. Possibly the most radical of these reviews resulted in the NHS and Community Care Act 1990 which led to the introduction of the concept of the internal market to health care services in Britain. Clearly this fundamental change in the way services were purchased and provided had implications for the delivery of nursing services. The introduction of trusts as independent financial units forced a reexamination of the most cost-effective means of providing services and this led to initiatives such as reengineering of the workforce, skill mix reviews and in many instances the development of new professional roles. Some trusts have introduced nurse-led preoperative clinics and rapid discharge programmes in an attempt to make services more efficient. In addition, new clinical roles such as nurse anaesthetists, nurse endoscopists and surgeon's assistants have been established. Some

The influence of professional and statutory bodies

commentators see these developments as evidence of the coming of age of professionalism in nursing, others have dismissed them as a resurgence of medical control over the profession and the epitome of the nurse as the doctor's handmaiden.

The White Paper *The New NHS: Modern, Dependable* (DoH 1997) emphasised the government's commitment to strengthening the nursing contribution to service delivery and certainly nurses and nursing seem to be becoming more visible in policy terms. Nursing representation is mandatory on the boards of trusts and primary care groups and some of the innovative personal medical services pilot schemes include nurses leading the delivery of primary care services and even employing salaried GPs.

NURSING: THE DRIVE FOR PROFESSIONAL STATUS

Since the end of the 19th century there has been a drive for professionalisation in nursing, which has increased in intensity since the 1970s in the UK. This commitment to changing the status of nursing has been articulated vociferously in the professional press and was encouraged by the establishment of degree courses in nursing (Davies 1995, Raffery 1997). The UKCC's *Project 2000: A New Preparation for Practice* broke with the traditional apprenticeship style of hospital-based nurse training and established a university-based diploma-level education founded on the concept of the 'knowledgeable doer' and a philosophy of health rather than disease (UKCC 1986).

Since the wholesale adoption of the new education system, however, concerns have been expressed in the professional and lay press about its effectiveness. For example, the 1999 Nursing Strategy notes that:

> Evidence suggests that in recent years students completing training have not been equipped at the point of qualification with the full range of clinical skills they need. (DoH 1999)

The government goes on to suggest that a stronger practical orientation to preregistration education and training is needed. On the other hand, the RCN has long been advocating degree-level preparation as part of its strategy for an all-graduate profession. And the Nursing and Midwifery Council (NMC), the body which currently holds the statutory responsibility for setting the standard, kind and content of nurse education, is currently reviewing preregistration education through its Education Commission chaired by Sir Len Peach.

THE RELATIONSHIP BETWEEN NURSES AND HEALTH CARE

The NHS has changed markedly over the last two decades but nursing has not always been ready for the changes that have taken place, particularly in the organisation and delivery of services. As a result the profession often appears to react too late. For example, as the case study in Application 2.1 illustrates, much of the debate about the desirability, preparation and evaluation of nurse practitioners came after their introduction into acute and the primary care services. Consequently, the profession was in a much weaker position to plan, manage and control the development (UKCC 1997). At the same time health care assistant roles are developing in all care areas in response to changes in preregistration nursing education and skill mix and reprofiling projects implemented as a response to the cost effectiveness agenda. Nurses' work therefore has increasingly become that of supervisor rather than hands-on carer yet the NMC has refused to allow membership of health care assistants and health care support workers. Clearly the existence of a large number of support workers who remain outside professional control has implications for safety, standards of care and ultimately the viability of the nursing profession. Indeed, serious doubts have even been raised about the contribution of various groups within the profession such as health visiting and school nursing.

In 1996 a report from the University of Manchester Health Services Management Unit on the future of the health care workforce argued for the creation of a generic health worker from which specialisms such as physiotherapy could emerge. Many of the duties that appeared to be expected of this generic health care worker seemed to closely resemble traditional conceptualisations of nursing. In 1997 the Lifespan Trust in Cambridgeshire fought a highly publicised battle to introduce the role of generic community health nurse at the expense of specialist health visiting and school nursing services, thus casting doubt on the sustainability of the eight 'specialist' community branches.

POLITICAL DECISION MAKING AND NURSING

Historically the nursing profession has been less involved in the political system than their medical counterparts. Nurses have been

The influence of professional and statutory bodies

lambasted by many commentators because the profession general-ly has seen being political as inappropriate. However, the situation is far more complex than it appears. It is important to note at this point that nurses are not a homogeneous group. Nursing has sev-eral ancestries that represent competing values and ideals; for example, the gentle, angelic, selfless woman epitomised in many portrayals of Florence Nightingale and the militant trade unionism which emerged from the asylums and poor law institutions (Owens & Glennester 1990).

Nursing is also split into subgroups by speciality and place of work. 'What counts as nursing may vary a lot, and sometimes even nurses find it difficult at first to recognise that what other nurses are doing is really nursing' (RCN 1992, p. 18). Similar barriers exist between and within practitioners, educators, researchers and man-agers. Each group possesses different values which are often in conflict with one another (Cooke 1993, White 1984). Because of the imbalance of power between practitioners, educators, researchers and managers, in many cases these groups have not been united in their pursuit of common goals. The barriers of speciality, heritage, grade and perhaps even gender have frequently prevented the pro-fession from speaking with one voice.

For example, in the fight for registration in the early 20th cen-tury nurses marshalled political and social power effectively to meet their ends. Similarly, there were nurses within the women's suffrage movement. More recently, nurses working in mental health and learning disabilities, who were predominantly men, have fought successfully for power both within and without the profession. It is within general nursing that the non-political atti-tude has appeared most prevalent. There seems to be a fear that becoming political will damage the caring ethic, stability and respectability of nursing. For example, Alison Dunn, in the fore-word to Jane Salvage's seminal text *The Politics of Nursing*, wrote:

> Many nurses are uncomfortable with the word "politics". It belongs to a world that they do not feel, nor want to be part of. Politics is for others. Politics is a deviant activity in which no self-respecting pro-fessional should indulge. (Salvage 1985)

However, things may be changing. In the 1997 general election two nurses, Ann Keen and Laura Moffat, were returned as Labour MPs. Increasingly, too, nurses are playing a role in local government.

The RCN, via its combined professional association and trade union functions, aims to promote the interests of nurses. The RCN has steadfastly refused to align itself to any particular political party, believing its members' interests are better served by providing a source of objective advice on political issues to all political parties. At times this lack of political acumen appears almost reckless. For example, in *The Value of Nursing* (RCN 1992), a document that was intended to make policy makers aware of and respect nursing, 'government-speak' regarding such issues as cost-effectiveness and value for money receive a high profile throughout:

> Nursing consumes three per cent of all public expenditure. It is therefore legitimate to ask whether nursing is giving value for money. It is inescapable that nurses will be asked to demonstrate that they are cost-effective.

The Department of Health has long perceived the RCN as the chief source of advice on nursing issues so there has been very little participation or consultation with other health trade unions which include nurses, such as UNISON. Rafferty (1992) stresses the resulting lack of effective action by nursing organisations to lobby on behalf of their constituency and suggests that the stratification of nursing into levels and specialisms has made the issue of true representation difficult.

PROFESSIONAL ADVANCEMENT

The nursing development movement was established in the 1980s on the back of initiatives such as the nursing process which was intended to be not only a system of documentation but also a way of illustrating the unique contribution of nursing to health care. The nursing literature in the mid-1980s was characterised by pleas to regain the fundamental value of nursing. Arguments were constructed to illuminate nursing's therapeutic contribution in its own right. Jane Salvage, long-time member of the radical nurses group, was appointed as Head of Nursing Development at the King's Fund. In the late 1980s the nursing development movement grew rapidly and appeared to have a significant influence on the policy and professional agenda. For example, the Department of Health supported the establishment of 30 nursing development units as a means of encouraging excellence in practice. The self-confidence of the profession was manifest in the empowering rhetoric of primary nursing and the legislative support for educational change (Salvage & Wright 1995).

Many commentators believed *The Scope of Professional Practice* (UKCC 1992) to be the culmination of this decade of nursing eman-

The influence of professional and statutory bodies

cipation (Land et al 1996, Paniagua 1995). *Scope* allowed individual nurses to take responsibility for the expansion of the service they provide. It emphasised professional accountability and placed decisions about the boundaries of practice in the hands of practitioners (Redfern 1997). However, *Scope* could equally be seen as enabling the resubordination of nursing. It was launched at the same time as the drive towards a reduction of junior doctor hours and arguably has been used to justify and promote the development of new roles that supported the needs of medicine and management rather than the needs of patients and nursing development (Denner 1995, Dimond 1995). For example, nursing in *Scope* was described as a reactive/adaptive force bending and changing to others' changing circumstances rather than as a proactive social force:

> The reality is that the practice of nursing, and education for that practice, will continue to be shaped by developments in care and treatment, and by other events which influence it. (UKCC 1992, p. 8)

CONCLUSION

As we have demonstrated, nurses are affected in many ways by the relationship of statutory and professional bodies with the government and health care providers. Several World Health Assembly resolutions have urged member states to encourage and support the appointment of nursing/midwifery personnel in senior leadership and management positions to facilitate their participation in planning and implementing their country's health activities. However, most nurses have paid little attention to this aspect of decision making which affects nurses' daily work, controls what practitioners can and cannot do, dictates who receives nursing care and where that nursing care takes place.

We hope that this chapter stimulates an interest and awareness amongst nurses of the fundamental importance and relevance of decision making in policy and politics to their everyday practice. The development of a cadre of nurses who can competently and effectively analyse and influence the formulation of health policies to support nursing objectives is crucial. Nursing is a valuable resource which must be actively utilised in health care policy and planning. If nurses are restricted to implementing the decisions made by others and working under conditions established by others, they may feel that they have little impact on health care

The context of decision making

policy and provision. This in turn promotes a cycle of frustration, detachment and powerlessness (Tierney 1990).

In 1991, Robinson noted that 'Nurses are virtually never involved in concrete policy decision-making processes; what may pass as a nursing decision is in reality acquiescence to others' prior formulations'. If nurses are to gain and maintain autonomous control over the practice of nursing, they must be involved in defining the scope of that practice. And if nurses want to have an impact on access, quality, allocation and the delivery of health care they must make that impact through the policy-making process. An understanding of the key actors involved and of the policy process itself can enable nurses individually and collectively to influence those decision-making processes.

References

Cameron A 1999 The role of interest groups. In: Masterson A, Maslin-Prothero S (eds) Nursing and politics: power through practice. Churchill Livingstone, Edinburgh

Cooke H 1993 Boundary work in the nursing curriculum: the case of sociology. Journal of Advanced Nursing 18(12): 1990–1998

Davies C 1995 Gender and the professional predicament in nursing. Open University Press, Buckingham

Denner S 1995 Extending professional practice: benefits and pitfalls. Nursing Times 91(14): 27–29

Department of Health 1997 The new NHS. Modern, dependable. The Stationery Office, London

Department of Health 1999 Making a difference: strengthening the nursing, midwifery and health visiting contribution to health and healthcare. The Stationery Office, London

Dimond B 1995 UKCC's standards for incorporation into contracts. British Journal of Nursing 4(18): 1045–1046

Ham C 1992 Health policy in Britain: the politics and organisation of the National Health Service, 3rd edn. Macmillan, Basingstoke

Hart C 1994 Behind the mask: nurses, their unions and nursing policy. Baillière Tindall, London

JM Consulting 1999 The regulation of nurses, midwives and health visitors: report of the review of the Nurses, Midwives and Health Visitors Act 1997. JM Consulting, Bristol

Land L, Mhaolrunaigh MA, Castledine G 1996 Extent and effectiveness of the Scope of Professional Practice. Nursing Times 96(35): 32–35

NHSE 1999 Review of the Nurses, Midwives and Health Visitors Act: government response to the recommendations. HSC 1999/030. NHSE, Leeds

The influence of professional and statutory bodies

Owens P, Glennester H 1990 Nursing in conflict. Macmillan, Basingstoke

Paniagua H 1995 The scope of advanced practice: action potential for practice nurses. British Journal of Nursing 4(5): 269–274

Rafferty AM 1992 Nursing policy and the nationalisation of nursing: the representation of 'crisis' and the 'crisis' of representation. In: Robinson J, Gray A, Elkan R (eds) Policy issues in nursing. Open University Press, Buckingham, pp. 68–83

Rafferty A 1997 If the past was tense, can the future be perfect? Nursing Times 93(5): 28–31

Redfern S 1997 Reactions to nurses expanding practice. Nursing Times 93(32): 45–47

Robinson J 1991 Power, politics and policy analysis in nursing. In: Perry A, Jolley M (eds) Nursing: a knowledge base for practice. Edward Arnold, London

Royal College of Nursing 1992 The value of nursing. RCN, London

Salvage J 1985 The politics of nursing. Heinemann, Oxford

Salvage J, Wright S 1995 Nursing development units: a force for change. Scutari, London

Tierney R 1990 Strategies for empowerment. Nursing Standard 4(47): 32–34

UKCC 1986 Project 2000: a new preparation for practice. UKCC, London

UKCC 1992 Scope of professional practice. UKCC, London

UKCC 1997 The future of professional self regulation: submission of the United Kingdom Central Council for Nursing, Midwifery and Health Visiting to the government's review of the Nurses, Midwives and Health Visitors Act 1997. UKCC, London

White R 1984 Nursing: past trends, future policies. Journal of Advanced Nursing 9: 505–512

The context of decision making

Application 2:1

Abigail Masterson and Ailsa Cameron

Case study: the development of specialist and advanced practice roles

INTRODUCTION

This case study illustrates the roles that the key actors such as the RCN, the UKCC and the Department of Health, discussed above, have played in the macro-level decision making which is shaping the career options and educational opportunities available to nurses post registration.

BACKGROUND

Nursing is constantly evolving and changing. Nurses have always adjusted the scope of their practice to meet changing health needs; for example, both temperature taking and blood pressure monitoring used to be the exclusive preserve of medicine. Changes in health policy such as the shift towards a primary care-led NHS and community care for people with mental health problems, technological advances and increases in scientific knowledge demand that the health care professions develop in new ways. These changes have increased the skills and decision making required of all nurses and what was once unthinkable – nurses carrying out endoscopies, acting as specialists in diverse areas of care such as diabetes and behavioural therapy, working as first assistant to surgeons or running their own clinics in acute and primary care – is now becoming the norm. In all care settings the traditional boundaries between professional groups are being rethought and redrawn in response to practice development, local service needs and national policy objectives. Hence we have selected the debates around specialist and advanced practice as a case study for analysis because they are topical, current and have huge implications for the future shape and direction of the profession in the UK.

NEW NURSING ROLES

The clinical nurse specialist role in areas such as infection control, tissue viability, stoma care, continence and so on has existed informally since the 1970s. Clinical nurse specialists were seen as experts in a particular area of care or with a particular client group, with postregistration education and a research base firmly grounded in nursing. The title was not regulated and postholders usually achieved such jobs through extensive experience and appropriate postregistration courses. Clinical nurse specialists were usually managed within the nursing service.

Nurse practitioners developed first in primary care in the late 1980s and offered an alternative service to that provided by general practitioners or filled gaps in service provision, for example by providing primary care to homeless people. Nurse practitioners diagnose, refer, prescribe and provide complete episodes of care for clients with undifferentiated health problems and have usually been managed outwith conventional nursing structures. In the 1990s posts emerged in secondary care with the titles of nurse practitioner, advanced practitioner and advanced nurse practitioner. Such posts frequently involved nurses giving care or performing tasks previously done by doctors. For example, in some trusts advanced neonatal practitioners are replacing junior doctors on the senior house officer rota in special care baby units; surgical nurse practitioners run preadmission clinics and clerk patients and organise theatre lists; other nurse practitioners work across the primary/secondary care interface and prescribe within protocols for conditions such as hypertension, asthma and so on.

THE REGULATORY FRAMEWORK

The Scope of Professional Practice (UKCC 1992) and EL (92) 38 *Withdrawal of guidance on the extended role of the nurse* encouraged nurses to take on new roles and activities to adapt to meet changing health care needs. There are few tasks which nurses cannot undertake legally. As particular tasks have become commonplace, e.g. intravenous drug administration, cannulation, venepuncture and ECGs, they have been subsumed into the core of nursing and form the expected skills base of all registered practitioners.

In its *Post Registration Education and Practice Report* (PREP) in 1994 the UKCC set new standards for the postregistration development of all nurses, midwives and health visitors which were designed to improve patient and client care through matching changing health care needs with flexible, responsive education provision. A key philosophical change within this report was an acknowledgement that practitioners should demonstrate that they are continually maintaining and developing their professional knowledge and competence in order to remain on the register.

The PREP report also highlighted the need to identify different levels of practice beyond registration and the preparation required for nurses to function at these different levels of practice. For example, specialist practitioners were expected to demonstrate higher levels of clinical decision making and to monitor and improve standards of care through supervision of practice, clinical audit, the provision of skilled professional leadership and the development of practice through research, teaching and support of professional colleagues.

To prepare for a specialist practitioner qualification nurses must have an effective registration and experience as a qualified nurse to gain a deeper understanding of their area of practice. To obtain a specialist practitioner qualification, nurses must undertake an educational programme approved by a National Board to meet the UKCC's standards in four key areas: specialist clinical practice, care and programme management, clinical practice development and clinical practice leadership. Such programmes must be at degree level and of no less than one academic year in length.

Specialist practice courses in community health care nursing are arranged around a common core with specialist modules for each branch of community practice. The areas of clinical practice are: general practice nursing, community mental health nursing, community mental handicap nursing, community children's nursing, public health nursing – health visiting, occupational health nursing, community nursing in the home – district nursing and school nursing. Specialist practice courses in the other areas of nursing, such as nursing older people or critical care nursing, also often involve shared learning in core subjects such as research and professional issues.

MANAGING PUBLIC PROTECTION AND PROFESSIONAL ASPIRATIONS

The UKCC's activities since the early 1980s have been dominated by discussions related to the postregistration education arrangement for nurses, midwives and health visitors, the culmination of which was the publication and implementation of the PREP report in 1994 outlined above. However, even in the professional literature there is no consensus and little consistency in the use of the terms advanced

The development of specialist and advanced practice roles

practice, nurse specialist and nurse practitioner. Advanced practice, for example, is frequently used to describe both taking on a technical task hitherto done by another health professional and developing innovative nurse-led services that change the boundaries of nursing practice. Despite the UKCC's (1994, p. 28:10) intention that 'there is a clear difference between practising within a speciality and being a nursing specialist', specialist practice as operationalised in many areas has become the preparation for professional practice with a particular client group, such as older people, intensive care or forensic psychiatry. In addition, despite the UKCC's assertion (1996, p. 7:4) that 'Specialist practitioner intervention and leadership are likely to be needed in most areas of clinical practice... This will not require every practitioner to become a specialist', in many specialities the majority of practitioners are undertaking courses leading to the recordable qualification of specialist practitioner. This link between specialist practice and preparation for an area of practice rather than a higher level of practice has been compounded by the association of community qualifications, such as health visiting and community psychiatric nursing, with specialist practitioner status.

In response to lobbying from the RCN, and in particular the Nurse Practitioner Forum, and the proliferation of new nursing roles developing in a wide range of care settings, further work on advanced practice was undertaken by the UKCC. This year-long consultation with the key stakeholders concluded that Council should not set standards for advanced practice but instead reexamine specialist practice.

Council agreed in December 1997 (UKCC 1997), following another extensive consultation process, that practitioners with the titles of nurse practitioner or clinical nurse specialist could record the qualification of specialist practitioner if they met the standards for specialist practice as currently laid down. It was equally accepted that some would not meet these standards, based on the nature of their current role and responsibilities. This was in line with Council's original intention that the concept of specialist practice was about a *higher level of practice* when it determined that: 'There is a clear difference between practising within a speciality and being a nursing specialist' (UKCC 1994, p. 28:10).

HIGHER LEVEL PRACTICE

The specialist practice consultation exercise referred to above demonstrated that in order to provide greater public protection and meet the needs of patients, professionals and employers, further work was necessary because currently:

● there is no requirement for practitioners to record the specialist practitioner qualification

- there is no way of checking what qualifications a nurse/specialist practitioner has, other than the fact that they are on the register, or how up to date and relevant their qualifications are
- existing courses which prepare practitioners for specialist practice tend to concentrate on education rather than practice competence
- other bodies such as professional associations, trade unions and the commercial sector are developing their own highly variable standards for this level of practice.

Consequently Council developed proposals for the regulation of higher level practice (UKCC 1998). The ensuing consultation process on these proposals suggested that there was overwhelming support from consumers, practitioners and employers for the UKCC to regulate higher level practice in order to protect the public and meet existing and future health care needs. Consequently, in December 1998 Council agreed that discussions should be commenced with key stakeholders such as the Department of Health regarding the regulation of those nurses, midwives and health visitors who are working at a higher level of practice, that a consultation on a standard for a higher level of practice should be undertaken and that proposals should be developed for a pilot assessment process. The standard and assessment system has now been developed and is currently being piloted with the profession.

CONSULTANT NURSES

On 8 September 1998 the Prime Minister announced that the Secretary of State for Health would be asked to look at introducing nurse consultant posts. He said that nurse consultants would have the same status within nursing that medical consultants enjoy in medicine. They would be rooted in clinical practice, provide a focus for developing and supporting other nursing roles and offer nurses an alternative career path. This announcement was made at the *Nursing Standard* awards ceremony (*Nursing Standard* belongs to the RCN Publishing Company) and seems to have been a surprise to the statutory bodies and the nursing officers at the Department of Health. The UKCC has welcomed the Prime Minister's proposals because they should help to keep experienced nurses in clinical practice and they encourage the recognition of clinical expertise for the benefit of patients. However, Council has emphasised that prior to seeking appointment as a nurse consultant, practitioners should achieve a defined professional standard such as the UKCC's proposals for higher level practice in order to provide a guarantee of competence. The 1999 Department of Health (England) Strategy for Nursing and Midwifery *Making a Difference* has honoured this

The development of specialist and advanced practice roles

request, stating that consultant nurses, midwives and health visitors will:

> . . . hold professional registration and additional specialist-specific professional qualifications commensurate with standards proposed for recognition of a 'higher level of practice'.

The RCN has been a key player in all these debates but its responses and actions highlight the tensions inherent in its dual role as both professional organisation and trade union. It lobbied successfully for a rethink of Council's postregistration framework and has publicly supported the establishment of consultant nurse posts. It is in the process of setting up its own accreditation system for 'expert practice' which ties into its plans for the development of a faculty system with a function similar to that of the medical Royal Colleges, all of which are firmly within a professional agenda. However, the RCN's support of these developments has always to be accompanied by discussions around pay, terms and conditions and a proviso that any such changes in the professional career structure be achieved within a framework of total workforce development. This stance is linked to its trade union function where it must avoid accusations of elitism from the bulk of its membership.

CONCLUSION

It is tempting to view current development as necessarily correct. It appears, however, as Robinson (1991) argued, that nurses can often be the victims of the rhetoric of policy change. They are hoodwinked into believing that if they comply with certain policy initiatives then their concerns will be acted on yet nothing changes as the fundamental issues of power and resources within the health care system remain the same. These developments in postregistration education and practice are exciting and emphasise the value of pushing back the boundaries of practice. But the current focus on specialist, advanced and higher level practice, some argue, has inadvertently devalued being a registered nurse.

Managers, educators and practitioners have expressed concern that nurses are being pushed into doing degrees and collecting extra certificates through fear of being left behind rather than to develop their practice or because the service needs it. Although patients and clients should have access to specialist care all practitioners will not need to be specialists and there will always be a requirement for up-to-date and competent registered nurses in all clinical areas. There will also be a need to constantly redefine the boundaries between professional groups and such definitions will, of course, reflect the values attached to certain groups and activities. This does not imply, both within and between groups, a dominance or

The context of decision making

subservience of position, nor will any of the boundaries remain absolute over time and the critical analysis of the roles of the various stakeholders in past and future decision making is essential.

References

Department of Health 1999 Making a difference: strengthening the nursing, midwifery and health visiting contribution to health and healthcare. The Stationery Office, London

Robinson J 1991 Power, politics and policy analysis in nursing. In: Perry A, Jolley M (eds) Nursing: a knowledge base for practice. Edward Arnold, London

UKCC 1992 Scope of professional practice. UKCC, London

UKCC 1994 Standards for education and practice following registration. UKCC, London

UKCC 1996 PREP – the nature of advanced practice: an interim report. UKCC, London

UKCC 1997 PREP – specialist practice: consideration of issues relating to embracing nurse practitioners and clinical nurse specialists within the specialist practice framework. UKCC, London

UKCC 1998 Higher level practice project – phase II. UKCC, London

The development of specialist and advanced practice roles

Application 2:2

Leslie Gelling and Mary Cooke

The role of RCN interest groups in local decisions

This application turns to an exploration of the relationship between local and national decision making. As you read this, you will note that the agenda for the local group was wide ranging and there was an expectation that its relationship with the national group would facilitate this. Differentiation is also made between research nurses, usually involved in medical research, and nurse researchers who undertake nursing research. Potential problems and synergies here are explored and the RCN's increasingly political stance is presented. Finally, methods of enhancing the local profile of research interests are summarised.

MEMBERSHIP

Nursing groups find that their membership is often divided by personal and professional agendas. People join groups for a purpose, either altruistically to support the profession or to support their own personal advance in career. Leslie Gelling and a cohort of colleagues have recently made an effort to push the profile of nursing research forward in the Eastern Region of England.

The RCN has had a research interest group since before 1996, after which members were able to 'sign up' or register. This produced the largest membership group in the RCN (some 12 760 nurses over the UK), reflecting the national interest in research. Some reasons for such a large membership would be: research is now reflected in the necessity to underpin practice with evidence, to determine guidance for practice and to support all academic study done by nurses and midwives as part of their personal learning.

LOCAL REPRESENTATION

The need for local representation for research was explained by Leslie as follows.

1. The Eastern Region has only recently gained representation on the National Policy and Practice Group of the RCN Research Society. This fact is of interest when comparing health research activity across professional groups in the country.
2. Minimal original research is being undertaken by nurses and midwives in the Eastern Region and having a group such as ours is seen as a positive step towards raising the profile of nursing and midwifery research and, as a consequence, the numbers participating in research activities.
3. Local research ethics committees are extremely knowledgeable about research by scientists, medical staff, junior doctors and pharmaceutical companies concerning drugs, chemical and biophysical interventions in medicine and genetic 'blue-skies' research. They have less experience of appraising health and social services research that may adopt methodologies other than experiments or randomised controlled trials. Nurses encounter problems when submitting applications to the LREC where few non-medical projects are approved without difficulty. More nursing and midwifery research proposals being submitted to the LREC should force the committee to employ external reviewers with other, broader specialist research interests and abilities.
4. Nurse researchers and research nurses are different but they both have an important role to play in developing the potential for research within the region. The former, those involved in clinical trials as part of physician-led teams, should have more opportunity to build on their research skills. This would raise the research capacity of nurses in the region.

RELATIONSHIP BETWEEN LOCAL AND NATIONAL GROUPS

Reflecting on the ways in which the RCN Research Society (Eastern Region) works, it relates to the national RCN Research Society Policy and Practice Group where some decision making should be devolved to the regional group. In reverse, support for activities from the devolved group move through the formal and informal system where a sustained relationship exists with the centre – the RCN Research Society Policy and Practice Group. As a result, local decisions reflect activities regionally rather than centrally.

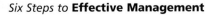

The Research Society is one of the largest RCN forum groups in the UK. Representation of local priorities and cultures will sometimes be difficult on a national committee, unless there is a forum in which attitudes, needs and strengths are collected, defined and disseminated. The Eastern Region is different from others, e.g. Scotland or Trent, because it is largely rural but with one huge university and three other smaller universities. This results in a transient scientific population but a stable local population.

The nursing and midwifery representation of the research activity of the region does not feature strongly because the emphasis in the health sector is on the existing and established medical, scientific and pharmacological fields of research. Therefore the sources of government, industry and health service funding are focused on the more high-profile and easily successful existing areas of research.

The academic nursing departments in the Eastern Region's higher education institutions have been largely research feeble. Therefore the RCN Research Society (Eastern Region) is seen as a method of supporting the nursing research that is ongoing and focusing the interests of isolated researchers by encouraging them academically and by sharing and disseminating skills.

Representation: is this easy? People will volunteer to join a local group but there needs to be a local representative at the national level. How this will be achieved has yet to be determined but it may involve regional groups electing a local representative to stand on the national Policy and Practice Group for the forum. The communication and dissemination of information in both directions, to local (sometimes individuals) interested people and from them to the national forum, can be time consuming but in research, networking is one answer to problems of isolation that may be experienced. A local person has a better view of local needs and should also represent the national view to the local group.

Recently (November 2000), the Nursing and Midwifery Research Unit (NAMRU) was launched at the University of East Anglia. NAMRU has many similar aims and objectives to the RCN group, so both groups are making a concerted effort to drive forward nursing research. Both groups believe that nursing and nursing research will be strengthened in this way. The two groups are seen as complementary rather than competitive and both are aware of the need to become more active in the region rather than passively assuming there is sufficient support for the practitioners.

THE SKILLS OF RESEARCH NURSES AND THE SKILLS OF NURSE RESEARCHERS

There is little original nursing research being undertaken by nurses in the community or in the secondary sector. The reason for this is that

The context of decision making

too few nurses have the necessary research skills and experience and the medical profession is supporting and moving its own members forward to take up funding for project work rather than sharing capacity building programmes. History could repeat itself.

Because of this we need to identify and justify the skills of research nurses gained through managing clinical trials. These skills include communicating with patients, recruiting people into trials, understanding methods of consent and the ethical considerations of participation. This important role is not always evident in research protocols but nurses do play an essential role in ensuring that many studies are more successful. Some nurses are involved from the outset of protocol planning. Good lead researchers are aware of the benefits of involving nurses in research projects from the initial stages to ensuring protocols are manageable and safe.

One of the most important events to occur recently, for nurse researchers, has been the election of Roswyn Hakesley-Brown as RCN President. Roswyn is a strong and long-standing member of the RCN Research Society. Obviously the RCN membership will now look to Roswyn to raise the profile of nursing research within and without the profession and to help push aside the barriers that have existed to date.

This view reflects the rise in political stance that the RCN has taken in recent years and that the membership require it to take. Pressure of competition for research funds, despite ability and skills, is frustrating. Nurses need open opportunities and a non-selective pathway to begin to appreciate how good our research is, and could be, especially if nurses in clinical situations are enabled to do it. This is why senior and experienced researchers, through groups such as the RCN Research Society (Eastern Region) and NAMRU, should support researchers and collaborate with clinicians.

ENHANCING THE LOCAL PROFILE

A further aspect of the Eastern Region's research group is that national draft or consultation documents can be commented upon by local people. We would otherwise not have an opportunity to so easily give feedback and be respected for our views. Local organisations can also attempt to influence local hospitals, through directors of nursing, to ask for a greater emphasis on nursing research to become the norm in clinical practice. One way of measuring the profile of a hospital and the impact of its strategy in research is to look at the presentations by its nurses and midwives at conferences. This record is poor for hospitals the size they are in the Eastern Region. The research interests and responsibilities of many senior nurses is low. One way of influencing these measurable outcomes would be to insist on restructuring the role of some nurses to take account of research interests and abilities.

The role of RCN interest groups in local decisions

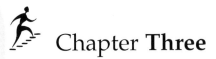

Chapter **Three**

Organisational culture and decision making

Margaret Todd

- Culture and performance
- Organisational culture – what is it?
- Transmission and maintenance of organisational culture
- Cultures and subcultures

- Managing organisational cultures
- Organisation structure, culture and decision making
- Management theories, culture and decision making
- Conclusion

The context of decision making

O V E R V I E W

Many different types of organisations exist. They could be categorised according to their ownership, such as private, public or voluntary organisations. Equally they could be classified according to the nature of their business, such as car manufacturers or health service providers. Many organisations can be found in the same line of business. In health care, the predominant provider is the NHS which belongs to the public sector. However, private enterprise is also involved in health care provision.

Despite the fact that these organisations are in the same line of business each organisation is unique. Each organisation has its own different ways of doing things; this is because each organisation has its own culture. This culture is reflected in the atmosphere of the organisation, the differing levels of energy and the degree of individual freedom (Handy 1985). It is believed that the culture of the organisation influences the behaviour of employees and that the culture develops over time (Beardwell & Holden 1994). The notion that culture influences employee behaviour raises the issue that the culture must influence organisational performance and its mode of decision making.

The effect of culture on performance is the first issue to be discussed in this chapter. In order to explore this, an attempt will be made to identify what the term 'culture' means and how it is transmitted in the workplace. Whilst the main focus is on the NHS many of the issues raised relate to any organisation. Following this, the relationship between organisation structure and culture will be examined. This leads to a brief exploration of two management theories and the effects of these on organisational culture and decision making. Finally the arguments presented will be applied throughout to national health care situations.

CULTURE AND PERFORMANCE

The notion of organisational culture and its effects on organisational performance have been the subject of much debate which remains inconclusive. It is said that they are inexorably linked. Research by Denison (1984, 1990) found that on the one hand an organisational culture which was decentralised and had participative decision-making processes had a good return on investment. Conversely, the culture was also found to have a strong relationship with below-average long-term performance. To date, research in the private sector has not found a relationship between organisational culture and profitability or performance. This may be due to the notion that organisations become stuck into set patterns of behaviour. The very culture which made an organisation successful, such as collective responsibility, consistency, quality and team spirit, which provide energy for growth, lead to the organisation becoming institutionalised. The organisation becomes locked into ways of operating and this stifles creativity and willingness to change. However, and perhaps because of the inconclusive arguments, the interest in the subject remains.

ORGANISATIONAL CULTURE – WHAT IS IT?

Many definitions of organisational culture exist. Anthony (1994) states that the culture provides shared meanings, obligations, expectations and understandings. Consequently organisational

51

culture influences the values and behaviours of its members. The organisational culture can be viewed as the shared rules which govern both cognitive and affective aspects of membership in an organisation. Thus employees are expected to have shared values, attitudes and beliefs (Kunda 1992). Schein (1985) also offers a definition which supports the notion that members of an organisation share basic assumptions, meanings, values and beliefs. Furthermore, it is claimed that without this it would be impossible to survive (Anthony 1994). Jacques (1952) defines organisational culture as the traditional and customary ways of doing things. This has some similarities to the previous definition. However, Jacques (1952) also states that whilst all members accept this, they do so to a greater or lesser degree. Thus the notion that disharmonious relationships can exist within an organisation is raised.

The majority of definitions of organisational culture focus on the individuals within an organisation. In contrast to this, it is stated that organisational culture is a catch-all phrase which incorporates all aspects of the organisation. This includes groups and individuals and provides a micro perspective. At the organisational level a macro perspective is provided. Thus culture can be considered at different levels of analysis (Wilson 1992). Here two levels of analysis are used: the interpretative level (micro perspective) and the structural level (macro perspective). When studying organisational culture it is necessary to take both perspectives into account. At the structural level of analysis the concern is with how roles are structured together to form a particular organisation design. The shape of the organisation becomes an important facet. The interpretative level is concerned with the ways in which individuals act out their role and maintain the culture of the organisation.

TRANSMISSION AND MAINTENANCE OF ORGANISATIONAL CULTURE

At the macro level, organisations communicate their culture to the external world; that is, they transmit their view of themselves to the outside world. This is achieved through a variety of methods such as advertising, company logos, furnishings and style of reception areas. NHS trusts also use some of these mediums, such as the promotion of a corporate image by ensuring that written communication conforms to the corporate style. Some trusts attempt to portray an academic as well as a health care culture. Here the image they are attempting to depict is one of excellence, indicating

The context of decision making

that the public will receive high-quality, research-based care. This is often achieved by including the term 'university' within the trust name. The corporate culture is also presented to the employees with the expectation being that employees will accept the corporate culture in preference to their professional culture (Anthony 1994).

At the interpretative level of analysis, culture is created and maintained through the use of symbols, language and ritual (Wilson 1992). Cultures are also maintained and transmitted through the use of a private language system. In health care terms this is achieved through the use of professional medical and nursing language. Story telling of past situations also maintains the culture of the organisation and reinforces the notion of the way things 'are done' or 'not done' here (Harrison & Stokes 1983).

The ways in which individuals act out their roles creates and maintains the culture of the organisation (Wilson 1992). If new members wish to be accepted by the organisation they must learn to accept the way things are done (Jacques 1952). Indeed, organisations regularly recruit people to fit into the organisational culture as this causes least disruption to the status quo (Pugh & Hickson 1989). Nurses and medical professionals are moulded into patterns of acceptable behaviour and then to a common set of attitudes and meanings. The logic of this is that it is easier to control people's behaviour than it is their values and attitudes. However, once the behaviour becomes routine it is hoped that the attitudes and values which are associated with the behaviours also become the norm for the employee. This is achieved through a process of rewards, sanctions and symbolic construction of outlook, including the induction process. This ensures that new recruits know 'how we do things here' (Anthony 1994). Thus individuals will be able to identify the kind of behaviour which is likely to be required by the corporate culture.

Through this process new members are socialised into the organisation and they are able to determine their own identity in the context of the organisation's culture. An example of this is when a student nurse observes her colleagues finishing duty late in order to ensure an effective handover of care from one shift to another or to finish delivery of care to a patient. The norm is that patients' needs are more important than finishing work on time, even though this 'overtime' will not receive a financial reward. The student nurse will adopt this behaviour and at a later date will form the attitude that patients' needs are of greater importance than finishing work on time. However, the process is unlikely to be this simple, as more than one cultural identity may be possible (Reed 1992). This is particularly so in health care where professional cultures also exist.

Organisational culture and decision making

53

CULTURES AND SUBCULTURES

Many different cultures can exist within a single organisation (Open University Course Team 1994). It is suggested that each part of the organisation should develop its own culture and that this will lead to organisational effectiveness. Furthermore, this culture should reflect the dominant type of activity performed by that department (Handy 1985).

Within the health service each professional group has its own culture. The differences between professional cultures and the corporate culture could be described as subcultures. Given the preceding argument this could be perceived as being good for organisational effectiveness. However, this perspective ignores the problems of subcultures. This multiplicity of cultures can result in disharmonious working relationships (Open University Course Team 1994). This is particularly so if the subcultures do not have an understanding of each other's perspectives. This is in evidence when doctors wish to use new and more expensive treatment regimens and the finance department opposes this.

The organisation's senior managers have a view of the culture of the organisation; that is, its values and vision. However, each professional group will also have a view of their professional culture (subculture) which may or may not reflect, either wholly or partially, the managers' view. It is suggested that managers need to understand all the subcultures within the organisation, which will enable them to analyse the likely responses of other groups to the decisions they make (Open University Course Team 1994). However, given that the interpretative approach personalises organisational culture, individuals will always ask what impact the decision will have on them (Wilson 1992). It is difficult, if not impossible, for managers to achieve this fragmented and personalised level of understanding. At the interpretative level of analysis it is only possible to understand what the culture means from an individual perspective.

MANAGING ORGANISATIONAL CULTURES

The notion that organisational cultures can be managed has been questioned. That culture can be manipulated continues to be a popular belief as it is perceived that changing values can be a quick fix to current difficulties. This notion ignores the complexities of organisational culture and that cultures grow and are established over a period of time. Indeed, the 1990 health care reforms could be viewed as an attempt to change the dominant professional culture to a culture of market responsiveness. The reforms ensured that a medical and nursing representative would form part of the trust executive board, thus adopting the management culture of cost effectiveness and efficiency. Furthermore, it was anticipated that they would be in a position to influence their colleagues to accept the managerial culture in preference to the professional sub-cultures. Thus managing the culture is concerned with managing the values of the organisation. However, attempting to manage the culture without addressing the structure of the organisation is likely to be ineffective (Anthony 1994).

ORGANISATION STRUCTURE, CULTURE AND DECISION MAKING

Whether culture influences organisation structure or is influenced by it is difficult to determine. However, research by the Aston Group (Pugh & Hickson 1989) found that the structure of the organisation was influenced by its size. Cultures differ not only between different organisations but, in large organisations, also between different parts of an organisation; that is, different clinical directorates can have different cultures. Organisation structure and culture affect decision making. They determine:

- who is empowered to make decisions
- the level and range of decisions which can be made independently
- the extent to which decision making is centralised.

Four main types of structure with accompanying cultures have been identified (Handy 1985) and will now be examined in relation to their effects on decision making.

Web structure: power culture

This culture is usually found in small organisations and it relies on a central source of power. This central power base influences every aspect of the organisation. Trust, empathy and personal communication are necessary for this culture to be effective. The recruitment of key people who think the same way as the centre is necessary to ensure that they can be left to do the job in the way that the centre would do it. Thus recruitment and selection of the 'right' people is an important means of control (Handy 1985).

Within this culture, decision making is the domain of the select few who are in positions of leadership. Subordinates are expected to be non-questioning and compliant and they are not expected to use their initiative or be independent. This type of culture can lead to a demotivated workforce (Harrison & Stokes 1983). This culture rarely exists within the health service as a whole because it is suited to small organisations, which rely on key managers for their continuing success. It is claimed that these individuals need to be risk takers who rate personal security as a minor aspect of their psychological contract (Handy 1985). Given that the health service is accountable to multiple stakeholders, such as the Department of Health, tax payers and patients, all of whom have opinions regarding the efficiency and effectiveness of the organisation, and that stability is of prime importance to these stakeholders, it can be seen that this culture is not suitable for the NHS. However, this culture may exist in some departments, such as research or training and development, or in some small private health care establishments.

Bureaucratic structure: role culture

Large organisations have features of bureaucracy. The larger the organisation, the more likely it is to have standardised procedures, highly structured activities, formalised documentation and employees who work in specialist functions, such as professional groups (Pugh & Hickson 1989).

Within this structure, the roles of individuals are clearly defined. Indeed, the role is considered to be more important than the person who fills it (Handy 1985). This role is specified in the job description and individuals are recruited and selected on their ability to fulfil this job description. Research by Jacques (Pugh & Hickson 1989) found that people needed to have their roles clearly defined and acceptable to themselves and others. Most large organisations, including the NHS, have strong elements of the role culture and this provides it with the stability it requires. It is claimed that this culture can be very efficient as much of the routine work can be subject to impersonal rules. This enables work to be delegated with the assurance that it will continue to be carried out without direct supervision from the manager. Individuals are expected to make decisions as they pertain to their role; that is, the decisions are within their sphere of operation such as nursing deci-

The context of decision making

sions relating to nursing care. However, the decisions should follow the organisation's procedures, protocols and rules. Thus individuals are discouraged from being innovative. Indeed, performance at a level above the required role can be disruptive to the organisation.

There are three main characteristics which are required for this type of culture to be effective (Handy 1985).

- Stable, predictable or controllable consumer demand.
- Long product life cycle.
- Monopoly or oligopoly supplier position.

The characteristics required for the role culture to be effective reflect the environment in which the NHS operates. The NHS is in an oligopoly position, operating in a relatively stable environment, with a fairly long product life cycle. Therefore this culture appears to be appropriate for the NHS.

However, role-oriented organisations are slow to adapt and make the necessary changes in order to ensure that they are doing the right thing. Thus they can become ineffective (Harrison & Stokes 1983). It is claimed that with rapidly changing technology, there is a need to move away from bureaucratic structures. Cultural transformation would result in bureaucracies being replaced with dynamic organic cultures. Responsibility would be pushed downward in the organisation in order to maximise flexibility. Employees need to be trusted and as they have the same values, goals and aspirations as the organisation, their judgement and decisions will be in the interest of the organisation (Anthony 1994). The notion of cultural transformation is seductive but it should be borne in mind that from the interpretative level of analysis, individuals accept the culture to a greater or lesser degree (Jacques 1952). Therefore not all their decisions may promote organisation well-being.

Matrix structure: task culture

The task-oriented culture is concerned with getting things done (Walton 1984). This culture provides people with opportunities to use their abilities and specialist skills in ways which are intrinsically satisfying or which advances a purpose or goal to which the individual is committed (Harrison & Stokes 1983). The opportunities for decision making are high and the individual is deemed effective if they achieve the required results (Walton 1984). The emphasis is on team work and the power of the group is used to improve efficiency and efficacy. Each of these teams has the decision-making powers they require and the individuals have a high degree of control over their work.

These cultures can flourish when it is perceived that the customer is always right and where speed of reaction, integration and creativity is more important than specialisation. There is little day-to-day management control in these organisations and little attention is given to how the work is done, as long as the outcomes meet expectations. However, when resources are constrained, that is, not available to all who can justify them, then managers feel the need to control how the work is done as well as the outcomes. The task culture changes to role culture under these conditions (Handy 1985).

Given that the NHS operates within resource constraints, it is difficult for the task culture to be sustained. However, this culture can be found within parts of the organisation such as when project groups are established to change or develop some aspect of service delivery.

Cluster structure: person culture

Within this structure a collection of individuals who share common aims and objectives work together to achieve their individual aims collectively. The culture holds the view that the organisation serves the needs of the individuals in it. Few organisations have this culture because they have objectives which are over and above the collective objectives of the individuals. In addition to this, management control is almost impossible (Handy 1985). However, some professional groups may value this culture. An example of this is where one NHS trust employed a clinical researcher to undertake research activity which was relevant to the trust's sphere of operation. At the end of the review period it was found that little of the work undertaken was of relevance to the trust but it was of interest to the researcher. Less overt examples of this culture can be found where hospital consultants and professors in education work to meet the objectives of their employer in order to retain their employment but they view the organisation as a means to achieving their own aspirations. They carry out activities which further their own interests and these indirectly add to the value of the organisation, such as having a respected 'name' on the staff team.

MANAGEMENT THEORIES, CULTURE AND DECISION MAKING

Organisational structures and cultures are not the only factors which impact on decision making. Management theories also influence the type and range of decisions found and how these decisions are made. Organisation structures and cultures are more supportive of some management theories than others. Indeed, it is claimed that imposing inappropriate structures on a particular culture will lead to ineffectiveness (Handy 1985). There needs to be a match between people, systems, tasks and the structure of the organisation in order to ensure effectiveness and efficiency. Values, which are part of the culture, are communicated by managers. Therefore, managers' beliefs about employees and culture are interdependent (Anthony 1994).

In any organisation there exists a set of beliefs about the way that people should be controlled and organised, how authority should be exercised and decisions made. Our basic assumptions inform our values and enable us to solve problems and make decisions. In everyday life and practice this is useful, as we do not explore problem-solving methods every time we are faced with a decision (Open University Course Team 1994). A number of factors influence our assumptions.

- How we understand reality and the environment in which we operate.
- How we understand our colleagues.
- The purpose of human activity.
- The nature of relationships.

Individual managers may have differing perceptions on these issues. However, it is likely that a core set of assumptions and beliefs exists at an organisational level (Mabey & Mayon-White 1993). These beliefs will be reflected in the style of management adopted and are underpinned by management theories. Differing management theories offer different perceptions on these factors and will influence the culture of the organisation.

Whilst many management theories exist, these can be placed on a continuum from no worker participation in decision making at one extreme (which may be commonly found in power cultures and role cultures) to full participation at the other (which may be found in task cultures, personal cultures and to an extent in role cultures). Whilst these two extremes will be discussed, it is not intended to suggest that either of these approaches is better than

59

the other but that the approach taken should reflect the structure and culture of the organisation and its operating environment. Thus the management approach should be contingent on the situation of the organisation and individual managers' behaviours should reflect this.

Classical management

The classical style of management predominantly reflects the steady state and fits with the role and power cultures. The concern is with allocating subdivided activities to individuals to ensure the most effective and efficient outcome for the organisation. Whilst proponents of this school of thinking have some differences, they have many areas of agreement, from which the following principles have been drawn.

- *Bureaucratic forms of control* – people in higher positions have authority and can delegate work to people in lower positions. There is a clear hierarchy in the organisation.
- *Narrow span of supervision* – each manager is responsible for a group of staff.
- *Clearly defined roles* – each individual knows what their role is within the organisation and they are not expected to undertake any activity outside this role.
- *Clear procedures and protocols* – which state how the role is to be performed (Buchanan & Huczynski 1985). This is in keeping with the notion that there is one best way to do the job. The job is broken down into its component parts and people are selected and trained to fulfil the necessary tasks. The supervisor's role is to get the work completed.

Employees have little discretion or freedom and they generally do not participate in decision making. This is seen as being the prerogative of supervisors and managers. This school of management has been criticised on several points, not least of which is that there is a lack of concern with the interactions between people and the conflict which may occur.

Human relations management

The human relations style of management predominantly reflects the task culture and is more in keeping with modern management thinking. Where the culture is based on this school of management, the supervisors and managers are employee

The context of decision making

centred. Managers concentrate on building effective work teams which set high achievement goals. This open participative style of management should ensure that jobs are designed in such a way as to enable employees to achieve their own personal goals and aspirations whilst meeting the goals of the organisation. Maximum participation in decision making is encouraged. The general belief of managers in this type of organisation is that employees find work fulfilling and rewarding in itself and consequently are motivated to achieve high levels of performance. Whilst this has a positive effect on motivation, attitudes and commitment (Pugh & Hickson 1989), it requires openness of information and dialogue, a clear direction (Anthony 1994) and a vision for the future.

Degree of involvement in decision making

If the culture is taken to mean the way things are done within an organisation, Table 3.1 indicates the degree of involvement in decision making according to the culture of the organisation and the positive and negative effects of this. It can be seen that the decision-making process can be participative, consultative or autocratic. All these processes may be applicable in some circumstances, such as autocratic decision making during crises situations. Thus the culture of the organisation is not the only factor which affects decision making.

In role cultures the majority of decisions made are routine and repetitive or a definite procedure has been identified to deal with them (Pugh & Hickson 1989). Decision making is also influenced by knowledge, skills and habit. An example of this is the actions which are taken when a member of nursing staff reports unfit for work. The first decision to be made is whether to replace the staff member or not. In health care terms this will be influenced by safety considerations; that is, are sufficient staff on duty to deliver safe and effective care to the patients? Some trusts may have specified the minimum number of staff required to ensure safety. In these situations the scope for decision making is low. If this is not the case the second decision relates to the grade of staff required. The final decision relates to how this replacement nurse will be acquired; that is, will the trust bank staff system be used or will a nursing agency be contacted and if so which one? All these decisions are routine practice and are governed by the trust policy. In relation to the final decision, most trusts have the expectation that in the first instance the bank staff will be contacted. If a staff nurse breached this expectation (thereby not conforming to the

Organisational culture and decision making

The context of decision making

Table 3.1 Involvement in decision making

Culture type	Decision making	Positive aspects of culture	Negative aspects of culture
Exploitative authoritarian	Majority of decisions are taken by senior managers	Can achieve high productivity. Decision making can be rapid	Communication is downwards. Managers gain compliance through the use of fear and threats. Employees have negative attitudes towards managers
Benevolent authoritative	Policy decisions are made by senior managers. Employees involved in decisions within a prescribed framework	Managers use rewards to gain compliance. Decision making can be rapid	Communication is predominantly downwards. Subordinates' attitudes are subservient towards superiors
Consultative	Policy decisions are made by senior managers but employees can influence these. Employees make specific decisions at lower levels of decision making	Managers use rewards to gain compliance. Some two-way communication. Some involvement in decision making	Occasional use of sanctions to gain compliance. Limited two-way communication. Decision making can be slow
Participative management	Full use of group participation and involvement in decision making	Two-way communication. High productivity. Improved staff–management relations. High level of job satisfaction	Employees need to understand group decision-making process and be prepared to sacrifice self-interest in the interest of the organisation. Some individuals will not do this. Decision making can be slow

culture of the organisation) and contacted a nursing agency to supply the required staff, they would find that sanctions would be brought to bear in order to ensure future compliance with the norms of the organisation.

CONCLUSION

It is suggested that less hierarchical approaches would lead to greater involvement in decision making. Recent changes in the NHS have reportedly led to flatter and less hierarchical structures. It is claimed that these changes have led to decentralised decision making and that there is now a greater degree of employee involvement in decision making. One of the factors which may have led to this is the notion that participation in decision making is correlated with improved employee commitment. However, one research study indicated that nursing staff did not feel involved in decision making which affected their jobs (Tourish & Mulholland 1997). One explanation for this is that, given the size of NHS trusts, they tend to have a strong element of the role culture. However, as stated earlier, each directorate can have its own culture within the over-arching role culture.

Given that different cultures can exist within one organisation, culture clashes can occur. Individuals have their own values and beliefs and these impact on the organisation's values and beliefs and vice versa. When the two are in harmony there will be agreement. If the dominant culture is one which stifles innovation, this will have an adverse effect on innovative staff. These staff will either adopt the values of the organisation or leave as sanctions are applied in order to gain conformity. Thus if decision making is perceived to be the remit of managers, employees will refer all decisions to the managers and thus become disempowered. This occurs as role-appropriate behaviours are reinforced, not only by formal mechanisms but also by less formal means such as non-verbal gestures indicating approval or disapproval.

Furthermore, each clinical area can have its own subculture which is influenced by the values and beliefs of the clinical area manager who is in a position to reinforce their notions of role-appropriate behaviours. This can be seen when each clinical area uses a different method for completing off-duty rotas and there is no uniform practice within the trust as a whole. In some clinical areas, nursing staff are fully involved in planning the off duty. Although they follow a preset system, such as numbers and grades

Organisational culture and decision making

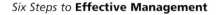

of staff required for each shift, they have a degree of flexibility regarding their off duty. This practice is in keeping with the human relations school of management. However, in other clinical areas the ward manager plans the off duty and there is little if any involvement by the staff. This reflects the classical management school of thought.

It can be seen that culture is a complex concept which impacts on every aspect of the organisation and is also shaped and influenced by the employees of the organisation. Employees are responsible for transmitting and maintaining the culture and they socialise new staff into the accepted behaviours, norms and values of the organisation.

References

Anthony P 1994 Managing culture. Open University Press, Buckingham

Beardwell I, Holden L 1994 Human resource management: a contemporary perspective. Pitman Publishing, London

Buchanan D, Huczynski A 1985 Organisational behaviour. An introductory text. Prentice Hall, London

Denison D 1984 Burning corporate culture to the bottom line. Organisational Dynamics Autumn: 5–22

Denison D 1990 Corporate culture and organisational effectiveness. Wiley, New York

Handy C 1985 Understanding organisations, 3rd edn. Penguin, Harmondsworth

Harrison R, Stokes H 1983 Understanding your organisation's culture. A users' guide to diagnosing culture. Administrative Science Quarterly 28(3): 399–407

Jacques E 1952 The changing culture of a factory. Tavistock, London

Kunda G 1992 Engineering culture. Temple University Press, Philadelphia

Mabey C, Mayon-White B 1993 Managing change, 2nd edn. Paul Chapman, London

Open University Course Team 1994 Managing your enterprise. Block 5: culture and innovation. Open University Press, Buckingham

Pugh D, Hickson D 1989 Writers on organisations, 4th edn. Penguin, Harmondsworth

Reed M 1992 The sociology of organisations: themes, perspectives and prospects. Harvester Wheatsheaf, London

Schein E 1985 Organisational culture and leadership. Jossey-Bass, San Fransisco

Tourish D, Mulholland J 1997 Communication between nurses and nurse managers: a case study from an NHS Trust. Journal of Nursing Management 5: 25–36

Walton M 1984 Management and managing. A dynamic approach. Harper and Row, London

Wilson D 1992 A strategy of change. Routledge, London

The context of decision making

Ann P Young

Reflections of organisational culture in managerial job descriptions

Although professional staff are not known for working closely to their job descriptions, there is no doubt that the job description and person specification are an important influence on appointments and do serve the purpose of flagging up key functions of the job. What is less often appreciated is the way job descriptions open a window onto organisational culture.

The job descriptions reproduced here are of two managerial posts at a similar level of seniority, with both postholders reporting to the general manager of a hospital or directorate within a hospital. However, one is from the NHS, the other from the private sector.

It is suggested that the job descriptions are examined for points of similarity and difference. Bear in mind that the deputy general manager does not manage the nursing staff and a nursing qualification was not essential, although desirable, for this post. The matron, on the other hand, had specific line management responsibility for nursing staff and had to have a nursing qualification. Although this has coloured the job descriptions, there are other interesting differences that seem to reflect culture rather than job content.

Box 3.1.1 Sample NHS job description

Post:	**Deputy general manager**
Directorate:	**Medicine**
Location:	**— Hospital**
Reports to:	**General manager**

Job purpose

The postholder will work to the general manager to ensure that the day-to-day operational management of the Directorate is effective. The postholder will be responsible for key groups of non-nursing personnel and will advise the Directorate team upon best utilisation of resources. The postholder will provide business management support in contract monitoring, support service developments and reviews undertaken on a regular basis. The post will provide professional advice to the Directorate management team.

Key areas

The postholder will:

- support the general manager in preparation of the Directorate business plans/Directorate performance charter and negotiate with internal and external parties over future service requirements
- monitor the Directorate's expenditure on staffing, supplies and equipment, advising the management team on potential efficiency measures
- monitor the workload in line with contracts and develop systems for handling fluctuations in activity
- ensure Trust policies and procedures are implemented within areas of responsibility across the Directorate and organise appropriate training and development for staff
- monitor compliance with Patient's Charter standards, develop and implement actions to ensure requirements are met
- monitor, investigate and collate responses to complaints, providing feedback to the management team quarterly
- assist the general manager with the development and commissioning of new services
- take responsibility for the overall management of the medical secretaries, support staff and key departments to be agreed
- work closely with the medical teams and ensure junior doctors' hours are met, intensity of work is monitored and systems developed for effective patient management
- take lead responsibility for health and safety management and compliance with Trust policies

(continued)

The context of decision making

(continued)

- produce business cases for new or replacement equipment in response to both patients' needs and advances in chemical technology
- work with the medical team to develop multidisciplinary clinical audit, research and use of evidence-based medicine
- establish an efficient multidisciplinary communication system for the Directorate
- develop a local risk management policy incorporating corporate risk profiling
- act as the lead officer for the transfer of services
- any other duties that may from time to time be delegated by the clinical director/general manager.

NB: This job description identifies the key aspects of the post. It will form the basis of discussion between the postholder and the manager to develop a set of annual objectives against which performance can be measured.

Person specification

	Essential	*Desirable*
Educational qualifications	Management qualification	RGN, degree, diploma
Skills, abilities	Excellent communication skills, strong leadership ability, ability to negotiate, challenge current practice, influencing ability, change management	Presentational skills
Experience	Minimum 3 years in senior nursing/management position	
Knowledge	Human resource policies, budgetary control	Contracts, business plenary, IT skills, standards for clinical care
Disposition	Assertive, ability to work autonomously	
Other requirements	Good attendance, ability to work flexibly	

The context of decision making

Sample private health care job description

Post: **Matron**
Reports to: **General manager**
Location: **— Hospital**

Job purpose

To provide overall clinical leadership and operational management. To promote a cost-effective, patient-focused, quality service for the continuing success of the company hospitals in an ever-changing competitive health care market. To provide a clear focus on business results, maintaining the balance between quality health care delivery and good financial performance. The job holder will deputise for the general manager in their absence.

Key accountabilities

Professional issues

- Monitor and maintain a safe clinical environment that meets local registration and statutory requirements.
- Develop and implement nursing and clinical strategy and business developments, supporting the general manager.
- Establish and develop consultant relationships.
- Represent clinical services on the Medical Advisory Committee.
- Advise on impact of local/corporate clinical issues, to business planning and achievement of annual operating plan.
- Identify opportunities to develop and improve patient care.

Customer care

- Act as patient champion and advocate.
- Empower clinical staff to achieve excellence in patient care.
- Regularly discuss care with patients, staff and consultants.
- Perform concurrent review of inpatients.
- Monitor the standards of patient care and clinical staffing arrangements.
- Develop patient care standards and staff involved in setting them.
- Ensure evidence/research-based best practices in patient care.
- Manage all clinical patient complaints and liaise with MAC chairperson (as detailed in handbook).
- Represent all patient issues in hospital forums, e.g. MAC, SMT, ensuring all business decisions are patient focused.

(continued)

(continued)

- Act as role model for all nursing staff; 'walk the walk'.
- Participate in clinical supervision of patient care.

Human resource management

- Act as positive role model, enhancing standards and professionalism.
- Establish an empowered environment in order to facilitate the delivery of first-class health care.
- Nurture an innovative thinking and creative culture.
- Promote appropriate crossfunctional teamwork, including multiskilling, with an overall emphasis on accountability and responsibility.
- Lead, develop and empower individual staff to realise their full potential for the business.
- Contribute to effective use of staff within multidisciplinary teams, e.g. skill mix.
- Be responsible for continuous learning for themselves and their staff, thus developing the competencies required to achieve business objectives, thus leading to continuous improvement in health care and customer service delivery.
- Ensure that resources are secured to enable the clinical strategy to be delivered and to maintain statutory requirements.

Quality and marketing

- Ensure that all clinical processes are designed to be customer driven, crossfunctional and value based and that they are fully applied and their clinical effectiveness monitored.
- Provide clinical expertise to the implementation and development of business processes.
- Ensure that the hospital provides the best solutions for its customers' needs in order to achieve business results, thus creating and developing strong relationships which will help strengthen the company brand name and create competitive advantage.
- Provide an excellent image of clinical services to customers.
- Achieve all targets set for patient/clinical areas and support the general manager in the delivery of achieving the AOP.

Information and communication

- Apply fact-based decision making, achieved through accurate and timely information.
- Be responsible for evidence/research practice and utilise information and quality systems to deliver cost-effective, quality patient care.

(continued)

Reflections of organisational culture

The context of decision making

(continued)

Person specification

A registered nurse with a robust track record in senior clinical management, with experience of change/project management. Preferably a graduate in health-related study who can demonstrate a sound understanding of clinical issues, Working life spent both inside and outside the clinical environment with experience of working in teams with other health professionals and non-clinical managers. Skills in diplomacy and negotiation will be needed to work effectively in teams, often in areas which challenge the status quo.

The job holder will need to be self-motivating and must have drive in starting and following through initiatives. Success in the job will demand perseverance and determination to carry to conclusion what may be fundamental changes in the clinical service.

An ability to provide a 'balanced' view is vital, weighing up costs of potential developments in relation to their value to professionals within the company, the hospital and patients/clients.

An ability to present concisely and effectively to senior managers to enable their decision making.

The job holder will be required to assimilate and utilise clinical data, information from external regulatory and educational bodies, academic literature and financial data.

The job holder will be required to be creative in driving initiatives within the constraints of company policies and practices. The job holder will have the authority to establish, implement and monitor clinical working processes and standards of practice.

The job holder must work within the professional, organisational and legal standards required.

NB: The job holder is operating within a 24-hour environment with on-call responsibilities, dealing with internal and external customers, inpatients and outpatients, critical and emergency situations.

There will be a pressure to work to strict deadlines on projects.

This job description is by no means exhaustive and may be altered at any time to meet the needs of the business. This will be in discussion with the job holder.

COMMENTS

Some common concerns colour both job descriptions and are typical of a post at this level. Both are operationally focused, require the postholder to work within and to implement agreed and imposed policies and procedures and have responsibility for health and safety. Specific to health care are aspects of dealing with patient complaints and the provision of professional advice and leadership. Both require a multiskilled and flexible person. Both include aspects of business management, reflecting the shift in the NHS towards a contract culture and financial efficiency already embedded in the private sector.

However, some of the differences between the two job descriptions are striking. The most obvious is the emphasis on customer care and customer-driven quality issues in the private sector whereas in the NHS a direct involvement with patient opinion is lacking. Quality issues here seem driven by government-imposed standards while in the private hospital there is scope to develop local standards.

The emphasis in the NHS job description does seem to be on monitoring, seeming to fit with a rather static and stratified organisational culture. Although the private hospital manager also has some responsibility for monitoring, there is a much greater emphasis on creativity, initiative and innovation, indicating an organisation that values a quick response to changing circumstances.

There is also a greater emphasis in the matron's job description on staff development than is found in the NHS. Finally, the job holder in the private hospital is expected to work on presenting a certain image to customers and strengthening the brand name of the company. Such requirements in a NHS job description at operational level would be highly unusual.

It might be worth thinking through some of these differing cultural issues. Obviously, the fact that creativity and initiative are missing from the NHS job description does not mean that NHS managers cannot act creatively or with initiative (see Chapter 11). The failure to emphasise staff development and ongoing learning should not lead the reader to assume that these are seen as unimportant to NHS organisations (see Chapters 12 and 15 particularly). The lack of any acknowledged customer drivers to quality issues does not mean that these are being ignored (see Chapters 7 and 8). However, their omission from or only brief mention in a job description does indicate an organisational culture that is slow to take these issues on board. This does make the job of the manager or practitioner attempting to introduce change much harder.

The other side of the coin should also be put forward. Just because certain ways of working do feature very obviously in the private care job description, their implementation by the postholder may not be as easy as anticipated. The broad range of key accountabilities seems to expect the postholder to 'walk on water' and may be unrealistic. A list of 32 key responsibilities compared to the 16 in the NHS job description may actually indicate a more prescriptive environment than assumed at first sight.

Reflections of organisational culture

Application **3:2**

Ann P Young

Interview with the manager of a unit for those with behavioural disorders

The context of decision making

As you read this interview, ask yourself the following questions:

1. What would you like about working with this manager?
2. What would you dislike about working with this manager?
3. What makes her successful in her role?
4. What are the drawbacks to her particular managerial style?
5. To what extent is the organisational culture at odds with this manager's style?
6. How does this manager's approach compare to your own and to that of some of your colleagues?

> I have been in this job for 3 years. My boss is the clinical director who is a consultant psychiatrist but informally I go to the chief executive. I will not take the clinical director's decisions on things.
>
> Networks are important to me. Internal networks are those you can get on with, those you can work together with, those that are mutually beneficial to each other in becoming powerful. People like the head of corporate development, in finance, in contracting, down to those who are trust administrators but because they have been there some time, they are quite powerful as they know everything and are very threatening to other people. Nursing networks are negligible. Networks are useful in order to get things done, to get them on your side.
>
> External networks – I've lost a lot of those. Regional ones were huge but largely disappeared. I have a link with the DoH nursing department. At the King's Fund, I did the nurse executive course because that's my ultimate aim, also on a learning set, all nurses, one
>
> *(continued)*

director of nursing, others like me, so we link regularly and have a facilitator. RCN is good in psychiatry. The private sector are our biggest competitors so I've worked on them, got to know people and got on with people so I know who I can ring up really. Networks are useful for a number of reasons, as a support mechanism, to get ideas in psychiatry, to get things done. I am doing an MSc course and one of the attractions was for the networks it was going to develop for me.

I see power as the ability to influence people and to ensure that people get things done and achieve. I definitely have power in my directorate. My ability with staff is very powerful and feared by a lot, I know. They are afraid that I'm going to change the culture of the trust – yes, I want to; it's one burning ambition I have. Things are changing. People I have clashed with or failed to get on with or they've done some rather untoward things to me, or tried to, interestingly have disappeared from the organisation.

I have a lot of influence in my directorate, particularly with the professionals, including the psychiatrists, psychologists – more than my clinical director. I'm clearly seen as being for the service and for the directorate and he is seen as having his own agenda. That's the difference. By influencing, I exert authority. I had some difficulty with a lot of new staff in one unit. They tried to test the system. So I took it over, had to be autocratic. I was suspicious of what was going on. I and others have started to influence change, particularly in one unit. I hope I am good at getting my staff on board and seeing me as the person to get on with. I'm not disciplinarian. I am against lukewarm discipline. If I have to discipline I'm afraid it's the ultimate. I believe that if I get my staff on board, they will be disciplined, they will work in a disciplined way. I have also got to show them that I have ability; I don't have knowledge of psychiatry, I have had to learn from them, but I showed them how to sell themselves, how to make things better. I had to have credibility. The fact I was a nurse was a plus.

I have limited scope, as a senior nurse in the organisation. I had more freedom as a ward sister than I have now. But if they take issue with me, I fight. One has to be cunning in the way one does it and one has to fight. Sometimes I do something and they know about it after the event. Now, I could risk getting myself disciplined but I am doing things that are good for the service, so I am proving myself. If they start putting the blocks on me, then I fight it but in a professional way. I mean, I never get into discipline issues. Some of the things I do – it's blackmail.

When I found myself at odds with senior management, I responded in two ways. First, I tended to go in and challenge, I'm used to doing that. Initial challenges worked, because I was succeeding where nobody had before, nobody questioned. Then the tide changed for all

(continued)

(continued)

sorts of reasons. And the challenges came. Now I make two responses. I might be almost submissive to it, seem to be submissive which I then have to convince my staff of why I am being submissive. I tell my staff that we have to not expect to get results in 5 minutes, I work way ahead. They see that those who have challenged me have gone, so that in itself says something. And the other side, I have to sit there and say, I can't accept this, on the one hand you are telling me I have to get staff, the other side you are putting blocks on me to do it. What do you expect? I don't challenge immediately, go away and fume, produce a document with a response of let's take this forward, e.g. to personnel. I make it abundantly clear that I am not going to be stepped on, I'm going to do everything to ensure the service is to a high standard. I don't get so angry now.

First, they just let me get on with things – as things changed around me, suddenly I started to get my knuckles rapped. My business manager said to me, you know why you're the one, because we upset others by our success.

I believe that rules are to be broken. I agree with some regarding safety around patients; around staffing – ridiculous, usually I get round them. We are most influenced by the targets, the requirement for break-even. We determine the targets. The success of the unit is its main fighting power.

I think I have changed. Yes. I'm probably more cynical. In the past, I enjoyed a lot of good fortune, a very different type of regime. I was a very dynamic innovative individual. I'm told I still am, but to me I'm not as much. I suppose because I'm not doing some of the things I was doing before. Nobody ever stopped me. I couldn't be a square peg in a round hole – it's been said, she's fine if given the freedom. But I survive. The reason I survive is I sit and grin and bear it, whereas other people walk out, I go away and fume, bang the wall and I know I'm a sticker, I'm a survivor through thick and thin, they cannot knock me and I think that has raised my esteem in the trust as well as my self-esteem. Less than a month ago, I went through a kangaroo court, my staff knew it, something I should never have lost. It was not about the issue but about me. I've survived, one of the panel hasn't.

Managerial roles have changed. I don't think the Trust understands what is required of a general manager whereas in my early days I knew I might have to work over the Easter period at home to put reports together for a deadline. In the NHS, more is expected of managers and there are fewer capable managers around. I think managers are not trained to an appropriate standard. I meet lots of managers and I can tie them up in business; I've long lived in a business environment, I grew up with business so the transition is relatively easy for me. Many managers are lost in the world of finance and marketing.

COMMENTS

You might have reached the conclusion that the manager being interviewed here gave some examples of useful skills but on the whole would have been a rather uncomfortable person to be close to!

For example, her ability to develop networks is a particularly useful skill. She takes a fairly instrumental approach to this and, as a result, has a wide range of contacts, both internally and externally. Note how she goes about building these networks and why.

She is also clear about her leadership role and not afraid of making unpopular decisions. Staff are likely to know where they stand with her although she can probably be a hard taskmaster.

Compromise does not come naturally to her and this probably reduces her effectiveness as a manager. It seems likely that she expects conflict and is therefore more likely to meet it. A more collaborative and cooperative approach might, in the long run, be more effective but is not one that comes naturally to her. She tends to interpret situations as win/lose, rather than win/win.

She herself admits to trying to change the culture. Her personal background is business orientated with a current job that involves managing profit rather than break-even. She is, not surprisingly, uncomfortable in a public sector organisation that is bureaucratic and carrying prescribed roles.

Her professional background has proved important in gaining credibility with other professionals. This seems to be a recurrent theme for all health care managers and underpins decision-making styles to a marked extent.

A number of these issues are explored further in the following chapters.

Interview with the manager of a behavioural disorder unit

Section **Two**

DECISION MAKING IN PRACTICE

OVERVIEW

Making a decision is not a simple event in a single moment of time. Instead it should be viewed as a complex activity. Decisions range from those that seem to be totally operational with short-term consequences to those that can be classified as strategic that will in due course trigger a whole range of subdecisions that, in turn, become increasingly operational. A decision, any decision, can be assumed to have wider consequences than the immediate and the practicalities of decision making highlight this. Also, the way people decide to approach decisions is influenced by the type of people they are, their background and experience and the particular day-to-day circumstances in which they find themselves. Making decisions is therefore a very practical activity and this underpins the emphasis of Section Two of this book.

Sandland's chapter on the characteristics of decision making provides the theoretical backbone to this section. He presents in a very clear and easily assimilated form a number of models of decision making set within the realities encountered. Categories of decisions, decision-making processes, some tools for analysis and choice and the importance of learning from the consequences of decisions provide a broad-ranging base for the following chapters and applications.

Chapter Five focuses on the interface between practitioner and management skills. A move from practice to management and a move into a combined practice/management role are explored. Smith and Young argue that an examination of managerial skills alongside the skills that the health professional develops through practice shows some important synergies. The practical nature of decision making is continued in Chapter Six where the effect of group processes and networks on decisions is explored.

Having concentrated largely in Section Two on the part played by the practitioner/manager in decision making, we then turn to the wider and politically sensitive issue of the health care user's involvement in decision making. This is seen as such an important issue that the whole of Section Three is given over to this debate.

Decision making in practice

Chapter **Four**

The characteristics of decision making in health care

David Sandland

- **The parallels between individual and organisational decision taking**
- **Categories of decisions**
- **The planning process**
- **The mission**
- **Objectives**
- **Strategic analysis**
- **Strategic choice**
- **Strategic implementation**
- **Review and evaluation**
- **The learning organisation**
- **Rational and incremental decision making**
- **Conclusion**

Good judgement comes from experience, and experience comes from bad judgement. (Barry LePatner, cited in Boone & Lichtenstein 1999)

Effective management always means asking the right question. (Robert Heller , cited in Boone & Lichtenstein 1999)

O V E RV I E W

The title of this chapter refers to the health care industry that has seen, and will continue to see, many changes. These affect the nature of the organisations in the industry, their remit and the political and social environment within which they must operate. With this background against which decision making is the subject, it seems right to take a wider focus, examining:

s and analysis
making

than only that of the health care industry.
iscinating subject, with areas of
from:

iourist approaches
iate decision
j-term strategic decisions
in individual decision maker to the
ip decision making.

At one extreme, it is possible to entertain the concept of logical, rational decision making whilst recognising that the other extreme is a poorly structured, non-logical choice. The former implies the provision of all necessary quantitative information and analysis skills whereas the latter indicates a much more imperfect system. In reality, decision making is an amalgam of the two. There are areas that lend themselves to rational, informed decision taking but, equally, there are areas that preclude this luxury.

Whatever role the decision maker fulfils or whatever the timescale is, the primary function of decision making is to create a suitable scenario for the *future*. This basic requirement questions whether any decision can be truly rational since trying to provide for the future means that the decision maker will never possess perfect information and so a completely rational decision can never be made. Whatever the circumstances, the identical scenario has never been encountered before. Some aspect will be different from the last time a similar decision was taken. Often, of course, the difference will only become apparent with hindsight. Obviously, the more repetitive and routine the style of decision making, the less likely it is that the difference will be of any significance in the outcome.

THE PARALLELS BETWEEN INDIVIDUAL AND ORGANISATIONAL DECISION TAKING

Decision takers are people

Probably the most obvious but also, possibly, the most overlooked. People take the same skills, knowledge bases, foibles and scruples

to both individual and organisational de
to make mistakes in whichever capacity they

Decisions come in different forms

Whether personal or organisational, decisions come in di
categories relating to the:

- term
- expense
- risk
- number of people involved
- complexity
- degree of influence on future decisions.

There are numerous categories but the list here will adequately illustrate the parallels.

Take a few moments to reflect on the decisions that you have taken recently. They may have involved some of the following or similar.

- What to have for breakfast.
- Where to go on holiday.
- Which car to purchase.
- Do you accept that job offer that is 300 miles away from home?

The first example is routine, commonplace, risk free (usually), non-consequential and affects no-one except the decision maker. It does not merit a great deal of attention, time or skill. It may not even be thought of as a decision. Nevertheless, it is and is seldom without its own features. Do you, for instance, have a free choice of what to have for breakfast or are you constrained by what is in the cupboard? Corporate decisions that are routine, day-to-day decisions only affecting limited parts of the organisation for relatively short periods before being overtaken by the next decision fall into very similar categories. Equally, these operational corporate decisions will be constrained. The decision taker will not have a free choice in the matter but will often follow previously devised rules and procedures.

The second and third examples are more complex and, necessarily, receive more time, skills and effort. They may involve:

- research
- more than just the decision maker
- a greater level of expenditure
- a greater risk of an unsatisfactory outcome.

The characteristics of decision making in health care

ls to Effective Management

sions. They are as likely to be making decisions.

erent

ly say they have made a ration-
very large number of 'off-road'
ars but are never driven off road
al decision taking involves simi-
ent decisions hinder organisation-
e decision is not unlike previous
nsiderable amount of high-quality
ecision taker but each decision is

ringing the alarm bells. A decision

- nav...
- carry a high degree ... isk
- involve many hours or days in self-debate
- lead to arguments
- involve a high level of stress
- have no clear answer however much research is undertaken.

The final decision is likely to be taken using imperfect information. A non-rational analysis is a time-constrained process that will in some part reflect the decision maker's attitude to risk. The above applies to many of the most important organisational decisions. They also suffer from difficulties in the formulation of the criteria on which to base the decision.

Decisions are not always rational

When faced with difficult decisions, the decision maker often addresses considerations that are peripheral but are treated as important and allowed to unduly influence the decision. Thus people can be 'protected' or the true facts of the situation avoided. Organisational decisions are vulnerable to similar occurrences; in fact, the problem is multiplied with each member incorporating their own private agenda, giving rise to the observation that the camel must have been designed by a committee.

Decisions can be delayed

'Delaying tactics' help to put off making the difficult and conse-quential decision, taking the form of easier, short-term decisions

Allows you to do further assessments, to rule out thin

that are suddenly very important. The major decision is sidelined while the short-term decisions are dealt with, allowing the decision taker to put off the evil decision with excuses that other matters are more urgent. Possibly they are but they cannot be used indefinitely to delay making that difficult decision without incurring severe penalties of some form. Organisational decision takers are no different in this aspect where the result could be a lost business opportunity or a deterioration in the situation.

CATEGORIES OF DECISIONS

The parallels discussed illustrate some of the difficulties decision takers encounter. To further this, it is necessary to provide a more formal analysis. First, a form of categorisation of decision types is presented.

Simon (1960) provided one of the earliest and most enduring categorisations with the concept of *programmed* and *non-programmed* decisions. This provides for the fact that many business decisions are routine and repetitive and are best handled by a rule-based procedure whilst others involve a much higher degree of complexity. A comparison between the two is provided in Table 4.1 Simon's categories provide the two extremes of a continuum of decision types. Some decisions will fall between these two extremes, with a *spread* of decisions from day-to-day operational aspects through to the strategic.

Gilligan et al (1983) extended Simon's two-category scheme to a three-category model.

1. *Short-term operating control decisions* – this category matches Simon's programmed decisions closely.
2. *Periodic control decisions* – here Gilligan et al introduced a category at some midpoint in the spectrum. These are not day-to-day decisions but are met on a regular basis, maybe every month, 6 months or every year. They are largely connected with monitoring the progress of the organisation, reflected in the chosen name – periodic *control* decisions.
3. *Strategic decisions* – this category closely matches Simon's non-programmed decisions.

Gilligan et al provide a more workable set of categories while reflecting the spread of types of decisions that are involved in the management of any type of organisation.

The characteristics of decision making in health care

Table 4.1 Programmed and non-programmed decisions

Highly programmed	Highly non-programmed
Concern the general operation of the organisation	Concern the future of the whole organisation
Undertaken by relatively junior members	Involve senior management
Involve little research	Involve detailed research
Require limited resources such as finance, labour, materials, time and only specific skills	Require significant resources such as finance, labour, materials, time and skills
Carry little risk for the future of the organisation	Carry significant consequences and risk
Routine by nature	Novel by nature
Relatively trivial	Complex
Straightforward	No clear structure
Involve certainty	Involve uncertainty
Rules and procedures to guide decision making	Few rules and procedures with which to approach these problems
Quick	Long term

Table 4.1 provides a framework for the further consideration of decisions using relative terms enabling a comparison to be readily made. In individual cases, decisions are encountered that cross these categories.

Operational decisions

These are the easier decisions, largely resulting from the rule-based nature of operational decision making, characterised by:

- repetitiveness
- relatively short timescales
- control rather than planning.

Within this framework, decisions acquire other characteristics.

- They are easily reversed, often because of the proximity of the next similar decision in the sequence.
- They generate much information useful for control and the decision-making process.

- They tend towards the quantitative, facilitating numerical processing.
- They involve numerate techniques and the degree of success is readily assessed, generating further information for the decision-making process.
- They require a number of simplifying assumptions about the 'real' world such as taking a restrictive view of the scenario. These are unlikely to be questioned whilst making the decision but must be reviewed in the wider planning process. Thus, managerial judgement, although not figuring significantly in operational decision making, cannot be too far divorced from these decisions.
- Objectives/targets, constraints and budgets will be clearly defined, usually in monetary terms but also by government-imposed requirements.
- They are addressed using a large number of techniques such as resource scheduling, capacity scheduling, stock control/purchasing, quality control and clinical audit.

Periodic control decisions

Gilligan et al's intermediate classification requires more managerial judgement in the decision-making process but the primary function remains that of control. These decisions share more features with operational decisions than they do with strategic decisions, namely:

- they are regular and repetitive, albeit on a much longer interval and not necessarily totally identical
- they lend themselves to numerical techniques
- they generate substantial quantities of information that aid future decisions
- they are part of the organisation's overall information system.

They differ from operational decisions in that a substantial part of their purpose is the review of the rules and frameworks for the operational decisions, including the allocation of new resources and the monitoring of those already allocated. This highlights two components of the decisions:

- forward planning
- review and control.

Typical techniques that may be relevant within periodic control decisions include:

- review of staffing levels and skill mix
- break-even analysis of the budget

The characteristics of decision making in health care

- longer term project control
- Patient's Charter analysis.

Strategic decisions

Gilligan et al refer to strategic decisions as:

> the most fundamental, often the most difficult but, paradoxically, the most frequently underestimated decisions encountered by business organisations. (Gilligan et al 1983, p. 154)

Strategic decisions are long term, both in their consequences to the organisation and in their formulation and implementation. They are always unique in that no identical situation can have been encountered before. They involve a high degree of uncertainty and a paucity of quantitative information. These last features are caused by the long timespan projecting into the future. This makes strategic decisions difficult to both formulate and assess in terms of their consequences.

Once a decision has been made, the course of action is selected and implementation begins. This takes a substantial period of time.

- The strategy is converted into detailed tactics.
- Tactics are converted into detailed campaigns.
- Physical resources are identified, e.g. location and equipment requirements.
- The workforce are recruited and/or trained.
- Communication networks are established.

Whilst these and the many other facets of implementation are taking place, the external environment has continued to develop and change. Against what should the outcomes of this strategic decision and implementation be measured: the criteria in place when the decision was 'frozen' or the equivalent criteria in the current climate?

Strategic decisions cannot be considered only in terms of deciding future actions. By their very nature and consequence, they also decide future patterns of managerial style, organisational culture and ethics. These decisions tend to change most aspects of the organisation and how people connected with the organisation work and relate. These cultural consequences add a further dimension and difficulty to decision making.

Established patterns of behaviour add further difficulties to strategic decision making. Reward systems for senior managers often include a substantial element based upon results. These

Decision making in practice

short-term rewards may interfere with the long-term decision-making process when the 'correct' strategic decision substantially reduces a decision maker's rewards.

The promotion mechanism within an organisation may also be a hindrance. Strategic decision making differs from operational and periodic control decisions, requiring a high degree of judgement. Usually staff demonstrating high levels of competence at the lower level decisions, requiring analytical skills rather than judgement, are promoted. Could it be argued that internal promotion is not the best way to equip an organisation with the strategic decision makers that it needs?

THE PLANNING PROCESS

All planning processes fulfil the basic purpose of asking two questions.

- Where are we now?
- Where do we wish to be?

Fayol (1949) defined the functions of management as: planning, organising, commanding, coordinating, controlling. It seems self-evident to say that planning should precede the remainder, being the mechanism for providing the framework within which the others operate. This was a major theme of Simon (1960), who was concerned that administration should place planning as the central focus to achieve effective action.

Drucker (1977, p. 28) added a further function to those of business managers – that of economic performance. This seemingly differentiates the manager's role in a profit-making organisation from that in a non-profit making organisation but the latter are more and more being driven by budgetary issues. Business managers must justify their actions in terms of the economic results. With non-profit making organisations adopting the management styles of the profit-making sector, these can be regarded as profit-allocating organisations rather than profit-making ones.

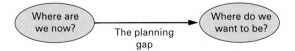

Figure 4.1 The planning gap.

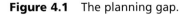

Just as most organisations have a management structure which is 'thinner' at the top, so the decision-making process in an organisation will form a hierarchy, seen in its simplest form in Figure 4.2. Like the organisation structure, this is pyramidal, the wider base representing the numbers of decisions involved.

Traditionally, decisions in the top layers of this hierarchy are few, less frequent and affect the whole organisation, being expressed in overall terms and lacking detail. This is progressively added as the process cascades down the pyramid. Decisions made at various levels within the pyramid become progressively more focused on to individual parts of the organisation, covering shorter timescales and becoming more detailed and quantitative in nature the lower the position in the hierarchy.

The lower levels of decisions in the hierarchy should not be made outside the framework provided by the higher levels. There is therefore a sequence of decision making with those setting out the mission of the organisation preceding all others. Decision making is inherently a *top-down* process. Senior managers can lose touch with the operational aspects of the organisation they manage, resulting in the possibility of strategic decisions being made that are operationally unsound. A bottom-up movement of information must inform senior managers on the operational aspects of the decisions they make.

Part of the implementation stage of a strategic decision involves the performance of many other tactical and operational decisions. These are put into practice to become the overall plan for the organisation.

Figure 4.3 is a model of the overall decision-making process incorporating the 'lower' levels of decisions within the corporate strategic decisions. At this stage, the feedback loop returns to all previous stages with the exception of the mission, which, by its very nature, should not be reviewed on a regular basis. This is

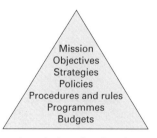

Figure 4.2 The hierarchy of planning levels.

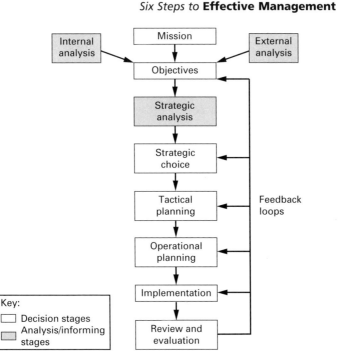

Figure 4.3 The decision-making process.

because it should be formulated in such a way that it applies for a substantial period of time without requiring review.

THE MISSION

The mission of an organisation is the starting point of all planning processes, being the long-term view of the organisation's purpose. The mission must be stable for it to be effective in providing the congruence for all the decisions taken within the organisation and therefore it should not be changed readily. To achieve this, it must be expressed in a general way that reflects the role and values of the organisation. It is 'The organisation's reason for existing: the identification of what business it's in' (Hellriegel & Slocum 1992, p. 247) or, more precisely, 'Establishing broad purpose and direction for the total organisation as in answering the question "what type of company do we want to be?" ' (Leontiades 1982, p. 3). Mintzberg (1976) refines this by suggesting it should be expressed in a form related to the organisation's products or services and Hannigan adds a further important dimension in that it should be 'The present view of the

The characteristics of decision making in health care

organisation's purpose without restricting future possible develop-ment' (Hannigan 1995, p. 122). A further element is given by Daft in defining the mission as 'A broadly stated definition of the organisa-tion's basic business scope and operation that distinguishes it from similar types of organisations' (Daft 1997, p. 218).

A wider definition is generally accepted, comprising four ele-ments.

1. *Purpose* – why the organisation exists. For most businesses, cre-ating wealth for the shareholders will take priority over any other component of purpose. For the public sector, the purpose may be enshrined in statute.
2. *Strategy* – the economic logic of the organisation in terms of:

   ● the nature of its business
   ● the markets it intends to operate in
   ● its own competitive advantages
   ● the devices it intends to employ.

3. *Policies and standards of behaviour* – an outline of those policies and standards of behaviour that should control everyday per-formance for the organisation, e.g. standards of service.
4. *Values* – an outline of the organisation's culture and the beliefs of the people who work for and on behalf of the organisation.

It can be readily appreciated that if any of these elements conflict, then the mission will fail to provide that degree of congruence needed for the organisation to prosper.

OBJECTIVES

In contrast to the mission, the objectives of an organisation should be specific and quantitative. Hellriegel describes the business goal or objective as 'a specific result or outcome to be attained; indicates the direction in which decisions and actions should be aimed' (Hellriegel & Slocum 1992). It is further defined by Brocka as 'a quantitative statement of future expectations with an indication of when it should be achieved (Brocka & Brocka 1992).

These definitions can be refined into the very useful acronym.

Specific
Measurable
Attainable
Realistic or results oriented
Time-bounded

Decision making in practice

In order to satisfy these, especially the measurable category, objectives are often expressed in financial or quality terms and have several functions.

● They enable the overall objectives of the organisation to be subdivided into clear statements of what should be done at each level.
● They provide clear statements of required action.
● They provide a focus for all activity.
● They facilitate the control of performance.
● They provide the basis for evaluating the success of implementation.

It follows that there needs to be a further hierarchy – one of objectives:

1. corporate objectives
2. functional objectives
3. team objectives
4. individual objectives

and as for the previous hierarchies, there is an ever-increasing number of objectives at each level. The timescale will also be shorter the lower in the hierarchy the objective falls. All objectives should be explicit, quantifiable, capable of being achieved and agreed by all the parties involved.

Corporate objectives should relate to factors that determine an organisation's success. Typically, these are long term. In the private sector, they are expressed in terms of:

● market share
● growth
● profitability
● cash flow
● survival
● growth in payments to shareholders (for profit-allocating organisations)
● customer satisfaction
● quality of the produced goods and services
● industrial relations.

In the public sector, objectives will include the last three on the list above but will replace the others with objectives expressed in terms of:

● commissioner/provider contracts
● budgetary control
● public accountability.

The characteristics of decision making in health care

91

Functional objectives have a shorter timescale and are specific to the individual units that make up the organisation. They might relate to a particular department or section and can be thought of as the tactical aspects of the organisation's activities.

STRATEGIC ANALYSIS

In order for any planning process to be effective, the decision maker(s) should be supplied with all the available information. They will not necessarily have all the information that they need, but they will be in the most advantageous position possible.

The vital strategic analysis phase involves information gathering. The analysis needs to be comprehensive and thorough, incorporating all aspects of the organisation and its environment. The health 'industry' is one where major contributory factors are the more general social factors such as population growth or decline.

The structure of the analysis is helped by splitting the environment into its two logical components, namely:

- the internal environment (of the organisation and its operations)
- the external environment (and its influences).

The internal environment

Good planning depends on a clear unbiased picture of the organisation's current position. This is a 'position audit' and involves an examination of (inter alia):

- skills
- resources available:
  - tangible assets
  - intangible assets
  - finance
  - labour

- services offered and current markets
- operating systems (e.g. communication)
- internal organisation (e.g. structure, management, culture)
- past and current achievements (e.g. specialist services, care pathways, management systems)
- identification of successes and failures with reasons for these.

Parts of this analysis can be carried out using 'value chain analysis' (Porter 1985). This method identifies those parts of the organisation that add value to products or services and those that do not. These non-value adding functions are the services (for example, the personnel department) not contributing to the 'output'. They help the value-adding functions do their work but are a cost to these functions. Value chain analysis should also identify the levels of value-add and cost of the various functions within the organisation.

The external environment

All organisations depend significantly on the environment in which they exist. To ignore external trends and events would be an act of 'suicide' for any organisation, profit allocating or otherwise. The external environment can be conveniently split into:

- the physical environment
- the social environment
- the competitive environment

and of these, the social environment can be further divided into 'PEST' factors.

- **P**olitico-legal
- **E**conomic
- **S**ocial–cultural
- **T**echnological

Some authors include further categories such as the weather, reflecting the growing globalisation of many organisations in all sorts of markets. They enlarge the 'PEST' acronym to 'PESTW'. For our consideration, this factor will be left within the physical environment.

It is impossible to enumerate in this chapter all the factors that need analysis under the categories for the external environment. It is sufficient to say that all categories should be investigated in a comprehensive and structured manner.

In his 'five forces' analytical method, Porter (1980, 1985) identified competitive forces that act on any organisation:

- the threat of new entrants to the market
- the bargaining power of suppliers
- the bargaining power of customers
- the threat of substitute products or services
- the threat of existing competitors.

The characteristics of decision making in health care

This framework may have seemed alien to the health industry some years ago but with moves to internal markets and the growth in private health care organisations, these forces are as relevant to the health industry as to commercial profit-allocating manufacturing industry.

However, in both public and private health care, there is a difficulty in defining the customer. Porter's model assumes that the customer and purchaser are one and the same whereas in health care they are often separate. This is always the case in the NHS, the patient being the consumer while primary care groups and local health authorities are the purchasers. In private health care, the consumer and purchaser may also be split with insurance companies acting as the purchasers. This does not totally invalidate Porter's model but does mean that it must be applied with care.

As must now be apparent, the quotation of Heller at the start of this chapter holds the key to the strategic analysis. The correct questions need to be asked.

STRATEGIC CHOICE

After defining the mission of the organisation, selecting the objectives and comprehensively analysing both the internal and external environments, the decision maker(s) are ready to make their choice.

The analysis procedures and objectives provide the information and the framework for the process of strategic choice which consists of three stages:

- identification of possible courses of action
- evaluation of these courses of action
- choice of the most advantageous of these alternatives.

A 'SWOT' analysis can contribute significantly to this strategic choice activity by breaking down all aspects of the organisation, its environment and its possible courses of action into four categories.

- Strengths
- Weaknesses
- Opportunities
- Threats

The first two of these categories will be identified by the internal environment analysis. The second two will largely result from the analysis of the external environment. The strategic choice should be based upon the concepts of:

- playing to and enhancing the organisation's strengths
- eliminating, or minimising, any weaknesses
- exploiting opportunities
- reducing the effect of external threats.

How the decision maker(s) make the decision based upon the information available and the defined objectives as criteria has been the subject of much learned work. This aspect will be returned to later in the chapter.

STRATEGIC IMPLEMENTATION

Implementation commences once the strategic choice has been made and the overall direction for the organisation as a whole has been decided. Implementation is a lengthy stage and involves:

- devolving the corporate plans into divisional, sector, unit, work group and ultimately individual plans
- implementing all these many and detailed plans.

As part of this process, decision making at various levels is still involved but these decisions will be 'easier', fitting within the now-decided corporate strategy – benefiting from a better defined framework for the decision making.

REVIEW AND EVALUATION

The result of the planning process should be assessed against the objectives that were set at the outset. Figure 4.3 shows this review procedure feeding back information to all stages of the planning process. This perhaps reflects the theory rather than the practice.

THE LEARNING ORGANISATION

In Figure 4.3, feedback is included from the review and evaluation stage to several of the previous stages in the model. If the review and evaluation stage and feedback loop were removed, the process would become a 'closed-mind' system as Figure 4.4. This model of the decision-making process has no stages beyond implementation. The individuals and the organisation will learn nothing from the outcome of their decisions. If the review and evaluation stage is incorporated, then learning begins. The individuals and the

The characteristics of decision making in health care

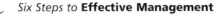

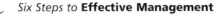

Six Steps to **Effective Management**

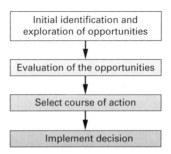

Initial identification and exploration of opportunities

↓

Evaluation of the opportunities

↓

Select course of action

↓

Implement decision

Figure 4.4   A closed-mind decision-making process.

organisation as a whole will benefit from the experience of the decision. In some cases, the results of the review and evaluation will be a modification of some feature of the implementation stage; it is possible, for instance, that some aspect of training may need to be revisited.

Argyris (1965, 1977, Argyris & Schon 1978) advanced the concept of single- and double-loop learning. In this concept, if the implementation of a decision or the planning stages (see Fig. 4.3) are reviewed and modified, the organisation is operating single-loop learning. The further back in the process the feedback travels, the greater the learning will be. Double-loop learning exists if the organisation and the individual decision makers review and change the objectives forming criteria for the decision and learning becomes truly significant.

The incorporation of any review and evaluation stage, together with the subsequent feedback loop, changes the closed-mind system into an open system, turning the organisation involved into a learning organisation.

Argyris claimed that most organisations were only capable of single-loop learning and that to become truly competitive in a fast-changing external environment, they should adopt double-loop learning strategies. As LePatner (see quotation on p. 79) indicated, most people, including organisations, learn best from mistakes. But if the individuals and the organisation are to benefit from this learning experience, they must admit they got it wrong. Only within organisations with a complete structure of trust will individuals be prepared to do this. Trust throughout an organisation becomes the key to whether full learning can exist, allowing the organisation to question the criteria used for the decision-making process. Only with this culture will the organisation be able to exploit the opportunities the external environment may provide.

Decision making in practice

RATIONAL AND INCREMENTAL DECISION MAKING

Simon (1975) advanced the idea of rational decisions. The decision would be organisationally rational if oriented to the organisation's goals. It can be appreciated that the achievement of such a decision would be very difficult. The rational decision requires:

- the decision maker(s) to have complete skills as necessary
- the decision maker(s) to have all the necessary time
- the decision maker(s) to have complete and accurate information
- the goals to be defined and available to the decision maker(s).

Realistically this situation is impossible. Strategic decisions are intended to provide the plans of the organisation for several years. Complete and accurate information about the future is impossible, never mind any of the other requirements.

Recognising these limitations, Simon introduced a modified version of rational decisions – bounded rationality – in which the decision maker chooses an alternative intended to satisfy rather than maximise values. Under this definition, decision making is no longer an optimal activity.

Lindblom (1959) disagrees with Simon's rational decision-making model because it was not adapted to:

- the limited problem-solving capabilities of humans
- imperfect information
- the high cost of analysis
- dynamic variables

amongst others.

Lindblom argued that rather than take rational decisions, managers took a series of limited comparisons, limiting the number of alternative courses of action that are considered and the range of the alternatives so that relatively small 'step sizes' are involved. In this way:

- the analysis does not need to be fully comprehensive
- the knowledge of the alternatives is improved as they are closer to the current scenario
- the decision maker(s) are more likely to possess the necessary skills for the analysis
- the limited 'step sizes' avoid the possibility of major irreversible mistakes.

The characteristics of decision making in health care

97

Lindblom further argued that individuals and groups adjust the objectives as they go along. Described as the art of muddling through, it has the merit that, unlike the rational model, it adapts better to the ever-changing external environment.

Etzioni (1967) argued for a 'middle road' solution. He accepted the validity and merits of incrementalism, creating small step changes that can adapt to environmental changes. His theme was, though, that these small steps may not, in the longer term, add up to movement in the correct direction without the benefit of a longer term, 'guiding hand'.

Etzioni advanced a new model of decision making incorporating both series of limited changes and a fundamental decision that provided the overall direction. Likening his model to a camera with two lenses, one telephoto and one close-up, he called it 'mixed scanning'.

Etzioni's fundamental decisions depend upon very similar features to Simon's idealistic rational decision model and it is therefore logical that Lindblom's criticism of the rational model should also apply to this model.

CONCLUSION

In this chapter, in order to avoid preconceived positions, decision making has been studied in a general way with only some reference to the health care industry. It has looked briefly at the decision maker, both as an individual and in a corporate setting, and has touched upon some of the problems that decision makers encounter, either acting on their own or as a member of a team. Models of different categories of decisions have been advanced; an overall planning framework has been discussed along with different models of the decision-making process itself.

References

Argyris C 1965 Organisation and innovation. Irwin, Homewood, Illinois

Argyris C 1977 Double loop learning in organisations. Harvard Business Review September–October: 115–125

Argyris C, Schon DA 1978 Organisational learning: a theory of action perspective. Addison-Wesley, Reading, Massachusetts

Boone LE, Lichtenstein E (eds) 1999 Quotable business. Random House, New York

Brocka B, Brocka MS 1992 Quality management: implementing the best ideas of the masters. Irwin, Homewood, Illinois

Decision making in practice

Daft RL 1997 Management, 4th edn. Dryden Press, London

Drucker PF 1977 People and performance. Heinemann, London

Etzioni A 1967 Mixed scanning: a 'third' approach to decision-making. Public Administration Review 27: 385–392

Fayol H 1949 General and industrial management. Pitman, London

Gilligan C, Neale B, Murray D 1983 Business decision-making. Pitman, London

Hannigan T 1995 Management concepts and practices. Pitman, London

Hellriegel D Slocum JW 1992 Management. Addison-Wesley, Reading, Massachusetts

Leontiades M 1982 Management policy, strategy and plans. Little, Brown, Boston

Lindblom CE 1959 The science of muddling through. Public Administration Review 19: 79–88

Mintzberg H 1976 The structure of 'unstructured' decision processes. Administrative Science Quarterly June: 246–275

Porter ME 1980 Competitive strategy: techniques for analysing industries and competitors. Free Press, New York

Porter ME 1985 Competitive advantage: creating and sustaining superior performance. Collier Macmillan, London

Simon HA 1960 The new science of management decision. Harper and Row, New York

Simon HA 1975 Models of man. Wiley, London

The characteristics of decision making in health care

Application **4:1**

Jane Hubert and Jennifer Gosling

A day in the life of . . .

This application gives the reader the opportunity to apply some of the theory of decision making to the reality faced by two managers in different health care settings. The first is the manager of an outpatients department, the second, in a very different setting, a practice manager.

As you read their accounts of a typical day, you will probably empathise with them as crises and operational tasks crowd out any possibility of concentrating for any length of time on longer term and more strategic decision making. It is suggested that you read their accounts several times and ask yourself the following.

1. Using Gilligan's three-category scheme, what is the balance between short-term operational control decisions, periodic control decisions and strategic decisions?
2. Although Chapter Four presented a framework for strategic decision making that included planning, analysing, choosing, implementing and reviewing, to what extent was such an approach applied to the shorter term decisions described by the two managers? Would it have been useful to apply it more consciously? Did the managers find themselves picking up just part of the strategic decision-making process?
3. Theoretically, objectives can be divided into corporate, functional, team and individual. Considering the managers' descriptions of their 'day', how would you put these categories in order of achievement?

THE OUTPATIENT DEPARTMENT MANAGER

Background to my role

The title of my role is Clinical Nurse Manager, Outpatients (OPD). I have responsibility for 35 nursing staff, both qualified and unqualified, as well as a specialist nurse and 60 clerical staff ranging from junior clerks to clerical supervisors. The whole team have responsibility for providing a service to patients attending new and follow-up outpatient appointments. I work closely with the service manager for medical records and other service managers across the trust. The role is very varied.

The day commences . . .

07.30
Arrive at desk, review diary and plan the day. Commence paperwork previously allocated for the day, i.e. respond to letters of concern and complaint from both patients and medical staff. These often reflect the problems associated with outpatients, for example shortage of staff due to sickness and vacant posts.

Complete termination forms for nurse who has submitted her notice. Write advert for replacement, complete relevant forms to submit request to finance department for replacement of staff member.

08.00
Attend weekly one-to-one meeting with manager. I provide feedback on issues such as vacancy rates, staffing and skill mix levels and highlight any concerns I may have. We discuss changes in practice, ideas for improvement and I ask advice on issues I am unsure about. My manager informs me of divisional plans and changes.

09.00
Attend all areas of responsibility, communicate with staff addressing any problems. For example, in orthopaedic outpatients today, the busiest day of the week, there is only one permanent member of staff in attendance out of a usual four. I telephone other areas of OPD and ask staff to come and assist. I also telephone external agencies to obtain temporary staff.

Further on my 'walk round' of OPD I find a clinic without a clerk based on the reception desk. I discover that the clerk is away due to ill health and the supervisor is reallocating the team to provide cover. I remain at the reception desk assisting patients until the clerk arrives.

I attend a further clinic and have a conversation with a member of the nursing team regarding setting up a training session for qualified nurses on taking blood pressures following medical staff concerns regarding disparities on recording of blood pressure readings. A health care assistant requests my advice and assistance on a forthcoming interview for nurse training. I give her a number of names of people who may be able to assist her and arrange to see her later in the week.

I collect my post.

10.45
I telephone the plaster technician from orthopaedic OPD to find out why she hasn't informed me of her absence. I reiterate the trust's

procedure/policy, then write to her confirming this conversation and the trust policy.

I return telephone calls received when I was out of the office, then commence the compilation of weekly monitoring forms that depict agency usage and absence for the finance department.

11.30
Appraisal meeting with a new specialist nurse. This is a new post so we discuss our plans for the post and where we envisage it proceeding in the future. I document the appraisal and agreed objectives.

12.45
I request information from the finance department before going to the canteen. Whilst there the senior nurse for renal disease approaches me to discuss care provided by the qualified nurses in OPD to renal patients. We agree that we should meet with the nurses involved and set some objectives for improving and enhancing the service.

13.15
I return to my office and commence compiling the figures for the contracts department on waiting times in clinic.

14.10
I attend a clerical team meeting. Issues discussed include the perceived poor service currently supplied to the OPD clerical teams by medical records in providing notes in time for them to be prepared for clinic, a bid for funding made by the assistant general manager for outpatients for an OPD telephone bureau and the fact that some patients seem to have more than one hospital number.

15.00
Attend a meeting with a member of the projects team to discuss the development of an endoscopy suite specifically for OPD, which will provide a 'one-stop' service for patients. Funding has now been granted and we review the plans and the schedule of works and set dates for future meetings in line with the schedule.

16.00
Return to my office. I continue with the Patient's Charter monitoring and review the work I have allocated myself for today.

I am informed that £4000 worth of equipment has arrived from an order cancelled 3 months ago. I telephone the supplies department and ask them to investigate.

16.40
I receive a call from the dermatology OPD stating that although today's clinic was cancelled due to absence of medical staff a patient has turned up expecting to be seen; the patient is dissatisfied and would like to speak to the manager responsible. I attend the dermatology OPD, spend 20 minutes apologising to the patient, rearranging the appointment and arranging transport home for them.

17.00
I return to my office and commence opening my mail. I find:

- literature on courses, which I review and send on to appropriate staff
- minutes from meetings missed during my annual leave, which I put into my briefcase to read during the journey home
- statements previously requested from staff regarding incidents that have occurred on clinic
- letters of concern and complaint from both medical staff and patients which I plan to investigate tomorrow.

17.30
I write up an agenda for the sisters' meeting at 08.00 tomorrow and deliver it to all relevant areas on my way out of the hospital, checking that clinics are closed or about to close and all staff are happy.

17.40
I leave the hospital.

THE PRACTICE MANAGER

A practice manager is much like a GP – a generalist in many areas and a specialist in a few. Although rooted in the NHS, general practices are in fact independent small businesses, run on a for-profit basis. The practice manager is key to running that business and ensuring it makes enough profit to pay the doctors and staff and provide all the services one would expect to find in a modern general practice. Practices vary quite widely in size, from the single-handed GP to the partnership of 10 or more GPs, but the practice manager's job is basically the same regardless of size.

A typical day

9.00
Arrive and check my in-tray for stuff that has arrived since I left the previous evening.
 Check that all the reception staff are in, no-one has called in sick, that everything is generally OK and that there were no problems last night.

9.15
I retreat to my office to check my diary and day folder to see what needs doing.

9.20
Begin generating short letters which need to be sent:

- slap-on-the-wrist letters to patients who have not turned up for three appointments in a row
- to patients who have moved outside the practice area, to ask them to find another GP
- then a letter to the Health Authority asking them to remove the patient from the list (this can only be signed by a GP)
- letters to patients asking them to confirm their address, triggered when the Health Authority has written to the patient and had the mail returned undelivered; we hope to prevent them being removed from the list.

9.30

The temporary secretary needs instruction in the format of letters, where to find information, the spelling of doctors' names and so forth.

10.00

I start tackling some of the bigger projects I have scheduled for today:

- working on the text for a health leaflet we are going to send out to all teenagers
- updating the practice nurse's job description and person spec, ready to begin recruitment of a new part-time nurse
- thinking of questions for the receptionist interviews tomorrow lunchtime
- re-reading the minutes of last month's partners' meeting and working on the agenda for this month's meeting.

10.30

The builder arrives to look at a problem we have at the top of the stairs. I leave him to take up the carpet and check it out.

10.45

I'm asked by the builder to come and inspect the hole in the floor. The underfloor joists completely fell away when the floor was taken up and are revealed as a dangerously bodged job by the company who redeveloped the building and put the staircase in. This was an extremely dangerous structure. The builder heads off to get the materials needed to put it right, recommending that we take photographic evidence. His mate is left behind to ensure people coming up the stairs are guided safely over the gaping hole in the floor.

Phone calls to and from the architect follow at regular intervals. The architect wants to come and see the hole himself or get a structural engineer to view it, but neither can attend until tomorrow morning.

11.00

I am called to reception to speak to a patient who wants to make a complaint. This is a misunderstanding that is soon sorted out.

11.30

The doctors have finished surgery and are upstairs reading their post. I explain the situation with the floor.

11.45

The builder returns and is unhappy to leave the floor as it is, so we have to call the architect again so builder and architect can talk technical. Fortunately the builder is qualified to write a report on what was found and it is agreed he can go ahead and fix it today.

12.30

Work continues to the background noise of sawing, hammering and drilling. With the numerous conversations with builders, architects and partners about the state of the floor, I have completely lost the thread of my paperwork.

2.00

I remember I am supposed to be at the Commissioning and Performance Management Committee meeting at the PCG. Unfortunately this is at the offices in Waterloo so I will arrive late. Luckily I am able to stock up on tea and biscuits while I'm there, remembering, again, that I haven't had lunch yet.

3.30

I stop off at the administrator's office to book a room for our clinical awayday, then head back to the practice. On the way back I detour to a local restaurant to book a table for lunch for the same meeting.

3.45

Back at the practice, the builders are just finishing up. I can now start taking old computer terminals downstairs ready for Lambeth Council to collect them.

4.15

Finally back at my desk, my in-tray has filled up again with letters, notes from doctors and telephone messages to return. I prioritise the pile and put some things in tomorrow's day file.

I return what phone calls I can and deal with the paperwork that can't wait.

4.30

I abandon the teenage leaflet until I find a time when I can concentrate on it. I sketch out an application for funding to provide locum cover while one of our doctors is on extended leave.

I update the nurse's job description and put it in tomorrow's file to check and pull out the last set of interview questions we used for receptionists for updating.

Finally I make a list of outstanding items from last month's partners' meeting and timetable them for completion before the next. I check the budget implications of employing an extra receptionist.

5.30
I start tidying up my desk despairing about the accumulated filing.

5.45
I speak to the cleaners (diplomatically!) about the standard of cleaning in the consulting rooms.

6.15
I have a brief chat to the evening receptionists before I leave to make sure the evening surgery went OK and they are happy.

6.30
Head for the tube!

COMMENTS

How these two managers face a range of decision-making situations shows some marked similarities in spite of differing contexts. They are both largely driven by operational crisis or demands, either staff sickness or Health & Safety issues. However, both managers do spend some time on 'periodic control decisions', for example, relating to staff recruitment, patient waiting times, budgetary review or confirming patient addresses. These short-term and periodic operational decisions tend to crowd out a more strategic approach. Just a few of this latter variety can be identified. The OPD manager is a member of a project team. The practice manager makes several attempts to work on a health leaflet for teenagers although in the end she sets it aside for another day.

A more strategic approach to short-term operational decisions is demonstrated by the OPD manager in relation to staff sickness and vacancies. She has identified that staff training and appraisal might help to reduce absence and her implementation of this strategy is demonstrated. For the practice manager, any expectations of converting operational difficulties to a more strategic approach seemed to disappear along with the floor!

Both managers give illustrations of implementing strategies decided elsewhere. For the OPD manager, an important task is collecting and collating figures on patient waiting times as part of contractual requirements. The practice manager also has to operate within a framework set by statute, for example, the removal of patients from the GP list.

A final area of consideration is the nature of the objectives driving decision making. These may not necessarily be expressed. For example, the practice manager sees an important role as the defusing of patient complaints, an area of importance at a corporate level. For both managers, the functional nature of many of their objectives is clear.

The OPD manager seems to operate within a larger number of groups than the practice manager. Some group objectives may or may not fit corporate objectives. For example, the clinical group that the OPD manager wants to set up with the senior renal nurse seems driven by professional objectives but whether the cost implications will enable a match with corporate objectives remains to be seen.

Finally, neither manager expresses any personal objectives that may need to be addressed separately. Whilst this is not surprising as they may only be visible infrequently, it is to be hoped that the two managers illustrated in this application remember that personal development is an important component of a satisfying and successful career.

A number of threads illustrated so forcibly in these two 'days in the life of . . .' are addressed more fully in other parts of this book. Section Five, on managing risk and crisis, seems particularly relevant while Section Four, on the implementation of strategy at local level, explores the ever-present interface between planning and action, autonomy and control.

A day in the life of . . .

Application 4:2

Mary Cooke

Evaluating decisions: a case study from a rural practice

This application explores some of the particular differences and challenges of decision making in a small rural community. The documented processes of decision making usually assume an organisational setting where a number of individuals communicate with and relate to each other in a fairly structured way. But what particular problems are encountered by the practitioner working in an isolated setting with little contact with other professionals?

The case study presented here looks at how a practice nurse in a rural setting deals with some critical issues. Management of clinical supervision, evaluation of clinical effectiveness and evidence-based practice and involvement of the local community in decision making are described. The value of a specialist perspective may seem obvious to the practitioner but ways of inputting this knowledge and then persuading others to act on it have to take account of the isolated position of the practice nurse and the difficulties others might have in relating their experience to her specific focus.

CRITICAL ISSUES IN A RURAL SETTING

Introduction

Patient care has to occur in all settings but the training and education of nurses may not. The nurse, after learning how to practise in a mainstream hospital and urban or even a city type of 'community', will normally be unprepared for work as a practice nurse in a rural area. Health and health care as viewed by the people who live and work there are often very different and not always the rural idyll that many people associate with a village of about 2000 population, almost all of whom are registered with one practice.

One of the most outstanding differences will be the distance travelled in a series of home visits, for instance. Some rounds can be up to 200 miles in a day, yet only three or four people have been on the list! The GP practice will also be relatively isolated. This means that pharmacy products will be dispensed from the practice as it is more than 2 miles from the nearest chemist of any description where prescriptions can be taken for preparation. (Even the main supermarkets cannot cover all places in the UK!) So in considering management decisions about patients and delivery of care in this type of setting, there are several models that would be the 'norm' in other communities but cannot be considered in a rural practice.

Clinical supervision

One area we can think about is clinical supervision. Where would you look for this precious necessity for good practice and reflective learning? You may find that there are some district nurses associated with the practice who could be approached, but frequently they do not have time to spend outside their own team to support anyone else. You may look to the local health visitor but their responsibilities are different and in some areas of England, e.g. Cambridgeshire and Huntingdonshire, these posts have been dissolved and reduced in function, so there will be a loss of inter- and intraprofessional support too, even for those health visitors and school nurses who remain.

One practice nurse used networking as a method of supervision, by email, by telephone and by infrequent meetings. Another practice nurse has developed a relationship with one of the patients on the practice list, who was a nurse tutor and willing to meet up in a social context as well as being able to objectively discuss confidential aspects of a practice nurse's work and personal decision-making problems. So professional isolation is a real difficulty in a rural situation.

Clinical effectiveness and evidence-based practice

Keeping up with the clinical effectiveness and evidence-based interventions is another area we can think about. In a rural setting this practice nurse could be relating her decisions in a way that is led by the GP rather than using nursing-focused guidelines. It takes a strong personality to ensure that, for example, the patient is supported and heard in a situation where a GP will want to make decisions associated with funding of the practice rather than the longer term health and social well-being of that patient and their family. The knowledge base of the practice nurse needs to be extensive to cover economic and political decision making as well as clinical in these situations.

Community-orientated decision making

One practice nurse kindly gave some time and words to a research project; these are used with permission. She talked about two local committees that she became involved with and how the community got drawn into that.

> The strength of my position at work was that I knew a lot of people in the village. When I was on the lottery committee, I was also on the HImp committee (health improvement committee*). I was able to network with those people. Yes at one point we were getting a bit low on people and we needed some energy put back in. So we sat in one meeting, went through the different roads in the village (and I know where everybody lives) and we came up with a list of about 20 more people whom I then approached. So in a way I sort of head-hunted, more successful than not doing it because it is not a very big village, we don't have middle-class people and those that have stayed here are of one sort, and then there are those who have arrived from London.

> Well, 10 years ago, there was a very stable group of people in the village and they had a traditionally rural background even though they had moved away from agriculture but the background was still there. Tradition carried on. Things have changed an enormous amount now, the list size has doubled in the 10 years.

The issue of control and power was acknowledged and differences between the two committees highlighted.

> . . . unfortunately I came off the HImp committee when borders changed, because, you know, I was just a nurse and I was not important enough to retain a position on the HImp, once it had got thrown together with all these other big and important people who have power . . . it was interesting watching the two because I was in control of (being Chairman of) the lottery committee, I chose how I wanted to operate it and it was started off in a very democratic way, there was a lot of shared decision making, I set out to do that very purposefully and was very caring of all my committee members.

* Commissions for Health Improvement – these were set up in 1998, in particular areas associated with bringing together representatives from local authority, Health & Safety, police, social services and other multiagency team workers to improve the health of people in towns, cities and other communities in England.

Influencing and evaluating decisions from a specialist perspective

The potential isolation of the rural practice nurse has to be addressed if her voice is to be heard.

> I've been to several things over the last year, where you think oh sod this, I'm not going to do this any more because I just can't tell if what I'm saying is any use, in any other context. When you work in isolation you can't tell what you are like. For instance, you can't tell if what you are saying is of any use to the people that you are talking to, I mean I've been asked to comment twice on the development of nursing in my patch, but they didn't make any reference to my comments at all. Maybe it's not what they wanted to hear.

However, by contrast, as a respected professional, she was asked to contribute to a new training course for practice nurses. Initially her knowledge was not fully appreciated. This may have been because the trainers were not in contact with practice as they should have been, in order to understand the ways in which nurses work in community settings in the new NHS.

> Then I was invited to an education committee, planning. I've actually managed to swing things round the way that I wanted to in this 'practice nurse induction course curriculum development committee', which I got shoved onto because there was nobody from my locality on it. It was a working group to set up a course and they wanted to know how to do it. But their approach was going to create a highly taught task-orientated nurse, which I felt was a really missed opportunity. There were a couple of trainers who were too focused because when I said 'What is needed is input on depression and mental health', and the trainer said, 'Oh we don't do that', I said 'What about HRT?', she said 'No, never done that, don't need that in it at all'. She didn't have the basic grasp of the idiosyncrasy of employment by different general practitioners either. Somebody else just wanted ear syringe, injections, you know, task orientation, now what I wanted this course to contribute was to develop an exploration of the context of general practice, 'The scope of professional accountability', and all the other areas, like health promotion, you know, safe practice, infection control, all of that stuff and I wanted a much more global approach to your role, as a nurse in general practice.

The practice nurse decided to draw on some support for her approach.

So before too much went further awry, I was in touch with a lady who was on a PCG. Between us we offered her services in the local School of Nursing so that the course was on a sounder footing.

By now, the practice nurse had a very real input into the committee and was also influencing a course curriculum because of her superior knowledge. She had managed the learning context too.

> I ended up explaining how community work happens to one of the trainers. They really have to take account of the National Service Frameworks and the Mental Health one. You have to know which people you need to deal with immediately or otherwise, such as when a person comes into the surgery, and you say 'You're not right, you need to go to the GP or do you want to talk to me about this?'. This is the responsibility, family health care. It is first contact. That's the reason nurses are not regarded as authoritarian and being more approachable and so on. You've got a nurse who just gives you blooming injections, fine, but that person may be suicidal. So it could be that an opportunity is lost and a life may be lost because the nurse is not able to spot depression.

CONCLUSION

This was a practice nurse working in isolation in a rural practice who had to acknowledge that she might not always win the argument with a GP. However, she could define the principles of practice, the needs of the local community as individuals and as a group and could skilfully manage the outcomes of an education committee by facilitation of the situation externally. These acquired managerial skills are professional and political.

Evaluating decisions: a case study from a rural practice

Six Steps to **Effective Management**

A final comment from the practice nurse emphasised the need for practice nurses to be accountable across a wide range of practices, even when having to function within numerous, and sometimes conflicting, imposed frameworks.

> Nurses need to be seen as skilled resources and the trouble is that now today, we have a lot of top-down need, particularly from the National Service Frameworks. Also from the GP's point of view from targets, you have to be accountable for immunisations, you have to be accountable for following up smears. I'm not expecting new practice nurses or anyone else to appreciate or to know the whole lot all at once but if you have an accountable practice, you will extend it gradually into areas where you are safe.

Chapter **Five**

The practitioner as manager

Elizabeth A Smith and Ann P Young

- Becoming a manager
- Role transition
- The manager's role
- Management skills from practice

- The practitioner as manager
- Sources of conflict
- Identifying and planning career directions
- Conclusion

O V E R V I E W

This chapter explores the transition of the practitioner to manager. Although written from a nursing perspective, the theoretical framework is applicable to any setting in health care where employees start as practitioners in a field but progress to adopt management roles. It is interesting to consider at what point a practitioner becomes a manager as many of the skills that managers require are similar to those used by a practitioner, although the context may vary. Practitioners have a variety of career options open to them. Management is one of them but increasingly research, education or some combined role is an alternative. It is essential that practitioners explore these in light of their own strengths and choose appropriate pathways.

This chapter presents a summary of the skills needed for management and how these may emerge from experience as a practitioner and identifies the potential for conflict in shared management/practitioner roles.

BECOMING A MANAGER

In nursing there has always been a career pathway from practice to management. This pattern has also developed in other related health care professions and, most recently, the creation of clinical directors in some trusts has resulted in medical staff assuming management roles.

This progression is not marked by any particular professional or personal development, which poses the question 'How does practice prepare an individual for management?'. Nurses are novices (Benner 1984) but over a period of time become competent in their role as practitioner. This happens through a combination of formal and informal education, guided practice and role modelling. As they develop into competent practitioners, they begin to learn the skills of time management to be able to organise their own work. The organisation of nursing work has increasingly become team led, so that practitioners may be responsible for named patients on a shift, working with one or two others. This type of organisation results in nurses learning skills of people management. The involvement of staff in service changes is a popular approach to change management and as a result nurses are increasingly experiencing negotiation and bargaining, working in multidisciplinary and multiagency teams, and involvement in budgetary decisions.

There is evidence that nurses do not recognise that they have these skills as a result of working in practice and do not realise that they are transferable to management. In addition, nurses at lower clinical grades may not appreciate that there is a management component to their role (Smith 1997).

ROLE TRANSITION

Practitioners who become managers may find their work is very different from their previous role. Handy (1985) discusses the idea of role definition where a role may be defined by cultural expectations and outward signs of the role, such as uniform. This applies strongly to the practitioner role but the role of manager is much less clear and this may lead to role ambiguity (Handy 1985). In this situation, the new manager may retreat back into the more comfortable practitioner role. It is essential for new managers to spend some time defining their roles and responsibilities to reduce this ambiguity.

Decision making in practice

Increasingly, a combined practitioner/manager role is being adopted in health care. In these roles, clarity is even more important because practitioner/managers need to review their practitioner role in order to delegate some responsibilities to others, creating space to take on new managerial aspects of the job. An example of this type of job role development is explored by Robinson et al (1992) who describe an associate charge nurse (ACN) role developed in Australia. This role was defined as having substantial clinical experience, being capable of advising nursing staff on technical or ethical issues as well as having an operating knowledge of varied managerial procedures. In their study, they found that the ability to adopt a managerial role was also affected by the perceptions of others. Nursing staff expected that the ACNs would be available in the clinical area as a resource to support their clinical work and that when the postholder did not comply with these expectations, the nurses often responded with various forms of censure.

These difficulties can be overcome by clear job descriptions and clearly defined roles, objectives and responsibilities, together with a recognition that role transition is a process with which a new postholder must engage in order to become competent as a manager.

THE MANAGER'S ROLE

Much has been written about the role of the manager and the emergence of management as a profession. Studies date back to before 1900 in attempts to define principles and practice of good management. Findings are presented in the underlying philosophy of the time and started with a very scientific approach to management, focusing on 'observation, quantification, analysis, experimentation and evaluation' (Taylor 1947). These values are clearly evident in the 1990s business culture of the health service. Fayol is credited with developing the process approach, looking at what managers do (Fayol 1949). He described the role of management as being to forecast and plan, to organise, to command, to coordinate and to control. These ideas have pervaded management ever since Fayol's pioneering work and are sometimes called the 'classic view' (Child 1984). In the 1930s and 1940s, the people component of management started to be investigated with the famous Hawthorne studies into motivation and other research into group behaviour and management styles (Likert 1961, Mayo 1933).

In the 1960s and 1970s, the advent of computer technology led to the development of 'management science', with consultants

The practitioner as manager

offering operations research such as computer modelling, simulations and risk assessments. These ideas still exist in a much more complex form but they are accompanied by an awareness that human behaviour is an unpredictable variable and that such models, whilst appearing objective, incorporate judgements which are inherently subjective (Drucker 1987).

The *systems approach* was developed in this period (Beer 1980). It emphasises the interconnectedness of departments in whole organisations and the reliance of one organisation on another. The importance of monitoring systems was stressed as was identifying the links between functions so that focused problem solving could occur. The current interest in standard setting and audit reflects this monitoring approach and ideas like 'seamless service', 'inter-agency team working' and 'primary care teams' are examples of the reliance of services on each other to meet patients' needs.

This period also saw the development of the *organisational approach* which tries to harness individual and organisational goals to move together in one direction (Peters & Waterman 1982). It considers the behaviours that people adopt individually and in groups, what motivates them and how they respond to internal and external influences. This approach also looks at the way an organisation is structured and whether that enables effective working together.

Finally, the *contingency approach* has emerged which takes the view that organisations develop in different ways and develop different approaches to management according to circumstances (Mintzberg 1979). As a result, large organisations may have different approaches in different areas that meet individual department needs but may not work well together at a corporate level.

Therefore, the practitioner developing a management role not only has to explore that role at an individual level but will also need to determine the style and culture in their own work area and the organisation as a whole. The clinical supervision and reflective practice may help practitioners who become managers to identify this in advance of adopting a management role. The increasing focus on succession planning as a human resource strategy may enable practitioners to complete management training *before* they become managers. This will also provide increased awareness of skills.

MANAGEMENT SKILLS FROM PRACTICE

Management is multifaceted and complex, as already stated, but it has several key components, for example, planning, directing, organising and controlling. Many writers and researchers have tried to define management but no definitive view exists. Mintzberg (1973) described three areas of management: interpersonal, informational and decisional. He then described 10 managerial roles within these areas.

- Interpersonal   figurehead
                            leader
- Informational   liaison
                            monitor
                            disseminator
                            spokesperson
- Decisional   entrepreneur
                            disturbance handler
                            resource allocator
                            negotiator

These roles require some key skills. Strategic skills would include creative/logical thinking, having a vision and being able to operationalise it by objective setting, decision making and planning. Operational skills would be about actioning and prioritising decisions and problem solving. Skills for reviewing would involve monitoring and evaluating. Communication skills would include networking and making presentations. A cluster of self-management skills would include speed reading, time management and stress management.

Katz & Kahn (1966) also described managers' basic skills and identified technical, human and conceptual components. The following discussion suggests how professionals develop some of these through their practice.

Technical skills incorporate prioritising, decision making, record keeping, planning and scheduling. In an average working day, experienced nurses will certainly plan the shift and prioritise their work and that of others, deal with a variety of unexpected events that require quick decisions, plan, deliver and evaluate nursing care for patients and record this in some detail. The skills are certainly transferable to a management role.

Human skills will include team working, both with individuals and with groups. These skills are also learned in practice but are often informal rather than formal. Reflection and guided practice of chairing meetings, appraisals and interviews would make transfer of skills to a management role possible.

Conceptual skills involve being able to see the organisation as a whole and the role of individuals, teams and departments within it and to identify the key elements of integration, dependence and conflict within these relationships. This is an area where practi-

The practitioner as manager

117

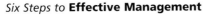

tioners may be at a disadvantage as they often become focused on their own work area and do not perceive how it links with others. However, some practitioners would claim that their role brings them into much more frequent and wider contact with the other workers in the health care setting than experienced by other professionals. This particular cluster of skills can be developed by participation in activities that cross boundaries into other departments and by taking opportunities to reflect on the differing perspectives and objectives in each area.

The emphasis on patient-focused care, care pathways and interdisciplinary working to enable health professionals to be more involved in the organisation as a whole will facilitate development of these skills in the future. The move towards college/university-based student experience may also make nurses more conceptually aware as they have the opportunity to learn and mix with others. Joint training initiatives will make this more explicit.

A further category is included here, that of political skills. These are not included in Katz & Kahn's categories but need to be added for them to be relevant in this new century. Health care has become a highly political arena and nurses must be aware of government focus and understand legislative requirements and objectives in order to promote the role of nurses in its provision. As Witz (1994) points out, senior nurses must be proactive in progressing the national agenda. They also need to be aware of local political influences and the power relationships within an organisation. Nurses have traditionally been apolitical so these skills are less likely to develop in practice. They need to be encouraged from the start of nurse education and continue through a nurse's career in order to become embedded in the profession.

THE PRACTITIONER AS MANAGER

The previous section suggests that the practitioner should be able to transfer some skills from practice to management but will also need to develop some new ones. It may be helpful to consider the advantages and disadvantages of an overlap of skills and activities if the roles are combined. However, it may be difficult to determine which work activities are management and which are practice. This creates potential areas for conflict unless they are harmonised by objectives that coincide.

The practitioner may need to release control of some areas of practice by delegation to others in the team or to a deputy. This can be a difficult transition if the practitioner is very experienced or a

Decision making in practice

specialist in that area of care, as they may wish to retain high-profile input in the care area. However, it is impossible to fulfil both roles effectively unless the practitioner becomes less enmeshed in day-to-day practice and has the space to achieve a more objective overview of the area.

The following is a summary of both the benefits and challenges of combining practitioner/manager roles. Benefits are:

- maintenance of clinical credibility
- maintenance of clinical competence
- management awareness of the reality of practice
- problem solving and decision making based in the reality of practice.

These benefits result in more realistic management of the environment and the staff. Staff may be more willing to change and develop practice if they recognise the manager as a credible and competent practitioner.

Unfortunately, the benefits are not always evident as practitioner/managers find it difficult to maintain an appropriate balance between the two roles. Difficulties encountered may include:

- lack of visibility in the practice area
- lack of organisation of routine activities
- conflict between the immediacy of practice and the strategy of management
- overload in one or both parts of the role
- lack of clarity about role boundaries.

Robinson et al (1992) noted that although there was a broad idea of the combined role in the setting in their study, there were implicit assumptions that were not explored and clarified. These included:

- an assumption that practitioner/managers knew what to do
- an expectation (from other managers) that practitioner/managers would do both roles simultaneously
- an expectation (from staff) that practitioner/managers would be available in clinical areas.

These challenges were experienced as censure from clinical staff and as lip service to help and support the practitioner/managers from other managers, demonstrating a lack of understanding of the role and the potential for conflicts within it. It is likely that combined roles will persist in both public and private health care but the first step to succeeding is to question the rationale for the post.

The practitioner as manager

The number of clinical practice specialist roles has rapidly increased over recent years and often they have been linked to management responsibilities. However, nurses who are clinical specialists often do not see themselves as managers (Smith 1997). It may be that services need to devise a different management structure, with a practitioner/manager, who is more generally focused and able to be objective across the interdisciplinary team, working alongside a clinical nurse specialist.

Once the need for a role has been established, it must be clarified from both a practice and management perspective. Research suggests that this should focus on boundaries and what is *not* in the role, rather than what the job is (Robinson et al 1992). Finally, the staff affected by the post need to be educated as to the person's role, especially if this is an internal change or promotion, otherwise the postholder will be expected to continue as before and conflict will be inevitable (Smith 1997).

There appear to be some inherent conflicts in the role of practitioner as manager. They revolve around issues of:

- important versus urgent
- demonstration of competence versus development of other staff
- own area versus organisation as a whole
- patient focus versus business culture
- subjectivity versus objectivity
- work versus 'real' work
- local power versus organisational power.

These areas will now be explored further.

SOURCES OF CONFLICT

The conflict between urgent and important is one faced by many staff, whatever their job. It does, however, particularly become a problem in the manager role where operational issues demand attention and longer term decision making gets pushed to one side. When the operational issues are associated with the clinical area, their urgency becomes impossible to ignore. For example, when faced with staffing shortages in the clinical area, the practitioner/manager's initial reflex decision is to provide cover for the shortfall by working the shift personally. Clearly, a brief input might be essential but the problem will not be solved in the longer term by such action. A more managerial approach is needed to both organise cover in the short term, by reviewing workloads elsewhere and redeploying staff or employing agency workers, and then reviewing the whole issue of manpower and resources in a wider context. However, there are times when the operational responses of the practitioner/manager do throw into relief these wider resourcing issues and might then be used as an additional argument for more resources.

Most managers in the clinical area will argue that a professional background is an important factor in gaining the respect and therefore the cooperation of staff when introducing change. A demonstration of this competence can very quickly bring people on line. It might therefore be tempting for the practitioner/manager to overuse this tactic. As already highlighted, it is often comfortable to return to this role. For example, in the A&E department, the manager might ensure that she is around to help in a major accident situation but, in order to allow other staff to develop their competence and confidence, the best option is to allow them to take the lead. The practitioner/manager can provide support and approval of decisions taken and still demonstrate competence, without undermining the upcoming clinical experts in that area.

It is often thought that the move to a business culture will inevitably undermine a focus on the patient. This is because in the NHS a business perspective is equated with cost cutting rather than a wider view of what constitutes good business. In the private sector, quality issues are seen as also important and very much part of the business ethos. While moves in this direction have started in the NHS through the frameworks of clinical audit, they are not yet well established. Professional and financial accountabilities are still seen as separate (Young 1999) but the practitioner/manager is in the unique position of being able to argue for some reinterpretation of both. A review of priorities that can be agreed between these two perspectives would be a way forward.

The practitioner role is often linked to a more subjective approach to work than the seemingly more objective manager. However, the practitioner/manager can demonstrate that clinical work is underpinned by certain objectivities based on research and well thought-out problem-solving processes. The manager should also take on board that the managerial role is scarcely 'scientific' as it involves working with relationships and issues of differential power. However, the assumption tends to persist that to be a manager, the postholder needs to be 'hard', while the practitioner is seen as more passive and 'tender'. The gendering of the professions is partly to blame for this, with the caring professions being largely female and management still male dominated (Halford et al 1997). The development of a new managerialism that is more

The practitioner as manager

people orientated still has a long way to go in the health care sector (Pollitt 1990).

Management is still considered not to be 'real' work by those that have not been managers! A manager may not be able to point to clear measurable outcomes on a daily basis nor link the activities undertaken to obvious benefits. For example, for many managers, their day revolves around preparing for meetings, attending meetings and actioning the outcome of meetings. Much of the work is about facilitating others and setting the wheels in motion for longer term outcomes that may not even be directly attributable to the manager concerned when they eventually reach fruition. It is therefore not surprising that practitioners may be critical of their perception of the manager's role. Managers need to have confidence in what they are doing and be clear of the staging objectives that make up the journey to the more distant destination. They also need to communicate some of this to their subordinates.

The final area of conflict is around power. Many managers will reflect that they had more power when in their clinical role, being a large fish in a small pond. The move into management immediately opens up the wider relationships that the individual will have within the organisation as a whole. While the potential for influencing others is greater, the networks of power found are complex and the practitioner/manager has to develop new sources of power through alliances and identifying specific expertise that is valued by the whole. However, the possibilities for individual growth are also greater. A small fish in a large pond can always grow larger!

IDENTIFYING AND PLANNING CAREER DIRECTIONS

The changes to basic nurse training from a certificate level course that qualified the nurse in a general, mental or child illness-related area are well established, with nurses now having a much broader based diploma course with specialisation not taking place until halfway through training. This broader base might seem more compatible with the move into a more managerial role but the reduced amount of time spent practising skills does emphasise the importance of Benner's arguments (1984). In addition, there is considerable pressure to move quite quickly into a specialist area of practice on completion of training. Previously, most nurses would move between a number of specialisms before deciding where to settle and, in practice, the older generation of nurses often have a

Decision making in practice

bigger pool from which to draw appropriate skills than those who have been through the Project 2000 route. However, this latter group may be at an advantage with a broader academic base.

The financial pressure to specialise early also has some unexpected spin-offs. There seems to be some evidence that the type of specialism carries with it a certain status. This tends to occur in any profession and is noticeable in both medicine and nursing. The ITU or theatre nurse tends to have a steeper career trajectory than the nurse who has spent more time in care of the elderly or on night duty. The situation tends to work against those with family commitments where work opportunities that fit with home requirements can be restricted. With the current shortages in nursing, this situation may change but it is difficult to envisage any major alteration to the status of different types of nursing work as these tend to run parallel to the medical profession (Larson 1977).

The final point to make is the existence of the glass ceiling in professional/managerial careers (Marshall 1995). Although there are some clear geographical variations, the overall evidence underlines the better career prospects for men over women. A disproportionate number of men reach senior and executive positions in health care when compared to the percentage actually entering the nursing profession (Hugman 1991). In spite of skills identified in the practitioner profile that are also valuable to the manager, the ability of the female practitioner/manager to argue this for promotion is limited by the cultural mores of the organisation that still see men as better suited to positions of seniority. This then becomes a vicious circle as, until more women hold the most senior posts in health care organisations, the norms will remain unquestioned and accepted.

The above points suggest that career progression is not simply a matter of ensuring that certain skills are developed. The need for a more political approach has already been highlighted and practitioners should be aware of learning and applying these skills in relation to their careers as well as the performance of their jobs.

CONCLUSION

This chapter has explored the route taken from practice to management. It has summarised some key thinking on the content of the manager's role and drawn from this a comparison between the skills of the practitioner compared to those of the manager. It has concluded that there are many areas of commonality between the two although there are some gaps that the practitioner will con-

The practitioner as manager

sciously need to develop. The particular difficulties of combining the practitioner and manager roles have been examined in some depth and a final comment has highlighted some of the issues in career planning and progression. The overall conclusion is that the practitioner is well positioned to take on board a managerial role as long as certain issues are acknowledged and managed.

References

Beer M 1980 Organisation change and development: a systems view. Goodyear, Santa Monica, California

Benner P 1984 From novice to expert: excellence and power in clinical nursing. Addison-Wesley, Menlo Park, California

Child J 1984 Organization: a guide to practice and problems. Harper and Row, London

Drucker P 1987 The frontiers of management. Heinemann, London

Fayol H 1949 General and industrial management. Pitman, London

Halford S, Savage M, Witz A 1997 Gender, careers and organisations. Macmillan, Basingstoke

Handy C 1985 Gods of management. Pan, London

Hugman R 1991 Power in caring professions. Macmillan, London

Katz D, Kahn R 1966 Social psychology of organisations. Wiley, Chichester

Larson M 1977 The rise of professionalism. University of California Press, Los Angeles

Lickert R 1961 New patterns of management. McGraw Hill, New York

Marshall J 1995 Women managers moving on: exploring career and life choices. Routledge, London

Mayo E 1933 The human problems of an industrial civilisation. Macmillan, London

Mintzberg H 1973 The nature of managerial work. Harper and Row, New York

Mintzberg H 1979 The structure of organisations. Prentice Hall, London

Morgan G 1997 Images of organisation, 2nd edn. Sage, London

Peters T, Waterman R 1982 In search of excellence. Harper and Row, New York

Pollitt C 1990 Managerialism and the public services: the Anglo-American experience. Basil Blackwell, Oxford

Robinson J, Gray A, Elkan R (eds) 1992 Policy issues in nursing. Open University Press, Milton Keynes

Smith E 1997 Staff development through role exchange. Unpublished paper, Addenbrooke's Hospital, Cambridge

Taylor F 1947 Scientific management. Harper and Row, New York

Witz A 1994 The challenge of nursing. In: Gabe J, Kelleher D, Williams G (eds) Challenging medicine, Routledge, London

Young AP 1999 The bed crisis of winter 1995–1996 in the British NHS: an illustration of accountability issues. Nursing Ethics 6(4): 316–326

Decision making in practice

Application 5:1

Samantha Lawrence and Mary Cooke

Managing staff and residents in a nursing home: conflicts in decision making

Managing a nursing home can be daunting in today's climate of continued revision of regulations, pressures from hospitals to move elderly and disabled residents from NHS to community accommodation and the lack of regularly staffed teams of health carers.

Samantha Lawrence has managed nursing homes for the elderly in Dorset, North London, the East End of London and East Kent over the past 15 years. This variety of experience has enabled her to understand the conflicts that can occur between staff, relatives and residents and also as a result of policy change. These experiences force flexible thinking in assessing short-term and long-term effects of decisions. The several examples of decision making brought to you here provide ethical conflicts where several answers to the dilemmas can be right but the outcomes of each decision could be diverse.

ETHICAL PROBLEMS POSED BY RESIDENTS

One such example is of a couple who became resident in a home, who had previously used separate rooms and wished to continue to do so. They were accommodated similarly, in separate rooms in the nursing home, and the husband visited his wife on occasion in her room. Their privacy was maintained on these occasions, but after the visits, the wife was reported by the health carers as having bruising on her body consistent with physical abuse. The husband was found to have been hurting his wife in this way as a part of their relationship for over 40 years. Bringing their relationship into the 'open' in a nursing home was possibly naive of the couple but to decide that their relationship should change may not be the responsibility of the staff although, at a personal level, they might want to intervene to protect the wife. A professional viewpoint might argue that the wife has 'consented' to this treatment and to leave well alone.

A second example is a familiar story to some practitioners: a stroke victim was in the stages of physical and nutritional decline, having had a dense cerebral vascular accident, being aphasic and having other multiple pathologies. The family, as is customary, were informed. Several interested factions in the family had to make decisions with the health care staff as to the best outcomes of care for the man. One daughter who had looked after him for some time in his home wanted him to be able to die peacefully. The other daughter demanded that he be kept alive using a percutaneous endoscopic gastrostomy (PEG) tube and enteral feed. This decision posed a conflict of interests. Care of other residents was reduced because of low staff ratios and the level of care needed for this man. To the practitioner, the preservation of life might seem to have precedence but the manager's concern had to be with the wider population of the home.

PROBLEMS IN MANAGING STAFF

An example is given of a dilemma in the management of teams working in the close confines of nursing homes.

A patient was defined by a long-serving member of staff as becoming 'difficult'. The resident accused the staff member of abusing him. This apparent breakdown of relationship can be exacerbated by a manager who does nothing or one who wades into the argument and makes some heavy-handed decisions that benefit one side only to the detriment of other staff or residents. After enquiring about the accusations, several methods of resolving the matter can be chosen. A strategic way of dealing with the matter can be to take the staff aside to discuss issues of 'difficult residents'; another can be to ensure that the resident does not have contact with the staff member. The former, if handled well, can work; the latter can be awkward if staffing levels are low.

CONFLICTS BETWEEN STAFF AND OWNERS

Other issues of nursing home management are associated with the owners. Some owners can be unscrupulous, denying the residents adequate food. In one situation, staff had to bring in food for the residents to ensure they were fed properly. No-one said anything about this situation for fear of the owner and of getting a poor reference on applying for another post. The owner would pick up the peelings of the potatoes, weigh them and accuse the staff of cutting too much off the potatoes. They would then take the newly cut peelings to their restaurant and sell the peelings as a dish, cooked and dressed with a sour cream and chive dressing! This case was eventually taken to the health authority but it was several years before the home was closed.

The lack of qualified staff in homes has proved difficult at times for those staff in charge of care. Some home managers faced pressures whatever decision they took: loss of job if unacceptable staffing levels were referred to the registration officers or continuing to work 70 hours a week to cover for lack of qualified staff. It is hoped that this situation may change. Recent modifications to the regulations will require homes to have less than 20% of their rooms as double rooms, the rest to be single accommodation. The ratio of staff has to be raised. However, this leads to fewer available spaces due to many homes closing through loss of profits.

ETHICAL ISSUES WITH EXTERNAL AGENCIES

Conflicts with external decision makers can also occur. Social services care managers who assess the elderly for their suitability for either care home (non-nursing care accommodation) or nursing home accommodation (qualified nursing staff in attendance) may well decide in favour of care homes, because of lower costs. The health needs of each potential resident are not always considered.

These examples demonstrate some of the conflict-ridden decisions that have to be made in community care homes. The manner of care giving for the elderly in any society is a reflection of the culture of that society and, as such, should provide an insight into how we in the UK could have better standards of care for vulnerable people.

Managing staff and residents in a nursing home

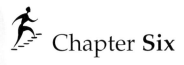

Chapter Six

Affecting decisions through networks and group processes

Debbie Lee

- Theories of group and relationship power

- The functioning of committees in the workplace

- The importance of networks for managers in public and private health care

- Conclusion

OVERVIEW

For those working in health care, the role of the manager has shifted from one emphasising control to one that is about dealing with change. This shift of emphasis means that managers need to develop different skills from those that were sufficient in a fairly static bureaucracy. Effective management relies more and more on a project approach to work, often with transient groupings of more equal partners than heretofore. Repeated restructuring of the workplace has broken down longstanding relationships, usually of a superior/subordinate kind. While a move away from a rule-bound role culture is to be welcomed, for a number of reasons these changes can lead to isolation which, in turn, must be managed.

This chapter presents two particular techniques for effective management: decision making in groups and networking. The

Decision making in practice

first part of the chapter outlines some broad issues about working in a group setting before moving on to examine some particular features of a formal group approach, that of committees. The example of a clinical audit committee is presented. It then argues that for a number of reasons, groups are also useful at the informal end of the spectrum in order to find creative solutions to 'wicked' problems, for example through brainstorming.

The next section introduces some of the issues relevant to networking. It presents both some of the functions of networking and some techniques to use.

The final part of the chapter presents a short case study of how a problem to do with patient records was solved by a specially convened project group. The members of this group had an important role to play in representing their particular professional group, communicating with them and gaining their commitment. Good networking skills were vitally important here as well as the ability to function well as a group member.

THEORIES OF GROUP AND RELATIONSHIP POWER

A group is likely to bring a range of complementary expertise, experience and knowledge to problem solving and the generation of workable ideas. Group members can provoke further ideas in the team by means of feedback and brainstorming. It is hoped that group decisions will lead to the more thorough evaluation of a situation and, because members have full participation in the process, that a decision gained in this way is more likely to lead to commitment on implementation.

Group norms and cohesiveness

A group of staff coming together as a group for the first time will set itself group norms even if they have never met each other before. A popular model by Truckman (1965) described the development of a meeting as going through four stages of development: forming, storming, norming and performing.

- *Forming* – this is the initial formation of the group and testing out each individual's position and influence within the group.

Affecting decisions through networks and group processes

Six Steps to **Effective Management**

- *Storming* – this is where the group gets to know each other better. Any major disagreements are brought to the surface and hopefully resolved.
- *Norming* – after having disagreement and debate the group members will now establish guidelines and standards to which they can all subscribe.
- *Performing* – with the methods of working agreed and a cohesive structure in place, the group can now work effectively to achieve the goals they have set themselves.

The formation of any new group begins with the expectation that the group will be able to cooperate in order to achieve the results expected. Working within a cohesive group can be a rewarding experience and can raise the morale of a unit. The outputs of a cohesive group will conform to the standards accepted by the group (Milgram 1965). A cohesive group is also more likely to increase staff satisfaction, reduce staff turnover and reduce absenteeism (Argyle 1974). When setting up any new group to aid decision making, thought must be given to a number of factors which will impact on the cohesiveness of the group (Stewart 1996).

Membership

- *The size of the group* – the larger the group, the more difficult it is to ensure total group cohesion. This is difficult to achieve if the group exceeds 10–12 members. More than this in a group can lead to fragmentation and setting up unplanned subgroups.
- *Compatibility* – shared interests, values and backgrounds all make it easier to establish group cohesion.
- *Performance* – establishing a team can take time. Cohesion and group relations are more likely to take place over a period of time.

Work environment

- *The nature of the task* – where the task brings people together this will instil group cohesion, by giving everyone a common focus.
- *Physical setting* – when a group is geographically working close to each other this will generally promote cohesion, as they are likely to communicate more frequently.
- *Communications* – the more freely group members can communicate, the greater the cohesion. Every opportunity should be taken to encourage both formal and informal communication.

Decision making in practice

- *Technology* – this can be very beneficial when establishing a group. It may be as simple as using the technology for communication such as using the e-mail system or sharing a website. It may be sharing common databases or utilising the same decision support systems.

Organisational

- *Management and leadership* – there is no doubt that the style of leadership and the overall management of the group will impact on group cohesiveness. The leader will need to guide, provide opportunities for all to participate and minimise any potential conflict.
- *Success* – success will help to maintain a cohesive group. Working to high standards, achieving goals and getting recognised for a job well done will all contribute to this.
- *External threat* – this can often pull group members closer together and give greater clarity of roles between group members.

Reasons for joining a group

There are many reasons why an individual decides to join a group (Jones et al 1996). However, it is important to consider some of the reasons that have motivated an individual to want to join. It may be that someone joins because they admire the group and want to be associated with its work. The individual may just want to be with their friends and not be interested in the subject area. The leader of the group needs to be aware of this as it may impact on the delivery of the group's objectives.

Being a member of a group may help an individual advance their career. Such a person is likely to contribute actively in the group tasks to raise their own personal profile.

Sometimes someone will want to join a group to seek protection from threatening surroundings. Joining the group may offer them a higher official status or greater influence due to the numbers of and positions held by the members.

Group behaviour and roles

Within any group there is a distribution of roles. Some of these roles will be formally established as the group is set up. Many will

Affecting decisions through networks and group processes

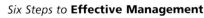

be adopted as members with specialist skills are exposed. Different roles of group members may include:

- *leader* – building the vision and initiating action
- *evaluator* – collecting and giving information
- *moral supporter* – encouraging the team
- *idea generator* – looks at very new and different ways of doing things
- *problem solver* – making practical suggestions for solution.

Not everyone's style will be the same and often group members will demonstrate a combination of roles within the group depending on their skills and background (Belbin 1981). The individual's role within the group is often influenced by their position within the structure of the organisation. For example, a staff nurse may have difficulty chairing a meeting where one of the members is a senior surgical consultant. In these circumstances mentorship and supervision will help to support the staff nurse in developing the necessary skills to establish the leadership position.

Conflict between group members

Everybody's style and personality are different. Conflict often arises when there is a lack of clarity of role within a group. In reality the way a person behaves is not always consistent with the expectations of the role. A number of reasons may lead to this.

- *Role incompatibility* – this will often arise when a person is inconsistent with their behaviour within a role. This occurs when an individual is trying to please two masters and is facing opposing expectations from each.
- *Role ambiguity* – when the role has not been defined the individual's expectations may be different from those in the group. This can often happen in a rapidly changing environment where there is uncertainty.
- *Role overload* – when a person has too many roles within a group, overload will take place. They will be unsuccessful in achieving basic tasks and dissatisfaction comes from quantity overshadowing quality.
- *Role underload* – this can occur when expectations of a role were perceived to be more demanding than in reality. Often it is felt that the role is not utilising many of the individual's skills and abilities (Secord & Backman 1964).

Team building

Many problems of integration within a group can be overcome by team building. This has been a popular approach to get individuals to work more positively in groups, avoiding conflict. The process of team building involves all members in the group, guiding them through all processes which can occur with that group. This will lead to a greater understanding of how to get the most out of the team, advancing both the team itself and the organisation (Adair 1987).

THE FUNCTIONING OF COMMITTEES IN THE WORKPLACE

The use of groups in the decision-making process in a fairly formal way is usually described as committee work (Lawton & Rigby 1992). A committee is a group of individuals that is appointed for a special function. A committee may have an advisory, information-al, coordination or decision-making responsibility. It very often acts as a way of facilitating change through an organisation by having members that represent different departments who can work together to solve interdepartmental problems. It can be a democratic way to involve all members of the team in the decision-making process. Committee appointments are an excellent method of developing skills in leadership and providing the opportunity to meet employees outside their normal environment.

When setting up any committee it is important to consider certain aspects to ensure that required outcomes are achieved (Bell 1990, Chang & Kehoe 1995). Some of these elements are outlined below.

Select the right members

A committee must have members that have the right skills and competencies from the relevant professional group. This does not mean necessarily having individuals from the top of their professional field but people selected must have the confidence and ability to cope with the workload and the demands of committee work. Members need to be selected with care in order to ensure that they are seen as credible by their peers.

The committee will also need specific roles to ensure that the work processed by the committee is efficient and effective. A key role for consideration is that of the chair, the person who will preside over each meeting. This individual may be voted in or selected by those who have commissioned the committee.

Fix the dates of all committee meetings from the outset

Ensure that the members have the dates set out for the year from the outset. This will help to reduce any absenteeism or disruption to the clinical staff's work. It may be necessary at times to change the date of a meeting but again, give consideration to members' other commitments by giving as much notice as possible.

Take action to ensure that expert advice is available

The committee will have members from a varied professional and skills base. There will, however, be times when further expert advice is needed that cannot be provided from within the team. Consideration needs to be given to what skills will be needed, whether the present committee members have these skills and if not, from whom they can be gained. The committee should decide this in a democratic way and an external expert coopted on to the committee.

Set up systems to ensure that the committee can make speedy decisions if necessary

There will be times when an issue of concern arises where it is necessary to set up an emergency meeting. There may be some major new evidence affecting care and the committee is not due to meet for a couple of months. In these circumstances the committee may seem negligent if it does not respond. Flexibility must be built into its procedures. In urgent situations, the committee may approve the chair's action later.

Ensure there is accurate record keeping

It is important that a factual record is kept of each meeting. This is to communicate the proceedings to those not present. The meeting needs to be minuted with enough detail to give the reader an

Decision making in practice

understanding of what has been discussed, the key decisions made and the reasons why those decisions were made. The committee also needs a clear procedure for checking accuracy of the minutes and a method for keeping a copy of relevant papers for reference.

Have access to the relevant information to aid decision making

In order for the committee to make informed decisions the team will need access to all relevant information. This may be research, trust papers or papers produced by committee members. To aid the decision-making process, where possible papers should be circulated prior to meetings.

Plan ahead and build in time for reflection

It is important to set agendas and monitor progress made towards meeting those targets set by the committee. Members will all have a busy schedule and will want to see the benefits of having a committee. Time should be allowed to reflect on progress made towards its objectives although sadly it is rare for this to be formally undertaken. Members should be involved in setting the agendas for meetings and mechanisms built in to enable staff to add items to the agenda when necessary.

Have a clear statement of purpose for the committee

Having clear terms of reference from the very start will enable the entire group to match the decisions made to the purpose of the committee. It acts as a useful means of communication to the wider organisation as well as a measure for a point in time. Some committees often have a remit to oversee a change and once that change is complete then the committee is disbanded. An example would be the commissioning of a new clinical service. Once the service is set up the commissioning group is no longer required. However, some committees are set up for ongoing pieces of work, for example committees on clinical governance. The specialist subject areas may change as new issues arise but the systems will be in place to improve the quality of patient care. A register should be kept of the names and terms and conditions of all those appointed

Affecting decisions through networks and group processes

to the committee. This will give the chair clarity on its membership and the rationale for the appointment.

Good reasons for using committees to aid decision making

Committees are a popular decision-making tool although sometimes seen as rather slow and cumbersome. The following list sets out the positive reasons for having a committee.

- It is a democratic way to set policies, establish objectives and design strategies.
- It helps to develop staff and build confidence by bringing staff into contact with colleagues outside their usual peer group.
- It is an effective way to promote ownership of change by having each professional/team/department represented.
- It is a structured way to make decisions.
- The outcomes can be measured.
- Often the committees have an official status within the organisation or commissioning body which may give the group more clout to implement change.
- It concentrates expert resources.
- It aids cross-boundary working.

The Clinical Audit Committee

The following illustrates how the remit of a committee might be drawn up.

Constitution

The NHS Trust resolves to establish a Clinical Audit Committee. This will be a subcommittee to the Clinical Governance Committee.

Aims

The aims of the Clinical Audit Committee are to improve the quality of clinical care and achieve clinical effectiveness.

Membership

The membership will consist of doctors, nurses, professionals allied to medicine. Clinical representatives external to the organisation shall attend the meeting by invitation only.

(continued)

Decision making in practice

(continued)

The chairman of the committee

The Clinical Directors of the Trust will appoint the chairman of the committee. The chair will stand for one year.

Frequency of meetings

The meetings will take place monthly.

Authority

The committee is authorised by the Trust Board to investigate any activity within the committee terms of reference. It is authorised to seek any information it requires from any employee and all employees are directed to cooperate with any request made by the committee.

   The committee is authorised by the Board to obtain outside legal or professional advice and to secure the attendance of outsiders with relevant experience if it considers it necessary.

Duties

● To undertake regular systematic audit that covers the work of clinical teams and enables all professionals to participate.
● To ensure that all audit work links effectively with other quality programmes and training and education programmes.
● To ensure that confidentiality procedures are in place.
● To take appropriate action where audit reveals problems related to treatment and care.
● To agree the annual programme with local managers.

Creative decision making in groups

It would appear that two models of decision making have evolved. First, there is the scientific or rational model. This process will involve a structured and logical analysis of evidence as demonstrated above in committee work. The second model of decision making emphasises a much looser process that relies more on stepping outside the normal decision-making conventions. Within a group setting, this is recognised as brainstorming (West & Farr 1990).

   The search for alternatives will identify that there are many different ways of solving a problem. The more alternatives identified, the greater change might be. Often the outcome will be a decision of a higher quality than one reached by more traditional techniques. The value of the group is in stimulating each other to generate more and more creative solutions.

A brainstorming approach involves members of the group producing as many ideas as possible. Everyone has the opportunity to contribute and think as radically and creatively as they can. There are a number of elements to consider when brainstorming.

- The initial emphasis should be on quantity not on quality of ideas.
- No ideas should be rejected or criticised.
- Individuals should be encouraged to elaborate on their ideas and bounce suggestions off each other.
- The environment must be right for a brainstorming session. The emphasis should be on capturing innovation and creative ideas so a location away from the work situation will get the best out of the group.

THE IMPORTANCE OF NETWORKS FOR MANAGERS IN PUBLIC AND PRIVATE HEALTH CARE

In today's health care environment participation in both formal and informal networking groups has become increasingly more valuable. The networking activity is aimed at much more than a group of peers getting together. It is not a hierarchical function, as it will often involve a cooperative relationship between peers, outsiders, bosses and subordinates (Fisher & Vilas 1996). Networking can be a quick and effective way to achieve clinical effectiveness through contact with those who have similar interests in health care. Network groups can be uniprofessional but, more increasingly, multiprofessional networks are being established as the concepts of patient-centred care are developed.

Functions of a networking group

The following list is not exhaustive but will act as a guide to the functions of a networking group.

- *Provision of access to new contacts* – a networking group will bring people into contact with those not normally encountered in their everyday working environment. New contacts will be invaluable

for obtaining diverse information on a given subject area which
will contribute to broadening and opening up new horizons.

● *Integration and a sense of belonging* – networks will provide the
opportunity to share ideas, experiences and information with a
group of people with similar interests.

● *Receiving guidance and advice* – this will provide the group members with valuable experience of feedback on some project or
issue on which the individual is working. The provision of literature such as good practice guidance is often generated
through network groups, particularly those which have been
set up nationally.

● *Assisting others* – a key benefit of networking is the motivation
of members to assist each other with practice development
issues. The provision of services and goods can also be coordinated through the network.

● *Opportunities to support others* – this may be in the form of emotional support and supervision or actual support with the task
or problem.

● *Fostering interdisciplinary and cross-boundary understanding.*

● *Maximising opportunities for staff development.*

● *The concentration of expert resources.*

Different ways of networking

Networks can be built in a number of ways.

● Join a specialist interest group. This could be a clinical or a professional forum.

● Attend a conference to meet people who may have common
interests.

● Attend a course to network with people with different backgrounds, experience and knowledge.

● Use the Internet for networks. This will provide a rich source of
information and contacts from an international pool.

● Consider shadowing someone more senior. This may give exposure to contacts not normally met.

● Look for a mentor who can be a useful link to broaden your networks.

● When a literature review is undertaken, note the authors and
contact addresses as they could be a useful resource.

● Keep a record of previous work colleagues and keep in contact if
you change jobs. You never know where colleagues will be in, say,
5 years' time and they may contribute a very useful network.

Affecting decisions through networks and group processes

- Build a personal directory of who is who. The list should include those working at national, regional and local levels.
- Have an open day and ask everyone to fill in a visitor's book. Send invitations widely. Some useful networks may result from those attending.
- Get something published. People will contact the author to share interests and new networks are made.
- Attend public meetings such as the open trust board meeting. This will provide a broader perspective on what is going on and again will be an opportunity to network with local people as well as some senior staff within the trust.

Influencing decisions through group processes and networking

The following case study illustrates how some needed changes were brought about through a specially convened group. The members of this group needed to work effectively with a wide cross-section of their organisation. They also had to ensure that networks were built and maintained so that the team's decisions would be implemented.

A project group of the Practice Development Unit

Background

The Practice Development Unit (PDU) at Seacroft Hospital, Leeds, was established in the very early 1990s. It provided a focus within health care for multidisciplinary practice development and research, making a key commitment to support the dissemination of good practice. The PDU operates beyond the confines of a unidisciplinary focus and addresses the pressing need to break down barriers at the interface of practice. Making decisions in groups was the norm. Participation in decision making was encouraged by all. It was not based on the traditional hierarchy but on innovation, motivation and abilities.

The issue

Staff were becoming increasingly frustrated with the fragmentation of patient records. Each profession had its own separate record, which was kept in different locations and maintained to different

(continued)

Decision making in practice

(continued)

standards. A multidisciplinary project group was established using a structured approach to problem solving.

The action taken

The following steps were undertaken.

1. *The identification of the problem* – the issue was raised through a communications forum by one of the staff nurses with support from the clinical nurse advisor and a consultant physician.
2. *The expression of the problem* – the multidisciplinary team met up to examine the issues more precisely in order to get a clear definition of the problem.
3. *Ownership of the problem* – once it was agreed that this was a problem to be addressed, the identification of the leads took place. This was based on individuals' motivation, skills, knowledge and abilities to tackle the problem. Due to the fact that all communication forums were multidisciplinary, obtaining ownership for problems that would impact on all professions was much easier. Individual members had a responsibility to link back into their own professional group.
4. *Formation of the goals* – the team agreed that there would be one single record kept at the patient's bedside. Clear goals were set in order to achieve this vision. This included the use of questionnaires to ascertain where the unit was now, establishing focus groups, undertaking a literature review and networking with any other unit that had developed health care records.
5. *Defining the current situation* – this part of the process involved the group identifying current deficits as well as aspects that were considered good practice, before any changes were agreed.
6. *The selection of the changes* – the project group not only needed to look at the issues associated with patient records but also any implications for the wider unit and trust. This part of the planning process would look at resource implications, timescales, opinions of key stakeholders and how to achieve the wider dissemination of results. Building on group members' existing networks made this feasible.
7. *Action* – the project group agreed a way forward and decided that ownership in the wider organisation would be achieved far more easily if there was a piloting phase. This would test out the processes and could refine the documents before there was a more comprehensive roll-out.
8. *Evaluation* – there was to be a written report on the project. This included an evaluation, which pinpointed any issues still to be

(continued)

(continued)

addressed when wider implementation of the single patient documents occurred.

9. *Dissemination* – it was part of the PDU's philosophy to share new ideas and lessons learnt within the trust and beyond. It was also customary to celebrate all achievements.

Outcomes

This structured approach to the implementation of a single patient-held health record was an important mechanism for the development of all staff working in the unit. Working together in a single multiprofessional group enabled rapid developments and an early success with a complex problem. By working together in a group and networking with the relevant stakeholders, there was ownership of the problem, a broader base for capturing innovation and creativity and the final document was more robust due to the richness of diverse skills and abilities in its creation. The new record was formally implemented by the PDU within 6 months of identifying the initial problem. It was rolled out throughout the whole directorate within a year.

CONCLUSION

In taking a very practical approach to the increasingly important part played by project and committee work in health care decision making, this chapter has set out a useful framework. It seems likely that most practitioners and all managers will be involved in this mode of decision making to some extent. The chapter also includes some aspects of networking that will enhance the quality of decisions made. Finally, the case study illustrates the interface between group functioning and networking, indirectly in how the group membership was decided and more directly in ensuring quality inputs and later commitment from the wider organisational environment.

References

Adair J 1987 Effective team building. Pan Books, London

Argyle M 1974 The social psychology of work. Penguin, Harmondsworth

Belbin M 1981 Management teams: why they succeed or fail. Heinemann, London

Bell G 1990 The secrets of successful business meetings. Heinemann, Oxford

Chang R, Kehoe K 1995 Meetings that work! Kogan Page, London

Fisher D, Vilas S 1996 Successful networking. Thorsons, London

Decision making in practice

Jones P, Palmer J, Osterweil C, Whitehead D 1996 Delivering exceptional performance. Pitman, London

Lawton P, Rigby E 1992 Meetings: the law and practice, 5th edn. Pitman, London

Milgram S 1965 Liberating effects of group pressure. Journal of Personality and Psychology 1(2): 127–134

Secord P, Backman C 1964 Social psychology. McGraw Hill, New York

Stewart R 1996 Leading in the NHS, 2nd edn. Macmillan, Basingstoke

Truckman BW 1965 Developing sequence in small groups. Psychological Bulletin 63: 384–399

West M, Farr J (eds) 1990 Innovation and creativity at work. Wiley, Chichester

Affecting decisions through networks and group processes

Application 6:1

Ann P Young

Networking by middle managers in health care

'Networking is joy!' So said one nurse manager working in a private hospital. 'It's good to get to know people,' said another from the NHS. Working collaboratively with others rather than in isolation is very much seen to be the way to develop ideas and achieve sound outcomes. However, in a research study covering both the NHS and private care, the extent and nature of managers' networking was found to be quite variable. The results of this study are now discussed and Table 6.1.1 summarises the main findings.

Managers were asked to describe their networks both within and external to their organisations. Internal networks within an NHS trust were sometimes quite difficult. A trust is a big organisation and managers complained of increasing fragmentation between directorates and of not knowing what went on 'along the corridor'. Internal networking had therefore to be consciously managed as isolation was a potential problem. Membership of certain decision-making groups and working in non-hierarchical roles improved communication across the trust. The infection control manager had set up link nurses in each of the clinical directorates to act as his 'eyes and ears'. The nature of his job also gave him wide-ranging access, as it did for the quality nurse manager. In the private sector, units tended to be much smaller, staff had usually stayed with the organisation for much longer and internal networking was strongly evidenced. However, here the danger, as perceived by the managers, was of professional isolation. Ideas could become entrenched, making change difficult and managers unaware of being out of touch with current reality.

External networks were again very variable. Here the extent of networking by the private care managers was much greater than those in the NHS. This seemed to occur for two reasons. First, the fear of professional isolation resulted in conscious decisions to build networks with other professionals, both across other private sector organisations and into the NHS through professional groups, such as RCN interest groups. Second, the executive of the private company

6.1.1 Networking

Interview code	Gender of manager	Level of networking	Type of internal networks	Type of external networks	Networks consciously developed by individual	Networks consciously developed by employer	Main uses made of networks
NN1	F	F	Mixed	Clinical	No	Some recent attempts made by the NHS trust for all groups of staff	I,F
NN2	F	G	Mixed	Mixed	No		I,O,F
NN3	F	F	Clinical	Clinical	No		S
NN4	M	H	Mixed	Mixed	Yes		S,O,P
NN5	M	F	Mixed	Clinical	Yes		S,C
NN6	M	H	Clinical	Mixed	Yes		I,O,P
NN7	F	F	Mixed	Clinical	No		S
NN8	F	L	Clinical	None	No		I
NN9	F	G	Mixed	Clinical	No		
NF1	M	F	Mixed	Finance	No		S,F
NF2	M	H	Mixed	Mixed	Yes		O
NF3	M	L	Finance	Mixed	Yes		C
NF4	M	G	Mixed	Finance	No		S,F,O
NF5	M	H	Mixed	Finance	Yes		S,O
NF6	F	L	Mixed	Mixed	No		O
PN1	F	H	Clinical	Clinical	Yes	Strategically set up by Head Office	I,S,O,F,P
PN2	F	G	Mixed	Clinical	Yes		I,O,F
PN3	F	F	Clinical	Clinical	Yes		I,S,C
PN4	F	G	Clinical	Clinical	No		O

Key
NN=NHS Nursing
NF=NHS Finance
PN=Private Nursing

Key for level of networking:
H=high, G=good, F=fair, L=low

Key for stated main uses made of networks:
I=information, S=support, O=achieve work objectives,
F=friendship, social, pleasure, P=prevent isolation,
C=career development

had set up specific networks across its hospitals to promote communication and shared practice. This was a strategic decision in order to enhance standardisation.

> The chief executive has been very clever. I think he knew exactly what he was doing. And while it smacked of Big Brother and upset a lot of people when the changes started, he has actually created a very effective machine . . . Without the networks making everybody talk to each other, you couldn't have introduced the bigger change.

External networking by NHS managers again tended to emphasise their professional remit but also included building contacts across a wider range where the managers saw their roles as facilitating a more holistic approach to care. For example, one manager thought it important to network with those commissioning care as well as those providing it and was quite prepared to build informal links with the authority commissioning child-care services. Again with child health, this same manager had consciously built networks with people in education and social services as being beneficial not just for problem solving, but for understanding each other's roles and promoting collaborative decision making.

Some moves had been made by the NHS trust to strategically increase networking across its different directorates. This had been facilitated by a programme run by the King's Fund. Groups were purposefully put together to create a mix of departments and professional allegiances.

> The King's Fund has been taking us away from the site and making people interact socially. You can only say it's positive, people talk about it, people talk about their experiences although it's all Chatham House rules.

Although it could only be run across a specified time period, it had had a marked effect on breaking down barriers. 'People will now interact and greet people in the passage who say hello to you and how are you and how are you getting on with your project?'

The main devices used by managers to build networks were by keeping in contact with colleagues from previous workplaces (particularly obvious with the NHS managers) and through the variety of training and educational programmes with which they had been involved professionally and managerially. How purposefully these networks were developed and maintained varied across two dimensions. As already mentioned, the private care managers acted more consciously to build networks to prevent isolation. However, there was also a difference according to gender. The male managers on the whole used networking more consciously, sometimes admitting to its use for career progression.

> In the last six months, some of the 'boys' have started playing football one evening a week. And various directors participate . . . they all happen to be male. So I suppose you could say I network with them,

it's fairly informal although I'm always aware of what I'm saying and I'm always beating the drum for my department.

The female managers were more likely to emphasise the support and social aspects of networking. One female manager actually expressed what she saw as an ethical dilemma in consciously building networks – 'I don't like to have a false relationship with people'.

The use made of networks was variable and mixed. Support, advice and assistance in achieving work objectives featured frequently; for friendship and pleasure came second; in order to gain influence or power was less frequently expressed. It is likely that motivations were, in fact, mixed. For one manager, the key issue of networking was sharing and communication.

> You can't get round personal contact, you just can't get round it. Even if we never take decisions at anything for 3 months, the important thing is that everyone has been in the same room together and had the chance to air any issues, to debate anything . . . that's probably as important as anything else.

A final fact to note was the marked individual variations in networking activity that were independent of context or gender. Here, Belbin's group roles were called to mind. Some individuals have a preference for this type of role.

> It's about personality to some extent. But it's also about building relationships. You don't build relationships in a month, a year or even two years. Sometimes you have to work, work, work with people.

Certainly, it seems that it is a skill that most managers should acquire to some extent in today's rapidly changing and overtly political climate in health care.

Networking by middle managers in health care

Application **6:2**

Ann P Young

Team roles and decision making

Increasingly, working in teams is seen as a key skill for managers and their subordinates. For professional staff with a nursing or other paramedical background, team working will have been an important part of their professional training but, as managers, a more conscious use of teams needs to be made in order to achieve required outcomes.

BELBIN'S TEAM ROLES

Belbin's description of team working has been well known for many years and is unusual in that it is strongly grounded in research. He identified just nine roles that are available to team members and found that effective achievement of tasks relied on having a balanced team with a mix of roles amongst its members.

Usually, an individual tends to have one team role with which she or he is most comfortable, but will also have a secondary role that can be used quite readily. The characteristics of each role are summarised below. As you read, think about which roles you feel most at ease with as well as those that are definitely not for you. Identify the team roles played by your work colleagues in one particular team with which you have involvement. Are team members being used appropriately? What improvements might be made to harness individual preferences? To what extent is success being promoted by the team having a cross-section of team roles or being put at risk by an imbalance in team roles?

The coordinator is mature, confident and trusting. She makes a good chairman, giving an opportunity to people to express themselves while maintaining some overall control. She will tend to clarify what has to be achieved and encourages decision making. She is not necessarily the most clever or creative member of the group but holds the group together.

The shaper is dynamic and energetic. He will focus on achieving targets and in order to do this, will challenge and pressurise those around. Determined and focused, he will find ways around obstacles and is unwilling to accept failure. He can be quick to anger if thwarted and frustrated.

The plant is the creative and imaginative member of the group. She will go for unorthodox and unusual solutions and is therefore particularly good at solving seemingly intractable problems. However, she is not usually particularly skilled in managing people.

The resource-investigator is the extrovert extraordinaire, very enthusiastic and an excellent communicator. He loves exploring a wide range of opportunities and developing contacts. Enthusiasms may be short-lived unless interest can be maintained and new opportunities and challenges presented.

The monitor-evaluator tends to keep a distance. She is the analytical and strategic member of the group who will examine all options before reaching a well thought out decision. Seeming to be a rather reserved and quiet individual, she works with others by calling on rationality rather than emotion.

The team worker is sociable, pleasant tempered and reliable. He likes to be accommodating and helpful, is a good listener and works to avoid friction. If faced with the need to make a decision, he will tend to be indecisive.

The implementer is a practical person who loves turning ideas into practical outcomes. She is reliable and efficient and is disciplined in her approach to work. However, at times, she may seem rather inflexible when faced with new situations.

The completer is painstaking and conscientious. He will examine what others have achieved for errors and put them right. Conscious of time constraints, he will deliver even if the costs are high. He is therefore prone to anxiety and worry and is reluctant to delegate.

The specialist contributes knowledge on a narrow front as appropriate to her speciality. Single-minded and dedicated, her focus tends to be narrow but deep and she is therefore able to supply knowledge that might otherwise be in short supply.

A managerial team

The particular managerial team described below illustrates the usefulness of Belbin's approach. The five people in this particular team were responsible for the administrative support systems of a training establishment. Penny was the formal leader of the group and line managed the other four as well as having responsibility for the non-pay budget. Martine was responsible for the recruitment, Julie for clerical support staff, Barbara for personnel issues and Jenny for communication. A current issue was how to build the marketing function within the organisation.

Penny had reasonably good coordinator skills and was able to clarify group objectives that reflected others' suggestions and not just her own. However, she was most obviously a shaper and tended to push for decisions, often at a faster rate than team members were ready for.

Julie, while having some shaper characteristics, was most notably an implementer. Not overly creative, she was excellent at translating an

149

initial idea into achievable action. She was a reliable and practical operator although occasionally impatient of low achievers and slackers.

Barbara was one of the quieter members of the group but missed very little and would comment thoughtfully and critically to Penny once meetings were concluded. Her judgement was usually good but she could be obstinate if decisions seemed to be made contrary to deep-felt beliefs. She was a fairly typical monitor-evaluator.

Jenny seemed to be the most passive member of the group. She rarely contributed any ideas but would go along with whatever was suggested. She liked working with figures and would happily produce monthly reports, although without showing any initiative at all. She seemed to demonstrate some characteristics of the team worker and the completer.

Martine was the most difficult team member to categorise. Her job required an organised and careful approach with some leadership skills of a small team of staff. However, she was not markedly competent in this role. Instead, the part of her job that seemed to light her up was the external visits she made and talks she gave. She was possibly a more natural resource-investigator.

One meeting of this group was set aside to address the marketing issue. Penny, realising that her shaper character tended to interfere with a free flow of contributions from the group, purposely kept out of the debate once she had set the broad direction. Martine suddenly started displaying a high level of creativity and had clearly been a 'closet' plant! With some support, Jenny moved closer to a team worker role but attempts to encourage initiative continued to fail. As expected, Julie encouraged application and Barbara facilitated some rethinking. A decision was reached that some expert knowledge on service marketing was needed and Penny agreed to invite somebody she knew who had been involved in marketing in a number of health care venues.

Lessons learned from acknowledging Belbin roles were as follows.

- There is potential conflict between coordinator and shaper roles. It has been suggested that the same person should not take both roles as conflict between social and task leadership is common.
- Other roles apart from leadership ones are important and essential for effective decision making to ensure that initial ideas are operationalised in the most effective way.
- Some staff may be stuck in roles that do not fit well with their natural team roles. Enabling them to widen their repertoire to include preferred roles should lead to better motivated and more effective staff.
- Knowing the limitations of individual team members in roles to which they are ill suited will reduce the risk of failed decision making.
- If essential roles are missing, additional team members may be needed for specific tasks.

Reference

Belbin M 1997 Changing the way we work. Butterworth Heinemann, Oxford.

Section **Three**

USER PARTICIPATION IN DECISION MAKING

OVERVIEW

The complexities of understanding how and even why there should be any social rights and responsibilities for citizens in the UK will be the subject of debate for many years. The academic arguments and theories support individual rights but deny the less political features of collective rights of groups and individuals. The continuous polarising of central and peripheral needs and rights contradicts the individuation required by the current Labour government to underpin their policies.

Some individuals do not exercise their rights, as users or consumers of health care, to singly or collectively make their needs known. The groups who wish to develop communication with the health care services have multiple agendas for changing the health service that as single groups, they have too little strength or power to do. Collectives, support groups, sufferer pressure groups, user support groups, consumers, carers, patients, grassroots organisations with voluntary, charitable and commercial/research backing are all concerned with raising the standards of health care, along with the government. The constraints of funding have become less apparent but the need to produce results for the collective majority is high in the agenda for trusts and ministers in return for the money invested in the NHS. Resources such as skilled staff, technology, buildings and other assets are not considered in this section but they are acknowledged as being a major consideration when making decisions in health care and planning for the future.

These three chapters review where the NHS has developed its identity against the stakeholders participating in using and providing the services in a private and public capacity. The ways in which governments politicise the NHS are accepted, the implementation of policies in accordance with local agendas is equally as interesting, so the debates review how this needs to change in line with any current government policy making. The theory chapters therefore cover the substantial documentation, strategy and implementation of change in involvement of consumers in the NHS. Historical pressure from the World Health Organization and the need to be among the leaders in the field of change in a technologically powerful health care system based on social welfare drive the government agenda. The countervailing pressures are from the professions, who are conservative in their vision of where they would like to see the NHS in its future, and the patients and support groups who need to lead some of the changes but do not want to lose any goodwill from the professionals. The triangle is complete but the answers are not available as to how it will happen, with which organisation making what moves and what losses and gains will be sustained from which side.

The Conservative and Labour governments have published documents, made Acts of Parliament, assured funding and supported a focus for change in the NHS that sustains their wish for further and deeper user and consumer involvement in planning health services. The New NHS Plan supports a focus for the NHS of empowered patients at the heart of the health service and a reconfiguration of provision in accordance with user needs, defined through involvement. Although these documents are set out in this section, it will become clear to interested readers that planning for and accommodation of needs cannot always be the precursor of action. Pressure groups are not normally in the public gaze or renowned for using their power. Consumers as individuals cannot become powerful overnight. Considerable risk is involved for all participants in changing to a democratic organisation from one which had defined but inconsistent and morally unrighteous leaders. Not only the risk but the dangers of wrong decision making should be shared among all participants. This is the challenge from the government, that stakeholders are welcome to make changes happen locally and nationally to the NHS but the consequences must be realised by everyone.

It is with personal and political interest that many people are observing how the National Plan for Health is implemented, gradually and incrementally through the health service in the first decade of the 21st century. Great words do not always make great deeds. However, dreams of real equity and equality of provision are available for anyone to sign up to and participate in working towards. It really is up to individuals as well as groups to see the opportunities, find the impetus to go forward rather than stay with the status quo (which is itself unsustainable) any longer.

User participation in decision making

Chapter **Seven**

Patient empowerment and the power of patients

Mary Cooke

- ● **The future health service based on the concept of participation**
- ● **Professional domination and domain**
- ● **Primary care and community development**
- ● **The future**
- ● **Endnote**

No-one would remember the Good Samaritan if he only had good intentions. He had money as well. (Prime Minister Mrs Margaret Thatcher)

Enemies are so stimulating. (Katharine Hepburn)

O V E R V I E W

This chapter looks at the health services from an alternative perspective, that of the user/patient/consumer/the carers/the public and receivers of health care. It may therefore challenge some of the current views of professionals who work in the NHS and the private and voluntary sectors where health care is provided. This is intentional, because although there will be many more years of health care provided via a system that does not consider the user/patient/consumer/the carers/the public, the chapter is written in the anticipation that health professionals may come to 'see themselves as others see them' in time.

This is the first chapter in the section about involvement in health care services by users or patients and their carers.

Participation by patients in consultations about their health and care interventions is another area of involvement covered elsewhere in this section. Participants have long been ignored as a part of the health care delivery system and as a resource for change in the structure and function of management in a public service. The government has now planned for their inclusion in decision making.

THE FUTURE HEALTH SERVICE BASED ON THE CONCEPT OF PARTICIPATION

This chapter reviews:

- current policy supporting users in groups and as individuals (all other references to patients, public, carers, stakeholders, etc. will call them users) – the Community Health Councils and how these have been superseded by the Patient Advocacy and Liaison Service (PALS)
- recent (past 30 years) history of how policy has influenced strategy in current thinking about the user movement (based on the complaints systems)
- where users will need to become more empowered to ensure their views are heard and acted upon in the clinical relationship

and looks at strategies for the inclusion of patients in planning health by reviewing the following issues:

- public accountability
- the funding of the user support processes
- how complaints feature as a means of user involvement
- public–private funding initiatives and the market pressure for change
- how medical professionals influence involvement
- the rights of users to maintain their cultural values in involvement
- predictors for future policy.

Governments have in recent times used 'think tanks' to draw together visionary people to generate ideas and debates. The 'visions' that abound are often exercises in thinking the 'unthinkable', moving away from the boundaries of consensus and building on the new ideas. Gradually, if discussed effectively in the public domain, the unthinkable becomes acceptable.

User participation in decision making

The lack of shared values in UK health policy results in a worried and disgruntled public, low morale among health care staff and indecision in health service management. The quality of service alters in response. The relationship that users expect to have with their health professional has not altered but the ways in which professionals relate to users have changed at the clinical interface.

PROFESSIONAL DOMINATION AND DOMAIN

Since the 19th century the medical profession has dominated health care, the processes of health delivery and the political stance taken by successive governments. This encourages other health care staff (managers, nurses, other therapists) to act on the opinions of the medical professionals, stating that they do so in the best interests of each patient. This consensual activity has developed into a wide and widening variation of practice standards in each area or specialism, promoting excellence in some acute specialties but with appalling standards of care in other less popular areas, such as mental health. Further effects are major differences in measurable outcomes of interventions between geographical parts of the country.

Variations in health outcomes, decrease in standards of care and slackness in providing equity of care (despite funding input and opportunity for improvements in community health and social services) to all patients across the country gave politicians the impetus to move into the arena of health services. Ratification has occurred through policies in support of funding 'disease-related' goals. National Service Frameworks for older people, mental health and cancer monitor and evaluate change through funding priorities. The goal was to raise standards across all specialisms but to provide funding in specialist areas that had received less money in the past, so that patients would get equality of care and equity of provision and therefore commonality of cost and effectiveness would arise. The government would be seen as supporting users in forcing the professionals to rethink their stance on service provision. Eventually, as budgets finally began to move into primary and community care-focused service provision, the new primary care organisations (PCGs and PCTs) benefited.

Most contacts between health services and users take place at the primary care level through a consultation. The quality and characteristics of the relationship are fundamental to users' experience of health care and dictate the extent to which it can be under-

Patient empowerment and the power of patients

157

stood as a partnership (Florin & Coulter 2001). In the 'patient participation' theories, a biomedical model approach puts the biomedical knowledge at the centre of the consultation. It is traditional and recognisable as focused on knowledge controlled by the paternalistic doctor and received by the passive patient. Several 'patient-centred' models of practice recognise to varying degrees the importance of patients' own views and often result in varying levels of compliance with treatment and the outcomes of future consultations. Interestingly, when the discussion papers around this subject are written by doctors, users are invariably referred to as patients.

One of the interesting features of all these models is that there is no universal agreement of the aim of consultation in primary care (Streeton & Cooke 2001). As Toon (1994) has noted, part of the difficulty in measuring quality in general practice stems from a lack of consensus (from the medical perspective) as to what general practice is for! (Toon 1994). Where users have been able to voice an opinion, they are clear about what issues are important, what care they expect and how they want the surgeries to be organised (Cooke 2001). Perhaps the real questions to answer are associated with patient-centred medicine.

1. Is patient enablement an aim in its own right or are other outcomes such as compliance, knowledge gain or sharing of experience important?
2. For whom is the consultation of most benefit – the GP, in keeping control over costs, or the user, in maintaining a positive contact with their access point to health care?

The effect of past policy

In the 1980s managers took over the leadership of the health service, acting in 'the best interests' of the customer or consumer (as opposed to the medical professionals). This led to the health service becoming a market-driven organisation with patients acting more directly as consumers making choices to help bring about change. The thinking behind the reconstruction of the service was to contain costs. The strategy failed. It increased 'postcode-biased' inequalities and alienated the public who preferred to understand the NHS as a service rather than a business.

More recently, a strategy to invoke primary care-led service was complemented by the White Paper *The New NHS: Modern, Dependable* (DoH 1999) which provides a written commitment to involving users. After this, *The NHS Plan* was published in 2000, focusing directly on the user as the centre of the service (DoH 2000, p. 17). In strengthening the power of the consumer, a further recent change in law that may affect the rights of individuals and therefore patients in the UK is the European Rights Act 1998, brought into force in the UK in October 2000. The alterations to people's lives that are reinforced by this Act are subtle in concept but could have a significant impact on how health services are managed and delivered in the future. Successful implementation of the Act will depend upon how health service users perceive themselves and their rights and how defensive of their rights they are in the current culture of the health service as an organisation. However, in their 2001 election manifesto, the Labour party decided to remove the patient support system of Community Health Councils (CHCs) and replace them with a trust-based Patient Advocacy and Liaison Service (PALS).

Public accountability and service users: user accountability by participation

The NHS is run by people who have been selected, not elected. Selection relies on patronage and inevitably favours people who are established and who are deemed to be 'experts'. This encourages sycophancy, personal philanthropy to support exclusive interests and a legitimised method of creating separately identified groups, arising from professional interests and (in patient terms) by disease or diagnosis.

This exclusivity has grown in a political and economic climate that requires inclusivity of treatment interventions by type and technology for equity, effectiveness and efficiency. Problems arise where users who are diagnosed with multiple pathologies (illnesses) cross diagnostic and professional boundaries that defy easy management and 'inclusivity' of interventions, unless users take more control of their plans for care. The medical profession justifies its status and power to control the separateness of the system in this way very well. However, where recent public and political criticisms have found the British Medical Association less than helpful in raising standards but supportive of professional chauvinism, the organisation has responded poorly in understanding where improvements to doctors' clinical skills, for example, can be made.

Users of health systems have had only two direct methods by which their opinions can be heard and, to a variable extent, acted upon: the CHCs and the complaints system (see below). The CHCs were started in the 1970s and will be disbanded by 2004. Their role has been superseded by PALS. Recent media discussion in the UK

159

and Europe has involved the concept of citizenship as a role for users. Health policies require direct involvement by citizens on committees to regulate professionals to define local need and commission health care (PGCs and PCTs).

In 1948 when the NHS started, the community health services were the poor relation of the acute and secondary services in hospitals. No lines of accountability were identified at that time for family practitioners, the GPs. Family Practitioner Committees replaced 'executive committees' in 1974 and were charged with responsibility for managing services.

By the 1960s some of the problems caused by the lack of lay involvement and accountability in the NHS were recognised. Women's groups and self-help groups had shown how little notice health services took of their users' needs and questioned the way health services were provided. Scandals in long-stay mental handicap and mental health hospitals had shown what could happen when there was little public scrutiny and how public trust in professionals could be undermined. As a consequence, both Labour and Conservative governments were involved in the introduction of the CHCs in 1974 as 'local watchdogs'. They were formed as a committee of lay people to safeguard patients and to sustain more public involvement and scrutiny. Half the membership came from local authorities, a third were elected by voluntary organisations and the remainder appointed by regional health authorities (these became regional offices of the NHS Executive in 1996).

This history of spasmodic involvement by the public and users shows no direct involvement in deciding health policy until 1997 when 'focus groups' were used to elicit citizens' ideas about their health system, in preparation for the Labour manifesto.

The CHCs developed as small offices in the High Street or in the local health authority or trust property. Members had statutory rights to visit hospitals, access to patient information, to attend HA meetings and to be consulted by NHS managers about changes in services. There was little guidance for HAs or managers about the function of CHCs and this resulted in disputes over interpretation of members' rights of investigation. These rights were unenforceable except by law; in some cases local authorities took action against health authorities on behalf of CHCs.

The White Paper *The New NHS: Modern, Dependable* (DoH 1999) put emphasis on accountability to local authorities. Health authorities gained stronger powers to improve the health of their residents through the development of health improvement plans, while PCGs and PCTs took over the existing commissioning and fundholding arrangements. These primary care organisations evolved into confederations of provider management and training. They are required to have clear arrangements for public involvement and are accountable through clinical governance-style agreements. Clinical governance offers NHS trusts responsibility for quality standards, management, user involvement and risk management in the same way as they have for finance.

The role of the CHC evolved. Advocacy schemes, self-help group support, community networks, surveys of users' views, research on the unmet needs of disadvantaged groups, development of patients' charters and provision of information and advice became the norm for their work as a result (Hogg 1999, p. 90). Many CHC chairs were visiting members of NHS trust boards in their locality and worked within trusts to develop service provision with users in mind. However, this has never forced any change in status or circumstance for user influence in service planning.

A community-based user body of representative people such as the CHCs or PALS must be independent and cannot be concerned with the agendas of the NHS or local authorities, so that their credibility with the public remains intact. Training and development of members need to be done under the auspices of the NHS but not by it, so the larger confederations of health management, PCGs and PCTs, have taken on this role.

Accountability was recognised as important. CHC members were accountable to no-one and became typical of most people to whom committee work is important: mainly white, middle class and middle aged or retired. Generating interest from a wider variety of people is difficult and a background attitude of 'managing' input from users leads to loss of sustainability of groups as cynical users begin to question the value and quality of initiatives they participate in.

Any community-based user group needs to have a remit that reflects the concerns that people have around health, health care and social care rather than historical organisational divisions.

The PALS initiative

This method of representation of patients began around July 2000. *The NHS Plan* (DoH 2000) announced major structural changes for the consumer movement, abolishing CHCs from April 2001 and replacing them with a tripartite structure of a PALS, patients' forums and citizens' forums. The final remit of the organisation will be devised after long and heavy debate in Parliament and the House of Lords. The government saw the role of the PALS as one of coordination of patient representation. However, at the time of going to print, it is not known whether the result will be a further reliance by the users on Citizens' Advice Bureaux – a (free to users) voluntary service provided by ex-public and private service professionals to give advice to members of the public.

Criticisms of user involvement

Allegations of counterproductivity to good user–professional relationships have been made, as follows.

- User involvement will raise expectations of the service and create an increase in demand.
- Participation and involvement will result in a reduction in user satisfaction as users become more critical.
- Users will make decisions about their own care that will prevent developments in medical treatment and are not sufficiently radical to change the system in line with government policy that drives management changes for target evaluations of the system.
- Trusts make arrangements to exclude users and others from their management decision-making processes.
- Private and voluntary health care has no system of accountability to its users.

Raising demand for health care has promoted a government-led policy of private–public partnership that links efficiency and effectiveness across the system. Research examples show that satisfaction is reduced with knowledge and professionals are not fully criticised for their part in any evaluation of care (Bernstein et al 1998) and that educational material tested on patients did not reduce their breadth of decision-making power to result in more conservative treatment options (O'Connor et al 1999).

In complying with user involvement arrangements, NHS trusts must hold at least one public meeting a year. An agenda, papers, the accounts and the annual report must be publicly available. Provision must be made for questions and comments to be put by the public. Public meetings must be held in readily accessible venues and at times when the public are able to attend but the public meeting is seen as a 'rubber stamping exercise' for agreed change that is planned in trust offices.

There is formal requirement for health authorities and acute and community NHS trusts to make publicly available a wide range of information about their activities and services. General medical practitioners are also required to give essential information for patients in the form of practice leaflets about individual

User participation in decision making

doctors' services. The patients' forum and citizens' forum need to be well organised to oversee all these activities as monitors of the system and advisors for change. They need training and education as well as knowledge and understanding of the health service system: this is not always funded by the trusts.

Private–public–voluntary commissioning arrangements for provision of services should drive the involvement of users through the purchasing systems. This will stabilise monitoring of health care in these sectors equally.

PRIMARY CARE AND COMMUNITY DEVELOPMENT

Community development offers primary care the benefits of individuals and community groups actively participating in their health care. The reasons for this are that:

- resources are used more effectively since it helps release and enlarge the community resources
- health goals are identified and health programmes become more relevant to local needs
- health care need is identified at individual level and simultaneously, ways of making care accessible are developed
- people's desire to take more responsibility for their own wellbeing is supported (WHO 1991, p. 5).

In 1997, the King's Fund developed guidelines for community-oriented primary care (COPC). This was defined as 'a continuous process by which primary health care is provided to a defined community on the basis of its assessed health needs by the planned integration of public health with PC practice' (Freeman et al 1997, p. 3). Since when, the government has raised funding and the profile of public health departments in health authorities to support the principle of local health planning being created by local demands (Cunningham 2000). Overall, government financial support for health care has arrived with the provisos and caveats of user involvement to support change. The result is that all stakeholders have had to adapt, redefine and renegotiate their roles and expectations.

Complaints as part of user involvement

The government made changes to the NHS complaints procedures during 1994 (DoH 1994). Since then there has been a sharp

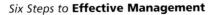

rise in the number and severity of complaints about a range of issues and practice in the services. The Labour government favours annual publication of lists of 'good' and 'bad' health authorities and trusts, resulting from the overall measurement of complaints in each trust and area of clinical practice. This punitive use of audit has fuelled obfuscation by trusts so that they gain higher places on the lists of results. The challenge to the trusts is that criteria for making judgements will alter annually to drive NHS change by the indirect effects of these paradoxical incentives.

Audit of outcomes of care is a feature of the recent developments in evaluation processes and openness in providing information about public services. Voluntary and private health services do not have a similar process of review.

The complaints procedure is intended to be a method of involving staff as well as users to effect a change to systems. Complaints are intended to be part of a learning cycle for this change. All the participants should be involved in making decisions about how to avoid the 'mistake' or 'problem' in the future. This ideal may not always be possible. Many professionals see the system as punitive and restrictive and defer an opinion about clinical experiences within an organisation to promote a local need. This method is intended to be empowering for both the users and the professionals involved but in practice remains outside the control of the user or their support group.

Little research has been accomplished to review the actual investment by managers or users in the complaints procedure. However, a visionary management will look on the procedure as an opportunity to implement change as a result of planned review and audit of the system.

The complaints system was altered in response to poor care by providers of health services. The previous system had altered in response to government reviews of health service complaints by the Health Ombudsman at Westminster, in particular and the Health Select Committee in general. Comments about the speed of conclusive outcomes to complaints were the concern of the Ombudsman specifically and annual reports consistently raised issues about lack of change in the system as a response to complaints. The aim of trusts continues to be one of dissipation of the direction of complaints and short-term avoidance of litigation. A minority of complaints result in legal activity and compensation payments to users can be an incentive to take the complaint to higher authority, but the trust, the PCG/T and ultimately users pay for this in the long term.

The power of the individual user and the influence of costs

At the most personal level, individuals who contact and interact with health professionals do so at their own risk. Professionals do not always recognise this fact. Since 1968, Torrance has written about a range of risk assessment decisions that users and professionals have to make concerning care. These decisions may affect their visit to the GP or the dentist, for example, and be made by the users and the professionals in partnership. They were then developed into the measures known as QALYs (Torrance 1986). For example, the individual consciously takes account of the cost of the visit to the GP or the hospital, travelling to the health service access point or the telephone conversation if telephoning NHS Direct. Further considerations include outcomes of the interaction with the professional, whether they will have a prescription and whether they can afford to pay to exchange the prescription for the medication. Other unconscious decisions are associated with anxiety over a possible diagnosis and the social costs of this to their family or work (Cooke 2001, Streeton & Cooke 2001).

The impact of the information age has influenced the way primary and community health services have changed recently and how users have learned to develop their potential for power. The most challenging change to current practice for the professionals is to understand the impact that 'being a patient' has on users of the service, whether they are involved in planning care or not.

Users' power in funding health services

Demand has grown for health care but the service is unable to cope with expectations. There is a continuing divide in health status between poor people and the rich, who have better access to health care, resulting in health gains. Waiting lists appear to have grown in proportion to the loss of hospital beds and provision of acute services nationally. The government uses these pressures to make the public aware that their health care is rationed. Options of user power can be most dramatic in the arena of private purchasing of health care by the rich, which has now been utilised by the government to alleviate waiting lists and use available services efficiently. This concept can be seen in diagrammatic form below.

Patient empowerment and the power of patients

Can't pay for private health care	**Can** pay for private health care
Will pay for private health care	**Won't** pay for private health care

Government translation of this concept is to involve the private sector in providing health care to everyone, paid for through the NHS funds in the community (PCGs and PCTs). An immediate source of health care is becoming available to the government, at cost price. This is one of the more subtle measures of power that users have over the NHS.

Funding of user involvement

Patients' forums are used as ways of involving users of services. They are associated with trusts in acute and community settings and funded by them. They are seen as a dissipating style of support rather than a 'one-stop shop' for users to promote their views of care, the way that professionals provide care and how the health service should alter to focus on their needs. Patients' forums are established in each trust and are composed of representatives from local patients' groups and voluntary organisations and other local representatives. Within their remit is the right to visit and inspect at any time any aspect of the trust's work and services to patients.

The PALS are also based within the NHS hospital and PCTs as services employed by the trust. Funding for the service comes from the trusts. This places the trusts in the strong position of controlling the activity of the PALS, the patients' forum and ways in which users' needs are met. This arrangement is criticised because it does not allow open scrutiny of the organisations by the general public.

Clinical governance and the medical professionals as intermediary for involvement by users

Within individual general practices and primary care teams, all staff will have a role in obtaining and using information for clinical governance – whether for maintaining chronic disease registers, promoting evidence based practice, improving the organisation of services, or reporting on the outcomes of care. In primary care groups and trusts, there is greater emphasis on improving the health of the population. This requires the collection and aggregation of information across practices to assess health needs, reduce inequalities, and monitor the quality of care in comparison to [sic] agreed standards. . . . In this paper we discuss the additional knowledge that will be needed by all staff working in primary care and the challenges faced by leaders of primary care groups and trusts. (McColl & Roland 2000)

There are many dimensions of clinical governance outlined by Rosen (2000) that highlight the wide range of information which primary care staff do need to use.

Effective clinical practice requires access to and use of evidence based guidance on cost effective care. To implement national service frameworks and local health improvement priorities, staff will need to understand what these priorities are and monitor progress towards agreed standards. (Rosen 2000, p. 872)

The culture that underpins the basis of the extracts is one of paternalistic and controlling rationalism. Doctors still see themselves as having the right of access to all information about their patients and their patients' bodies. It may be that patients may also have access to some of their recorded information but even if the facts about patients may be incorrect or incomplete, they are normally unquestioned by medical professionals. Patient organisations have had little impact in changing these arrangements.

Professional and patient relationships

Interpersonal relationships between users and health care workers have changed in their focus and outcome. This has occurred most remarkably over the past 10 years and can be said to be a result of political strategies associated with funding, personal and professional responsibilities and personal rights. The Nursing and Midwifery Council (NMC) (until 2001 the UKCC) is the official body acting to control aspects of nursing and midwifery practice. The rise in poor working relationships in the NHS and the reactions of nurses to both patient and management abuse have encouraged an awareness of personal rights in the workplace and rights to services by the users and patients.

Registered nurses, midwives and health visitors are responsible for ensuring that they safeguard the interests of their clients at all times. . . . The misuse of professional power within the practitioner–client relationship affects clients of all ages and in all settings. (UKCC 1999, p. 3)

Patient empowerment and the power of patients

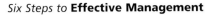

Six Steps to **Effective Management**

> ... the professional must treat the client and the client's decisions about their own care with respect. This involves identifying the client's preferences regarding ... care and respecting these within the limits of current standards of practice, existing legislation and the goals of the therapeutic relationship. (UKCC 1999, p. 4)

Although the code of professional conduct for nurses and midwives makes several statements about accountability and decision making and respect for the autonomy of the user as a patient and a person, the practice of nursing does not always empower the user or person receiving care indirectly as a carer. Decisions have frequently been made on behalf of the patient as a user of the health system, often without discussion or negotiation, and with only the needs of the professionals or the institution or the system providing and supporting the rationale.

Government policy identifies carers as supporters and partners in providing care. It is estimated that the ratio of carer to patient in a practice population is 120:1000 and it is likely that 40% of these will be men. The personal and emotional care that unpaid carers provide, including treatment and 24-hour supervision, is valued at around £34 billion per year (Nuttall 1994) and cannot be replaced by public services (Banks 2001). Nurses should be aware of this knowledgeable group as a source of understanding how carers receive information from them as professionals, use it in the home situation and empower themselves.

Users in minority ethnic community groups

Immigrants to the UK from countries where other health care beliefs and practices form the health system often have problems adapting to the culture of health care in the UK. Frequently, they cannot communicate well because of the language barrier, may not be aware of rights as well as responsibilities and may not be able to afford the costs of travel or prescription charges (Bowie et al 1995, NCC 1995, Popay & Williams 1994). The NHS has often been inflexible in its attitude towards this user population. Primary care professionals do not always make patients aware of the advice that is available to them from Citizens' Advice Bureaux or other advocacy services, with the result that some patients from minority ethnic communities miss out on potential health benefits and a rise in health status (Paris & Player 1993).

This group often resort to non-Western medicine. Muslims who use private health care in the UK expect and get separate accom-

User participation in decision making

168

modation for male and female visitors, carers and family, as they have in their homes. 'Complementary therapies' (complementary to the 'traditional' Western medical model of health care delivery), as used by many immigrants from Africa and Asia, have helped to reshape the ways in which medications are administered. For example, oil massaged into the body is an accepted method of administration for some herbal remedies. Homoeopathy is now becoming an acceptable method of treatment. Acupuncture forms a major part of Chinese therapy for 'loss of energy' in the body. This concept is alien to current medical beliefs in the UK but many practitioners are training in the skills and will therefore offer different treatments to satisfy user demand in recognition of the power of the balanced health care relationship.

Public participation and health promotion

User groups are now more politically organised than previously. Each group has had to recognise how they will work to support their membership of patients and carers. Many do not take up the support offered by groups and some people need to tackle their illness as individuals. For example, some 110 000 people have Parkinson's disease in the UK (about 10 000 new diagnoses annually) but only about 20 000 people belong to or are associated locally with the Parkinson's Disease Society. Larger and professionally managed organisations have public accountability and charitable status, have developed local and national links and lobby politically on behalf of members and non-members who are carers and sufferers of the diagnosis. The weakness of these groups is that they are defined by diagnosis and not by specified need. The medical power remains with the organisation of support.

THE FUTURE

Policy planners and researchers have begun to look into future strategies (Dargie 1999). Clear pathways for the future can never be accurately predicted, but many new initiatives can be expected. Methods of reviewing publications and evaluating activities in health authorities can support inclusion of users in planning services (McIver 1998). Often evidence for policies is not available and plans for new services are made on the basis of 'do it and see'. Now, as more evidence is required, it is supported by research and funded by special research funds. Research into this area of health care

Patient empowerment and the power of patients

is now mapping the process more effectively. It is a multi-personnel activity; all who are interested can join in.

ENDNOTE

> The reasonable man adapts himself to the world; the unreasonable man persists in trying to adapt the world to himself. Therefore all progress depends on the unreasonable man. (Shaw, *Man and Superman*, 1903)

Effective user participation centres on the user perspective. As a result control over decision making shifts towards the user. It is the failure to achieve this alteration of the balance of power that provides the main reason why many initiatives that attempt to build up user involvement falter. This is often because they incorporate user knowledge to support or develop organisational and professional priorities rather than addressing the core, direct concerns of users.

> Service agency discourse, not surprisingly, is primarily concerned with policy and services; with service organisation, management, efficiency, effectiveness and economy . . . service users' discourse is concerned much more explicitly and specifically with people's lives. (Beresford et al 2000, p. 192–193)

The power to make decisions and the control of accountability do not usually rest with users as a group.

> Consultation and participation are the usual ways that power centres think of involving other people – but these are usually attempts to enrol others in support of the priorities and agendas of the power centres themselves, in support of their own initiatives. (Wright 1999)

This is the fundamental weakness of *The NHS Plan* at present. Users could strengthen the outcomes of health care interventions and professionals need users to share their knowledge. Equity of value and appreciation of participants as stakeholders mean successful strategies. The stakeholders need to learn to work together for any success to be claimed by the new 'health teams'.

References

Banks P 2001 Carer's contribution in primary care. In: Gillam S, Brooks F (eds) New beginnings: towards patient and public involvement in primary health care. King's Fund, London

User participation in decision making

Beresford P, Croft S, Evans C, Harding T 2000 Quality in personal and social services: the developing role of user involvement in the UK. In: Davies C, Finlay L, Bullman A (eds) Changing practice in health and social care. Sage, London

Bernstein S, Skarupski K, Grayson C, Starling M, Bates E, Eagle K 1998 A randomised controlled trial of information-giving to patients referred for coronary angiography: effects on outcomes of care. Health Expectations 1: 50–61

Bowie C, Richardson A, Sykes W 1995 Consulting the public about health service priorities. British Medical Journal 311: 1155–1158

Cooke M 2001 Consensus of expectations through focus group – users' views of their General Practices in Corby PCG. Northamptonshire Health Authority, Northampton

Cunningham D 2000 Public health challenges for the new millennium. In: Hill A (ed) What's gone wrong with health care? King's Fund, London

Dargie C 1999 Policy futures for health: pathfinder. University of Cambridge in association with The Nuffield Trust, Cambridge

Department of Health 1994 Being heard: Review Committee on NHS complaints procedure. Stationery Office, London

Department of Health 1999 The new NHS: modern, dependable. Stationery Office, London

Department of Health 2000 The NHS plan – a plan for investment, a plan for reform. Stationery Office, London

Florin D, Coulter A 2001 Partnership in the primary care consultation. In: Gillam S, Brookes F (eds) New beginnings: towards patient and public involvement in primary care. King's Fund, London

Freeman R, Gillam S, Shearin C, Pratt J 1997 Community development and involvement in primary care. King's Fund, London

Hogg C 1999 Patients, power and politics: from patients to citizens. Sage, London

McColl A, Roland M 2000 Knowledge and information for clinical governance. British Medical Journal 321(7265): 871

McIver S 1998 Healthy debate? An independent evaluation of citizen's juries in health settings. King's Fund, London

National Consumer Council 1995 In partnership with patients. National Consumer Council, London

Nuttall SR 1994 Financing long term care in Great Britain. Journal of the Institute of Actuaries 121(1): 1–68

O'Connor A, Rostom A, Fiset V et al 1999 Decision aids for patients facing health treatment or screening decisions: systematic review. British Medical Journal 319: 731–734

Paris JAG, Player D 1993 Citizen's advice in general practice. British Medical Journal 306: 1518–1520

Popay J, Williams G (eds) 1994 Researching the people's health. Routledge, London

Rosen R 2000 Improving quality in the changing world of primary care. British Medical Journal 321: 551–554

Patient empowerment and the power of patients

Streeton R, Cooke M 2001 The patient's journey through primary care. British Journal of Community Nursing (in press)

Toon PD 1994 What is good general practice? A philosophical study of the concept of high quality medical care. RCGP Occasional Paper 65. Royal College of General Practitioners, London

Torrance GW 1986 Measurement of health state utilities for economic appraisal. Journal of Health Economics 12: 39–53

UKCC 1999 Practitioner–client relationships and the prevention of abuse. UKCC, London

World Health Organization 1991 Community involvement in health development: challenging health services. WHO, Geneva

Wright A 1999 Exploring the development of user forums in an NHS trust. In: Barnes M, Warren (eds) Paths to empowerment. Policy Press, Bristol

User participation in decision making

Application **7:1**

Mary Cooke

Empowerment of patients

Service users can be seen as passive recipients of care in the place chosen by the professionals and 'given' in the manner planned. This has been the norm over centuries, but:

> In a world in which cable television systems have fifty channels, banks let their customers do business by phone, and even department stores have begun to customise their services for the individual, bureaucratic, unresponsive, one-size-fits-all government cannot last. (Osborne & Gaebler 1992)

We can apply the same principles to the NHS, where the managed market type of non-profit-making organisation needs to adjust to changes happening in the external world. Illness controls a person by the manner in which it occurs, the symptoms and the prognosis take over the person's expectations of themselves and make demands on their family and close friends. In addition to this, loss of body image, especially when the illness is terminal, adds further tensions to those pressures applied by the health professionals who need to get their job done to targets and within margins.

Not all patients, users and carers have sufficient social or interpersonal skills to compensate for those missing in the repertoire of the health professionals. These extracts from a newsletter written by the Cambridge Cancer Help Centre offer an alternative view of coping together and a sharing of an illness process that support and self-help groups give to patients, users and carers to carry them through the illness experience. This insight into how groups work and how members support each other is unique to the Cancer Help Centre.

NOTES FROM A NEW GIRL TO THE GROUP

When I arrived in Stockwell Street, I was asking myself what I was doing there. Wasn't enough of my time already taken up with illness? I wouldn't know anybody and the only common factor would be illness. Depressing. And where exactly was the centre? Told at the

173

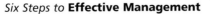

corner video shop that, no, they didn't know where 1A was, I was all for giving up. No, I would just stroll up the road and see what that notice was on the church door on the other side of the road and that's how I found the centre.

I rang the quaint bell pull and stood outside the cherry red door and waited. Margot opened the door almost immediately. I was welcomed as though I had been expected. The outside of the building had given me no hint of the tasteful, spacious room I was to find inside. It was lovely – comfortable and homely, a room I could enjoy. Here was the feeling of freedom. I could stay for a whole morning 'or drop in for a while', 'come alone or with a friend' and whatever my mood. I found the atmosphere supportive, so I could simply chill out or chat or leaf through a helpful book I found on the shelves. There would be opportunities to benefit from healing or I could join in the guided meditation planned for that day, put the forthcoming social events in my diary, listen to Pachelbel or . . . buy half a dozen free range eggs and have a slice of home-made apricot tart and a cup of tea. Relaxing! No pressure or demands. An empathy, acceptance and understanding. People there with time. Strong, courageous, positive people. There was a shoulder to cry on, a sympathetic ear, a helpful hand and the space to be – characteristics of the rapport that exists in happy families.

A group visit – the garden centre and restaurant

Sixteen of us met there, for lunch, chat and plant buying. Beautiful sunny day, but Ingrid argued with the garden hose and hit her head, cut her hand, twisted her ankle and smashed her watch and said she felt silly. Fran and the garden centre first-aider first-aided and Ingrid looked very fetching with a bag of frozen McCain chips on her head and frozen carrots on her ankle. So we stuck her in a wheel chair and gave her a cup of coffee – right as rain now, she says.

'So what if we didn't have a centre?' we asked ourselves after going through a particularly sad patch. Here are some of the replies.

- If this place wasn't here, I'd have nowhere to go.
- Where would we get a nicer group to go to the café with?
- We can be ourselves.
- We drop our defences and lose our pretensions of the illness.
- We wouldn't have a place where we not only receive support, but can offer help to each other. It's through giving that we receive and through helping others that we heal ourselves.
- A place where we know we are not alone.
- A place where we find that cancer may not be the big scary monster we thought it was.

SUPPORT GROUP ORGANISATION

Other support groups are organised differently. Some are associated at a local level with national organisations such as MIND, a mental health charity working for everyone with experience of mental distress to counter discrimination. This group started in 1946, campaigning for the opportunity to work and play a full part in the community. Since 1991, MIND has had a policy on user involvement which has been updated regularly. Volunteers who want to play a full part in the organisation meet regularly to talk about local issues. There are special programmes formed as a part of MIND such as Diverse Minds, set up with support from the Department of Health to make mental health services more responsive to the needs of people from black and minority ethnic communities. This was a result of a policy statement from MIND in 1993, highlighting concerns in relation to current services that included:

- the impact of racism on people's lives, on their mental health and on the services they receive
- the inadequate response to the varying needs of people from different cultural, religious and ethnic communities
- the high numbers of black people picked up by the police under section 136 of the Mental Health Act, compulsorily detained in hospital, diagnosed with schizophrenia and given high doses of medication; the underuse of primary and community care services by this group of people
- the differential experiences in relation to ethnicity, gender and social class
- high depression and suicide rates among Asian women
- the failure of services to meet needs, e.g. mixed sex psychiatric wards are often contrary to religious or cultural beliefs
- poor access to services for people whose first language is not English.

Professionals and managers have been helped to involve users in a meaningful way through video, leaflets and training resources produced by user-trainers. The first user-run sanctuary has opened in Lambeth. The three national user organisations – MINDLINK, the UK Advocacy Network and Survivors Speak Out – are regularly consulted by government and other decision makers.

Many other groups need members of these organisations to visit, to pass on their knowledge and expertise in representation. They could have an involvement in the local nursing training school and teach the students by sharing experiences with them from an original perspective. Local authorities invite users to planning committees and trust board meetings now. Each primary care organisation is required to have lay or user members to represent the non-professional perspectives on purchasing health, education of professionals and

Empowerment of patients

the delivery of services. The local and National Commissions for Health Improvement cannot work under the government guidelines unless they have users involved.

The Sainsbury Centre for Mental Health is another national organisation that involves local people who belong to or meet at centres. Recently, the Sainsbury Centre organised an exercise that trained users to interview participants for a national research project that evaluated mental health services over the country to demonstrate any differences in service delivery, outcomes of care and the user experience as expressed by patients and survivors. This involvement of users and carers seemed to be a resource that had not been appreciated previously.

The empowerment of users in this application has centred on mental health and the users and carers who have developed support groups in a particular way. This specialism has used its support well and has much positive experience in moving engagement and participation forward for involved planning and research of services in mental health.

References

Osborne P, Gaebler R 1992 Reinventing government. Addison Wesley, Reading, Massachusetts, p. 194

Application 7:2

Mary Cooke

Empowerment of users

This second application to Chapter Seven explores a slightly different perspective by looking at empowerment in the mental health arena and the potential for difficulties between users and carers.

Care managers are responsible for putting together the 'packages of care' for those receiving care in the community. It is therefore district health authorities and primary care organisations who exercise choice within the NHS internal managed market.

> In community care, there is a potential conflict between the customer, asserting her entitlement, by right as a citizen, to a particular service, and the care manager acting as a custodian of scarce public resources . . . Care managers, on the other hand, emphasise needs rather than rights, and have a wider responsibility to stay within a budget while ensuring the efficient delivery of services. Such an approach may prove particularly insensitive to the demands of disabled people and minority ethnic groups. Despite the 'user-led' language which has accompanied the introduction of community care, the pre-eminent tests of managerial efficiency are likely to remain resource centred and there is a clear danger that user pressure towards diversity of needs will not fit easily with cost effective managerial concerns. (Langan & Clarke 1994)

Politics of need as prescribed by the 'expert' professional are transformed through the process of diagnosis/assessment and delivery, even if users are encouraged to articulate their wishes. Users are drawn into the process of decision making through user panels and partnerships between users and assessors.

Some users play the 'game' of patient, lying or sitting still when being examined, keeping quiet when asked if they have any questions, answering the doctor with the responses needed to make a rapid and focused diagnosis. There is a positive outcome on both sides for this behaviour; the user is asked to return, their care is unquestioned, they participate by complying with all the needs of the health professionals, even joining the research trial for new drugs so that their care is of a better quality and more frequently assessed.

Other pictures of patient behaviour are of confusion in the system, not turning up for appointments, non-compliance with the medication (possibly because of uncomfortable side effects), asking awkward questions that require depth of knowledge by the doctor or nurse and even arriving at the consultation with up-to-the-minute information that the doctor does not know.

In all these cases, the patient's behaviour could be interpreted as being empowered. The reality is that the empowerment process occurs when all participants in the interaction or intervention are perceived by each other as having an equal part to play. The doctor respects the knowledge of the patient in the second case and also the patient's choice to keep quiet in the first case.

Where some difficulties occur is when the users get to control the setting and the circumstances in which all parties are working. One example of this is a user group of people who have mental health problems. The new government directives require that users, professionals and agencies are to work together to plan services for the future. Their schedule has them meeting for two hours every month for a 6-month project, funded by the mental health users forum budget. Doctors turn up because they are given bonuses to do so. Users turn up mostly because they want to make a difference, but also because their time is funded by the same budget. The first meeting starts quietly, then the doctors take over the conversation and talk using professional jargon not understood by the users.

The feedback from this meeting is poor, by letter and telephone, and the chair decides that there should be an opportunity for all the members to air their points of view in the next meeting. Each in turn, starting bravely with the users, tells of their embarrassment and anger at not having a chance to say anything in the previous meeting, that they felt used by the doctors and managers and that there was no point in continuing the process if this was the manner in which it would proceed. This is a positive move on their part, supported by the chair of the committee. It takes courage to come forward and tell your consultant how an experience is for you, especially as there has never been an opportunity to do so previously.

At the next meeting, a user puts forward a request: at a conference they had been to recently, there was an 'ice-breaker' exercise. She wants to use this now. Everyone had to give an example of one good event that had happened to them that day and one negative event. As she said afterwards, it was interesting to see some of the consultants squirm with embarrassment or to hear how their car did not have sufficient petrol to get to the station or that they had missed the train. This can be a futile exercise of interaction or there can be something positive arising from a small idea. It depends on how you view things: whether a cup is half full or half empty!

In taking opportunities to look at events objectively, members of a focus group of mental health users were discussing the way in which they were being overused to push through the government strategy of the new mental health framework for care. Their personal time had become taken up with some stressful events, there were few members to take on the voluntary work and even though they were given expenses, it was a burden they did not need. Then one suggested that, on reflection, there could be many reasons for this sudden involvement.

First, they were acting as unpaid social workers to push through government policy. Although each trust board chief executive was charged to ensure user involvement in planning health services, there did not appear to be any incentive for the users to do so. There were no expressed aims or objectives of the exercise.

Second, they were involved with many events but few of these would see the light of day once completed or they were becoming bogged down in interagency bureaucracy. It suddenly occurred to the group that they were being 'occupied' to achieve the targets gained by others and to prevent them spending time complaining. In this way the numbers of complaints would fall. The agenda of their next forum was used to discuss the implications of involvement for the users. Watch this space . . .!

Reference

Langan P, Clarke A 1994 Managing in the mixed economy of care. In: Clarke J, Cochrane A, McLaughlan E (eds) Managing social policy. Sage, London, p. 86

Discussion questions

- Does your organisation set aside time to meet any representatives of user groups and carer organisations in a formal way *to share their experiences of using your services?*
- If this happens, how are the users *invited or selected*?
- If it does not happen, *why do you think this is*?
- What are your feelings about your 'customers' discussing you and your manner of nursing/managerial behaviour *either with you or at a meeting where you are not invited*?
- If decisions were taken about how you would be employed from now on, at the meeting you attended or the one you did not, *how committed would you be to those decisions*?
- What could be the *incentives for users* to be involved in planning health services for themselves and *your incentives* to be involved as an employee of the provider?
- What *expertise* would you expect the users to have to be members of this planning committee?
- *Do you trust your patients? If not, why not? Why should they trust you*?

Empowerment of users

Application 7:3

Mary Cooke

Complaints and complainants

Mrs A was a woman in her late 80s, who lived alone at home until she had a fall which broke her left femur. The decision to operate and replace her hip joint was taken. She recovered from the operation but became less communicative, poorly motivated to mobilise and more chair-bound. Now unable to care for herself at home on her own, Mrs A was transferred to a unit dedicated to the elderly and infirm and for those patients in a longer programme of postoperative rehabilitation.

Mrs A had two sons. One, the younger, visited frequently; the other son was never seen until several months after Mrs A had begun living in the unit. He visited once and sent a letter to the manager of the unit that arrived 2 days afterwards complaining that his mother had not been looked after well, she could no longer walk and was not being moved around the ward. He also said that his mother had told him that she had fallen and hurt her other hip and it was painful.

Within 5 days, the manager was able to ascertain some facts.

1. Mrs A was taking medication for mild depression after her original fall and slow recovery.
2. The second fall was reported as an incident. X-rays had been taken but as the consultant had not visited the unit for 3 weeks, several locum doctors had been responsible for Mrs A's care in the interim. Clear guidelines for instigating treatment were not available and so treatment had not commenced.
3. The consultant was now requesting further tests and making decisions about Mrs A's care.

The elder son received a letter with this information, within the time limit of 10 working days. By this time, he had written to his MP, the trust chief executive and the trust chairman, demanding that the service should be critically reviewed. The elder son then began a campaign of letter writing, complaint and telephone calls that became abusive. Members of the trust offices dealing with these calls were briefed and supported with guidance on appropriate responses and what to do if the son were to call at the offices.

User participation in decision making

An external investigation was the next stage of the complaints system. A panel of experts external to the trust, comprising an experienced and senior nurse, consultants specialising in elderly care, psychiatry and orthopaedics and trust senior board members not implicated in the case, was convened.

All Mrs A's papers and records of treatment, her charts and all the correspondence associated with the case were sent to all the panel members so that they could begin to unravel the features of this business. There was time for the panel members to contact each other prior to the session and for them to be in contact with the chair of the panel, to be assured that they had all the papers and information necessary for the work.

The panel sat and discussed the issues with each of the 'witnesses' or people who had been asked to give information to the panel in order that it could make a fair and concrete decision. Although this panel has no power in law, it can make recommendations and will always make a report that will be sent to the Health Service Ombudsman, the panel members, the 'witnesses', the complainant, all trust board members and the Community Health Council.

One of the main issues was the intimidation of staff by Mrs A's elder son and whether this should be accounted for in any decision. Further discussion was about the role and responsibilities of the nursing staff for the care they provided despite the medical staff not being able to make decisions about Mrs A's care. Part of the main recommendations was about sufficient training, supervision and alternative cover for locum staff in the medical teams.

The panel's report was published within a month of the meeting and since then no communication by the elder son has occurred. Mrs A's younger son still visits as before. He did not want to be associated with his brother's complaint.

Discussion questions

- What are your first thoughts about this case?
- Are they associated with the role of the nursing staff or Mrs A's elder son?
- Are they to do with the responsibilities of the medical staff?
- What other comments would you make?
- Why do you think you began your analysis in this way?
- Are you defending other people and their role or what would have been your own?
- The nursing staff were ascribed no blame in this case; do you think blame should be shared across the unit?

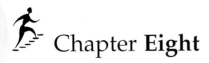

Chapter **Eight**

Consumer groups and community voices

Mary Cooke

- Introduction
- The potential for influence by user groups
- The history of user involvement
- Some theories of user involvement
- Ethics and policy

- The rationale for involving users in health care decisions (as user groups)
- The practical aspects of democracy in health service provision
- Endnote
- Conclusion

O V E R V I E W

People group themselves to justify and strengthen their individual views and support agreed activities. This behaviour is endorsed by recent shifts in local management of health and social care and is essentially political.

The World Health Organization has promoted consumers and their groups to become voices in changing the thinking about health care. Although the health service exists for the benefit of the patient or user, there are few occasions when users are invited to offer their views on their needs for health care. This means that each country's health service responds to the requirements of the professionals and the politicians. The 'voice' of the user or consumer continues to be lost in the political debate.

User and consumer groups allow the voice of the user to be heard within each group, but the rise and fall in their funding

User participation in decision making

182

(carers and users support the groups personally), membership (many groups are formed of patients in terminal care situations) and fortunes (some groups are not organised politically) mean that there may be little consistency in membership or drive to change their position. The government has had to make laws to ensure that users have a voice in the changes to health care.

INTRODUCTION

The NHS commenced with a political focus (Webster 1998) so that policy making and restructuring of systems and services in health care in the UK have developed since to reflect the political strength of each party in power.

Since the inception of the NHS in 1944 the fundamental object-ives of the government of the time for providing health care have not altered either politically, in their essential conceptual philoso-phy of universal coverage, or effectively, in the planning and devel-opment of strategy and the education of clinical staff. The main focus remains the equity of access to health care, according to need. The service was designed to be delivered through essential systems composed of three main elements: systematic service delivery, edu-cation and training of clinicians, and clinical research (Webster 1998, p. 15).

Ways in which decisions are currently made about the health service need further scrutiny. Looking at the NHS today, there are several ways in which it could be defined specifically as an organ-isation. One is the way in which the service is funded. Sources of funding give a perspective on the values of a society. Another is the way in which the political shifts in emphasis (the cultural develop-ments of the organisation) affect the health system in terms of edu-cation and training of clinical staff and developing priorities. A further approach may provide ideas about the ways in which soci-ety is driven (for instance, to involve its members in changing the health care delivery) and, as a response, makes its decisions about its public service.

Primary care groups and trusts (PCGs or PCTs) are composed of professionals and users (lay members of the public) and are the most effective method for users to have any impact in changing health service priorities. They have an explicit developmental mis-sion, part of which is to involve users through corporate commit-ment to establishing a pathway of communication between group/trust board and a user subgroup. These PCGs provide new

Consumer groups and community voices

opportunities for establishing users' place in local health economies. The PCGs use their subgroup members in defining guidelines for treatment and care decisions of patients and carers, user contribution to planning and monitoring services and citizen contribution to policy making (Barnes & McIver 1999).

The NHS also has a role as educator of clinical staff. Before the NHS, doctors obtained their income from private patients, who subsidised the public work they did in voluntary hospitals. Dr Julian Tudor-Hart describes this:

> Doctors traditionally recognised two kinds of patient. Paying patients, like other customers, were always right and therefore had to be humoured. Non-paying, public service patients were supposed to earn their right to care by having serious or at least interesting diseases, and to be grateful for getting any care at all; beggars can't be choosers. (Tudor-Hart 1994)

Little has changed in the attitude of medical care, in that the private health system allows doctors to treat people in the way they want while patients using the public health system are available for doctors to train with as 'interesting cases'. All other health professionals use the NHS patient population in a similar manner, to train and educate staff. Staff are then enabled to work in the NHS, the private sector and in voluntary and charitable organisations.

Another group of interested people who have opinions about the health service in the UK are described in several ways. Sometimes called patients, carers, consumers or clients, often ignored as survivors of the health service system, they are 'the users' of the health service. Some people would suggest that the opinions voiced by this largest group should be the most important when decisions about the health service are made. From other stakeholders' perspectives, users' opinions are seen as the least important in raising issues and making decisions. One method of ensuring that these otherwise disparate and unorganised groups of people are working for the benefit of their members, and of course now the government, is the fact they usually have national identities linked to local affiliation and involvement.

The World Health Organization issued a report in summer 2000 ranking health systems in 191 countries by a common set of measures. This list ranked overall health system performance and showed that health models not previously seen as successful were ranked highly, while other more highly respected systems ranked lower. France, Italy and Spain were seen as top Western health system performers. Canada, Germany, Sweden and Denmark, often cited as models to follow, ranked lower. This report was written on the information given by 'experts' who in some cases did not reside in the country they were reporting on. The rating was based on five composite indicators:

- overall level of population health
- health inequalities within the population
- overall level of health system responsiveness (a combination of patient satisfaction and how well the system acts)
- distribution of responsiveness within the population (how well people of varying economic status feel that they are served by the health system)
- the distribution of the health system's financial burden within the population (who pays the costs) (WHO 2000).

No patients were interviewed to establish these measures of health system performance; expert judgements were seen as being more reliable. Even in the organisation where user participation and involvement were established as democratic rights for planning and evaluation purposes, citizens' views and experiences did not carry weight in assessing a nation's health system performance (Blendon et al 2001).

THE POTENTIAL FOR INFLUENCE BY USER GROUPS

The UK has been absorbing different cultures and values with every immigrant and visitor to the country. Everyone who comes into contact with the health service has shaped it, from within, if they are a health care worker, or from outside the organisation, by using it. These changes are subtle and incremental and it is only recently that these influences have been seen as pressure on the organisation to change from within to accommodate the needs of the consumers of health care.

People's opinions about most things are intended to be heard freely in this country and in this way they shape the culture over-all, the ways in which decisions are made and the decisions themselves. The media in the UK play a strong role in raising awareness of issues but in an individual way, people rarely talk about the NHS unless they happen to be in contact with it. The political role of the NHS generally passes unnoticed by the public unless issues of economics or access threaten to alter its effect on individuals.

Horton-Smith (2000) looks at the phenomenon of grassroots associations that perform many functions. He defines them loosely as voluntary associations and in many respects they all started in that way, in both the US and the UK. Group members are almost always volunteers. Groups that are associated with a specific disease, such as the National Schizophrenia Society, the Parkinson's Disease Society, Cancer Bacup, Action on Smoking in Health, Association for Improvement in Midwifery Services or MIND (selecting a few representative organisations), provide the platform for people to voice their opinions and use them politically and personally. Other support groups may be formed specifically for a time-limited purpose by carers of people with disease or diagnoses. Carers provide the support by organising the group, running campaigns or supplying funds. Well-organised groups, such as those for cancer care or Parkinson's disease or arthritis sufferers, have a carefully constructed political arm through which they promote their concerns by employing professional people in the role of advocate at the political level. The benefits of this are a high profile in the press, in directing government funds and often in securing research monies and lottery funds to enable improvements to be made to services in a particular locality.

THE HISTORY OF USER INVOLVEMENT

The loss of participatory rights in health care decision making has evolved slowly with the rise in the 'science' base of medicine. The many parliamentary acts and publications since the 1950s can be seen as developing the strength of the patient as a consumer (rise in professional self-regulation, Community Health Councils, clinical audit) and as a result of events (e.g. NHS Health Advisory Service, Social Services Inspectorate, Medicines Control Agency, Human Infertility Authority, etc.). As different ways of providing care to vulnerable groups of patients were developed, the monitoring agencies grew to keep pace with them. Finally, the Labour government of 1997 defined the re-democratising of the NHS with *The NHS Plan*, in which users and consumers really are the central focus of the NHS, and by passing the Human Rights Act in 1999 that has determined the equality of participation in health care.

The recent government publication *The NHS Plan* (DoH 2000) centres policy on health service users and makes other stakeholders accommodate a method of involving and engaging users in the processes of decision making for service planning.

> The relationship between service and patient is too hierarchical and paternalistic. It reflects the values of 1940s public services. Patients do not have their own health records or see correspondence about their own health care. The complaints system in the NHS is dis-

User participation in decision making

credited. Patients have few rights of redress when things go wrong. (DoH 2000, p. 30 section 2.33)

The patient's voice does not sufficiently influence the provision of services. Local communities are poorly represented within NHS decision-making structures. Despite many local and national initiatives to alter the relationship between the NHS and the patient, the whole culture is more of the last century than of this. Giving patients new powers in the NHS is one of the keys to unlocking patient-centred services. (DoH 2000, p. 30 section 2.34)

SOME THEORIES OF USER INVOLVEMENT

As one of the major theorists who has written on change in health care as an organisational evolution, Lindblom (1979, 1982) discusses the rationale for change and calls it 'muddling through'.

> These two – big actions and comprehensive analysis – are obviously closely related and they come nicely together in conventional notions of 'planning'. Hence a choice is clearly posed. Is the general formula for better policy making one of more science and more political ambition, or as I would argue, a new and improved muddling? (Lindblom 1982, p. 25)

The ideologies of management for problem solving are well intentioned. Lindblom remarks that poor analysis of the problem prevents systems from helping themselves. There appears to be a conspiracy to consistently justify the reasons for not changing anything, in order to solve the larger problem of the whole system. Incremental change has been employed by governments to move their agenda forward. The involvement of users in consumer groups and networks of patient support groups (formal and informal) has been visibly and audibly growing since the early 1970s in the USA and since the 1980s in the UK.

One consequence of the medical professional's inability to reflexively listen to the realities of the illness experiences as expressed by patients and carers has been the 1997 Labour government implementing their strategies and commencing additional services such as NHS Direct. This was more to do with a government agenda to move traditionally held power and influence from the medical professionals. Politically, support groups have not missed the opportunities gained by sanctioning this promotion of their political involvement in change. Kempley (2000), in a letter to the *British Medical Journal*, suggests that NHS Direct meets the needs of an

Consumer groups and community voices

'information-hungry population' who, if it cannot get the information it needs, will turn to other 'less reliable or relevant sources'.

In recent policy developments, the 'user' of the health service has been seen as needing a method of support (formal advocacy services, as in mental health services) and the provision of a channel for their views to be heard in the most positive way, such as through the complaints service. The language of discussion between professionals, managers and users of health services has been ameliorated to accommodate users and to avoid confrontation through misunderstanding of priorities, obfuscation of facts and issues and ambiguity of intentions.

Theories of involvement are few and they are also diverse, suggesting that there is insufficient evidence to project the success of a programme by basing it on any defined theoretical foundation.

Arnstein's ladder of citizen participation (Fig. 8.1) provides a useful typology and evaluative measure with which to assess efforts to involve service users (Arnstein 1969). Here, citizen participation is seen as being linked to the redistribution of power and there is a critical difference between going through an empty ritual of participation and having real power to affect the outcome of the process. If power is not redistributed, the status quo will be maintained. Caution should be applied when taking this model to the real world (Leonard et al 1998). Distinctions between levels can be blurred and there may be further intermediate rungs in the ladder

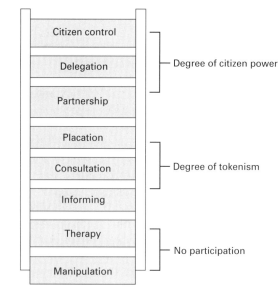

Figure 8.1 Ladder of citizen control (Arnstein 1969).

not expressed here. Different levels of participation may be operating simultaneously (Curtis & Taket 1996, cited in Leonard et al 1998). Arnstein's ladder has been used to analyse user involvement in health care settings and current literature may be reviewed to apply the principles (Dargie 2000).

Freeman et al (1997) have developed a guide to involving the community and provide a theory of community development in primary care. This guide assumes that there is sufficient communication in primary health care teams where staff (health and social and local authority) are enabled to work together to achieve health improvements. The reality is that more time and energy are spent in ironing out inequities of power among the agencies than in moving community care programmes forward to a successful evaluation. This is the real reason for the 'guide'.

Involving users and carers in making health care decisions requires an understanding about how demand and need are both incorporated into the planning process. Research and modelling associated with the relevance of lay concepts and experience of illness are balanced with understanding help seeking and health care as a social process. The basis of the UK welfare system is that health care is free at the point of delivery. This fact does not prevent people seeking help from lay people with some health knowledge (complementary health providers), networking with informal access to health systems (pharmacies) or self-medicating in accordance with past experience and family behaviours. These models do not qualify or quantify the impact that the media have on reactions to health issues. Much user knowledge arises from the media, as does their attitude formation about various sources of illness or remedies (Rogers & Elliott 1999).

An interesting theory proposed by Le Grand (2001, p. 48) looks at the manner in which people (society) behave in relation to social policy and changes in health provision. Le Grand uses Hume (1875) to describe the behaviour of the population as knights, knaves and pawns. Knights are seen as predominantly public spirited or altruistic, so that policy makers in health know that a proportion of society will behave in a way that is unthreatening to others in sharing out resources. Pawns are seen as passive or unresponsive recipients of charitable acts. Knaves will always respond to incentives from which they will benefit in some way. Over time, other names have been found for these groups – 'the reluctant collectivists' (Beverage and Keynes) and the 'democratic socialists' who included Marshall and Titmuss during the 1954–61 Labour governments. Democratic socialists assumed that the state and its agents were competent and benevolent so they assumed that the

Consumer groups and community voices

189

others were always working in the interests of the public. Professionals such as doctors and teachers were expected to work within their professional ethic and were concerned with the interests of the people they were serving. Politicians, bureaucrats, civil servants and managers were expected to define social and health needs and operate services to provide for them.

Taxpayers were assumed to be part of the collective view that progressive tax would redistribute welfare to the needy and social justice would be guaranteed by altruism. Individuals in receipt of benefit would behave accordingly and were also (naive) passive altruists.

Since the government of Margaret Thatcher and the allocation of new powers, as consumers, people have taken a considerable time to understand that as users their role is not passive but should be active, participatory and vociferous.

Few theorists have applied their thinking to how user support organisations and consumer groups devolve the work of their membership. The above definition of behaviour is one of the closest to voluntary and charitable organisations' structures. The application is more effective where those with altruistic attitudes work for others who will benefit passively. Many carers who belong to a support group (and whose relative/partner has died as a result of their illness) remain in the organisation. Social theories will analyse this as a social link with the memories of their dead relative. Others will understand that the support group was probably the only social life there was for people otherwise isolated with an illness. Members who are ex-carers are usually the most active.

Beresford et al (2001) discuss the effect of a worldwide development of service users' organisations. They cite people with learning difficulties, older people, psychiatric system survivors and people living with HIV/AIDS. The Disability Discrimination Act 1999 and the Community Care (Direct Payments) Act 1996 are both milestones for users challenging the system of health and social care planning and delivery.

Obstacles to user involvement in support groups will be associated with quality of services. It is in this arena that the government sees most benefit for involvement. Engagement in debate about services will centre on the user experience and how their expectations are not matched with reality. Unequal roles and relationships are central to the failure to engage and lack of communication. The service user organisations are crucial to the support for training and representation that members of groups require to meet on an equal basis and work with health and social care professionals.

Many of the national organisations can be categorised by their method of support. Some are professionally led, such as the British Diabetic Association, whose objectives are associated with research, support of professionals and information to patients. Another category is that of user and professional support group, who provide services, offer self-help information and support and also campaign for services. Examples of these would be Action for Sick Children, Parkinson's Disease Society, National Childbirth Trust or MIND and the Terrence Higgins Trust. The third category is composed of those groups that are user led. These are defined through their focus on self-help, information and support, as well as campaigning efforts and include, for example, Association for Improvement in Maternity Services, Survivors Speak Out, Radiotherapy Action Group Exposure, People First and the Cancer-Help groups.

Recently, the government has brought into its strategy the Human Rights Act 2000 which could be interpreted in many ways not experienced before. Many health professionals feel exposed to challenges through this Act, as common practices in health care delivery have had to be revised to accommodate the personal rights of users, carers and patients, rather than the current culture of focusing on the professionals' personal and/or professional rights. (You may need to stop and think about this for a moment and refer to Chapter 7 on user empowerment.)

Some groups have in the recent past been set up by influential medical groups. Philanthropic they may be but their aims are seen as autonomous and, with a cynical gaze, they may be viewed as inverted support for the medical profession and its own aims. An example of this is Healthwatch, set up in 1989 (formerly the Campaign Against Health Fraud), 'promoting assessments of new treatments and protecting consumers from fraudulent claims (in medicine)'. In 1979, the Coronary Prevention Group was set up by doctors who were critical of the approach of the British Heart Foundation. The argument was that the British Heart Foundation believed that coronary heart disease is a disease of diet and lifestyle and the doctors thought poverty was also a strong causative factor.

ETHICS AND POLICY

At the root of all policy making and decision making are issues associated with people's rights and duties; that is, the ethics of activities that occur in the provision of a public service where everyone has a stake in the outcome from a personal, a social and a financial perspective.

Consumer groups and community voices

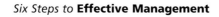

Six Steps to **Effective Management**

> Patients are the most important people in the health service. . . . too many patients feel talked at rather than listened to. This has to change. NHS care has to be shaped around the convenience and concerns of patients. To bring this about, patients must have more say in their own treatment and more influence over the way the NHS works. (DoH 2000, p. 88 section 10.1)

Systems of provision, power and decision making all have one common feature. This can be described as an ethical stance and may offer one of the strongest reasons for altering the focus of service to users as the central force for change in the new NHS of the 21st century (Midgeley 1992).

Figure 8.2 represents providers at the centre of health services planning; they are seen as being more important because they are employed by the health service and therefore have most to lose through devolving power to outside organisations. The users are beyond the margins of the system; they are not directly employed by the health services, yet they cannot be totally excluded because they are key stakeholders in service development outcomes. The paradox of this situation is that users will influence the service by not using it or their influence may become lost because of the potential rise in health status of the population. The idea behind this system is that everyone should be influencing outcomes of health in order to create health and therefore wealth for the country. The values should be common to all.

THE RATIONALE FOR INVOLVING USERS IN HEALTH CARE DECISIONS (AS USER GROUPS)

One of the Department of Health's medium-term priorities for the NHS in 1990 was to:

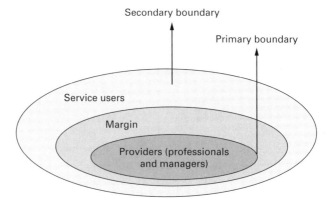

Figure 8.2 Midgeley's system boundaries (adapted in Thomson 1995).

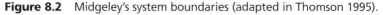

... give greater voice and influence to users of NHS services and their carers in their own care, the development and definition of standards set for NHS services locally and the development of NHS policy both locally and nationally. (DoH 1992, p. 7)

The government paper *Local Voices* (DoH 1992) made it clear that the government expected health authorities to take into account the needs and preferences of local people when purchasing services. It introduced the notion that health authorities should be 'champions of the people' and that:

... their decisions should reflect, so far as practical, what people want, their preferences, concerns, values. (DoH 1992, p. 13)

In practice, local authorities have interpreted *Local Voices* in different ways and there have been wide variations in the methods used and extent to which the public has been involved (Barnes 1997). For example, some health authorities and PCGs/PCTs have seen their role primarily as one of needs assessment and have carried this out using quantitative methods such as surveys or qualitative methods of enquiry such as focus group discussions. Others have used community development and modified community development approaches such as rapid appraisal and a general scoping of services with few decisions made as an outcome of the picture drawn in the scoping exercise (Cooke 2001). Other health authorities have interpreted their role as that of championing the people's health and have sought to collaborate with local agencies such as the Chamber of Commerce, city council and voluntary organisations to pursue this aim (as encouraged through the 1998 directives to Commissions for Health Improvement – CHImp).

Elsewhere, attempts have been made to engage the public in priority setting, using approaches such as surveys, workshops, health panels, discussion groups and citizens' juries (Bowie et al 1995, Lenaghan et al 1996, McIver 1995). Some of these activities were heavily funded (as a disincentive to the government to incorporate this strategy nationally) and most did nothing to improve the rate of decision making by involving users directly in the process. The current method for encouraging participation of users is through groups that offer an information service to their members, a support service for rehabilitation for users and carers and additional services to raise the quality of life of sufferers in ways that the NHS cannot (e.g. Cancer Bacup, the Arthritis Association, the Schizophrenia Society). Other ways of user groups becoming prominent is through their links with consultation programmes, such as the Sainsbury Centre for Mental Health, an organisation that involves consumers in planning research into specific mental

Consumer groups and community voices

health conditions and whose report helped to develop policy for the National Framework for Mental Health.

It is clear that public involvement serves various purposes and it is therefore not surprising that many different methods have been used in practice. It is also clear that none of them have had any firm influence on the management and planning of health care systems or the changes that are needed to focus on the patient as the partner in health.

THE PRACTICAL ASPECTS OF DEMOCRACY IN HEALTH SERVICE PROVISION

A wider debate about the nature of democracy in contemporary society does not normally associate with health service provision or involvement of patients and professionals outside the clinical situation. Some writers have argued that although the UK has a system of representative democracy this does not mean that the role of citizens or participants in health care system utilisation should be limited to voting in elections. If citizen participation is perceived to be limited or restricted, it could be argued that:

> It is as if the citizen is treated as not being capable of any involvement beyond deciding between conflicting parties on who should constitute the government. (Stewart 1996, p. 1)

From this perspective, users and participants in the health care relationship should take a more active role in the process of governing. As a consequence, they should have more opportunity to take part in decision making which results in changes to public services. In relation to the NHS specifically, it has been argued that the NHS is not sufficiently locally accountable to the public (Cooper et al 1995) and that the changes introduced as a result of the 1990 NHS and Community Care Act have further reduced local accountability (Coote 1996). It follows that action needs to be taken to involve the public in planning health services, in ways that go beyond lay involvement in the work of NHS trust boards, primary care groups and trusts and the CHCs. In this context an analytical distinction can be made between citizens and consumers. Citizens can have an interest in public services even though they do not currently use them. Beresford & Croft argued:

> It is not enough for service users to be conceived of as data sources or for our rights as citizens to be reduced to consumer rights. What is at issue is the responsibility of a democratic state to uphold the rights of its citizens. (Beresford & Croft 1993, p. 39)

User participation in decision making

You may not accept this argument as representing a view you recognise. It is clear, however, that a person's views may change, depending on whether they are speaking as a service user or a citizen. This means that the aims of consumerism and those of participative democracy may not always be the same. Rudolf Klein offers this view in relation to the NHS.

> In short, we have to be clear whether we are concerned about strengthening the responsiveness and accountability of the NHS to a wider body of citizens, or of strengthening consumers as an interest group within the NHS. Both may be legitimate aims of policy, but they are not the same or necessarily congruent. (Klein 2000, p. 20)

Indeed, since the 1960s a view has been debated about social action and methods of changing policy through understanding the ways in which market forces work. Hirschman (1964) offered a discussion that was taken up by Klein 20 years later and applied to the health service. Debates about 'exit', 'voice' and 'loyalty' in association with making views known have taken place in the context of social activity and analysis of market activity. The difficulty in applying this theory to the NHS is that people can only 'exit' by buying care privately, which restricts some people through personal resources and principles of payment. The 'voice' of the user has not had the greatest opportunity, even in a democratic environment, to be heard. Where incentives to involve users in giving their views are not available to professionals, this will become a problem for ensuring engagement and democratising of the power of stakeholders in the NHS. The public is expected to be 'loyal' to the NHS but in the late 1980s the Conservative government found that the NHS was seen as precious to users and 'not to be meddled with' (Klein 2000). This precarious hold on the tensions that control NHS reform accounts for the timidity of past governments to really upset the system of health care delivery and allow the NHS to become measurably more efficient and effective.

ENDNOTE

User participation in health services decision making requires a depth of understanding from all sides of the situation. The user's understanding of the manner in which decisions are made is seen by health service personnel as superficial (Hogg 1999). Yet, by understanding user needs valid deployment of resources can be

Consumer groups and community voices

agreed, within available funding arrangements. Users and their carers have a grasp of the way in which the disease affects them that they are not always invited to share with the professionals. The user's concept of recovery is not always the same as that of the professional.

Change in health service culture will be required to promote policies that encourage user involvement. Kurt Lewin (1951) has provided a sound method of understanding and analysing general change situations. According to Lewin, organisations achieve a state of equilibrium by the balancing of equal and opposing forces. Decreasing the restraining forces and increasing the facilitating forces can achieve the required change.

Value systems of the users of health care have not yet been taken fully into consideration in planning what care is required and what will be provided. Citizens' juries have been tested but derisory comments came from the medical professionals about the costs of ensuring that the users (citizen groups) had sufficient knowledge to participate fully in the jury and in decision making. Other difficulties arose from criticisms of representation on the jury – whether it was sufficiently broad; this provided little encouragement for the involvement exercise to continue and gave poor opportunities for the applications of findings from the social exercises (Barnes 1997, Cambridge Health Authority 1992, ESRC 1998, Kelson 1995, 1997, King's Fund 1996). The culture and health beliefs of the users have not been fully evaluated in relation to what is being provided at present.

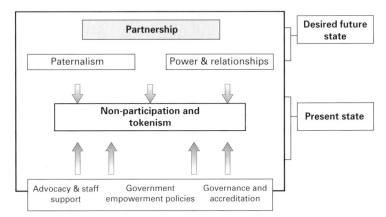

Figure 8.3 Forces driving and opposing user involvement.

CONCLUSION

This section has shown that until information about users' needs and beliefs about their health care demands is available and until users are more fully informed and involved in decision making about issues of health (their own as well as their communities'), the poor communication between all participants in the use and delivery of the NHS will be exacerbated.

It may be that the users, as citizens of the UK, will voice their opinions more succinctly and promote their views more forcefully. They will decide on whether and how they will fund and organise health care from a unilateral perspective of perceived need rather than the welfare system of provision for all regardless of need that we have become used to.

Alternatively, the health system could become more fragmented in accordance with the ways in which public needs are driving the structure of the health service. Maybe user groups will make a major decision not to be defined by their medical diagnosis but more by their collective needs. Maybe they will become so embroiled in the political system and promoting their own charitable causes that they will be diverted from complaining about the NHS and promote the NHS politically to deliver health measured by patient-evaluated outcomes.

In any case, public opinion about health care is destined to become incorporated more often into planning processes, whether the professionals want this to happen or not.

References

Arnstein SR 1969 A ladder of citizen partnership. Journal of the American Planning Association 35(4): 216–224

Barnes M 1997 The people's health service? Research Paper No. 2. Health Service Management Centre, University of Birmingham

Barnes M, McIver S 1999 Public participation in primary care. Health Service Management Centre, University of Birmingham

Beresford P, Croft S 1993 Citizen empowerment: a practical guide for change. Macmillan, London

Beresford P, Croft S, Evans C, Harding T 2001 Quality in personal medical services: the developing role of user involvement in the UK. In: Davies C, Finlay L, Bullman A (eds) Changing practice in health and social care. Open University Press, Milton Keynes

Blendon RJ, Kim M, Benson JM 2001 The public versus the WHO on health system performance. Health Affairs 20(3): 10–20

Consumer groups and community voices

Bowie C, Richardson A, Sykes W 1995 Consulting the public about health service priorities. British Medical Journal 311: 1155–1158

Cambridge and Huntingdon Health Authority 1992 Healthgain '92, the standing conference. The public as partners – a toolbox for involving local people in commissioning health care. Healthgain Conference, Eastern Region

Cooke M 2001 Consensus of expectations through focus group – users' views of their general practices in Corby PCG. Northamptonshire Health Authority, Northampton

Cooper L, Coote A, Davies A, Jackson C 1995 Voices off: tackling the democratic deficit in health. Institute of Public Participation in Research, London

Coote A 1996 The democratic deficit. In: Marshall M (ed) Sense and sensibility in health care. BMJ Books, London

Dargie C 2000 2000 report. Nuffield website online [http://www.official-documents.co.uk/document/nuffield/policyf/report2k.htm] accessed on October 16 2000

Department of Health 1992 Local voices: the views of local people in purchasing health. Stationery Office, London

Department of Health 2000 The NHS plan: a plan for investment, a plan for reform. Stationery Office, London

Economic and Social Research Council 1998 Conference proceedings: Economic beliefs and behaviour – efficiency, innovation and responsiveness in primary health care. ESRC, London

Freeman R, Gillam S, Shearin C, Pratt J 1997 Community development and involvement in primary care: a guide to involving the public in COPC. King's Fund, London

Hirschman AO 1964 Exit, voice and loyalty: a study of movement in organisations. Harvard, Boston

Hogg C 1999 Patients, power and politics. Sage, London

Horton-Smith D 2000 Grassroots associations. Sage, London

Kelson M 1995 Consumer involvement in initiatives in clinical audit and outcomes. College of Health, commissioned by the Department of Health Clinical Outcomes Group, London

Kelson M 1997 User involvement: a guide to developing effective user involvement strategies in the NHS. College of Health, London

Kempley S 2000 NHS Direct: doctors may gain time to use their true skills if people start using NHS Direct (letter). British Medical Journal 321: 446

King's Fund 1996 Grants for three health authorities to develop citizen's juries. News release October 29. King's Fund, London

Klein R 2000 New politics of the NHS, 4th edn. Longman, London

Le Grand J 2001 Knights, knaves or pawns? Human behaviour and social policy. In: Davies C, Finlay L, Bullman A (eds) Changing practice in health and social care. Open University Press, Milton Keynes

Lenaghan J, New B, Mitchell E 1996 Setting priorities: is there a role for citizens' juries? British Medical Journal 312: 1591–1593

User participation in decision making

Leonard O, Allsop J, Taket A, Wiles R 1998 User involvement in two primary healthcare projects in London. School of Education, Politics and Social Science, Southbank University, London

Lewin K 1951 Chapter 5. In: Lancaster J, Lancaster J (eds) The nurse as a change agent. Mosby, London

Lindblom CE 1979 Still muddling, not yet through. Public Administration Review 39: 517–526

Lindblom CE 1982 Still muddling, not yet through. An abridged version of the original article in Public Administration Review. In: McGrew A, Wilson MJ (eds) Decisionmaking approaches and analysis. Manchester University Press in association with Open University, Milton Keynes

McIver S 1995 Information for public choice. British Medical Bulletin 51(4): 900–913

Midgeley D 1992 Where ethics and politics meet. In: Thomson J (ed) User involvement in mental health services: the limits of consumerism, the risks of marginalisation and need for a critical approach. Research Memorandum No. 8. University of Hull

Rogers A, Elliott H 1999 Primary care: understanding health need and demand. National Primary Care Research and Development Centre Series, University of Manchester

Stewart J 1996 Further innovation in democratic practice. University of Birmingham

Thomson J 1995 User involvement in Mental Health Services: the limits of consumerism, the risks of marginalisation and need for critical approach. Research Memorandum No 8. The University of Hull

Tudor-Hart J 1994 Feasible socialism: the National Health Service past, present and future. Socialist Health Association, London

Webster C 1998 The National Health Service: a political history. Oxford University Press, Oxford

World Health Organization 2000 The World Health Report. www.who.int/whr/2000/en/press_release.htm

Application **8:1**

Mary Cooke

Grassroots organisations and user support groups

Users and carers, patients and consumers of health care may not all need to be in touch with organisations that 'stigmatise' them with a disease. Others rely on the coordination of support that exists through self-help and professional support groups where volunteers give such a great deal to others who can appreciate the availability of skills outside the NHS and private sectors of health care.

Below is a list of various types of organisations set up through charities or by users who had no support for themselves. Some groups started because they had needs that were not being met by the NHS or other agencies and in a support group they provided care for themselves, their carers and others who were similarly needy. Other groups are heavily supported by charities that supply funding for research, in addition to supporting users who may also be subjects of the research. This sounds like an incestuous relationship, but is significantly and sufficiently strong to enable support in various directions to be sustained. All types of group are represented here.

WEBSITES AND BOOKS

AIDS/HIV: the Terrence Higgins Trust
http://www.tht.org.uk/

Alzheimer's Disease Society
http://www.alzheimers.org.uk

Arthritis and Rheumatism Council
http://rheuma.bham.ac.uk/arc.html

Asthma and Allergy Research
http://www.users.blobalnet.co.uk/~aair/

User participation in decision making

BACUP
http://medweb.bham.ac.uk/cancerhelp/public/bacup

British Digestive Foundation
http://www.bdf.org.uk/

Deaf and Hard of Hearing
http://web.ukonline.co.uk/hearing.concern/

Dental phobics information
http://www.dentalfear.org/

Diabetes – adults
http://www.diabetic.org.uk/index/htm

Disabled Living Foundation
http://www.atlas.co.uk/dlf/

Epilepsy
http://www.atlas.co.org.uk/

Hepatitis Network
http://hepnet.com/

Institute of Psychiatry
http://iop.bpmf.ac.uk/

Marie Stopes Institute
http://www.mariestopes.org.uk/

Mental Health Foundation
http://www.mentalhealth.org.uk/

Multiple Sclerosis
http://mssociety.org.uk/

Parkinson's Disease Society
http://www.parkinsons.org.uk

Prostate Help Association
http://www.u-net.com/~pha/

Spina bifida and hydrocephalus
http://www.asbah.demon.co.uk/ifhsb.html

Twins and Multiple Births Association
http://www.surreyweb.org.uk/tamba/

Voluntary Organisations Internet Server
http://www.vois.org.uk/newhtml/about.html

Women's health – infertility
http://ferti.net/uk/index.htm

Patient's Pictures – a range of books containing clinical drawings for use by health professionals when describing medical conditions and treatments to patients. Covering basic anatomy, disease progress,

Grassroots organisations and user support groups

investigations and treatments. Available from the Sales Office, Royal College of GPs, 14 Princes Gate, Hyde Park, London SW7 1PU.

ORGANISATIONS

Centre for Health Information Quality
Acting as a source of expertise and knowledge for the NHS and patient representative groups on all aspects of patient information, to improve the NHS's capability, competence and capacity to provide good evidence-based patient information.
Centre for Health Information Quality, Highcroft, Romsey Road, Winchester SO22 5DH.

College of Health
A national charity founded to represent the interests of patients. The College publishes a range of research reports, guidelines and packs based on independent research.
Publications Unit, College of Health, St Margaret's House, 21 Old Ford Road, London E2 9PL.

Help for Health Trust
Aims to provide people with the information they need to make healthy choices. It provides a freephone health information service (0800 665544) for patients and carers in central/southern England. It produces a database selection of consumer health information and has a specialist health information research unit.
Help for Health Trust, Highcroft, Romsey Road, Winchester SO22 5DH.

King's Fund
An independent health charity that promotes the health of people in London through policy analysis and development and information about health and social care. Five major programmes of policy and development work: community care; effective practice; health systems; primary care; and public health. Key themes include promoting cultural diversity, tackling health inequalities and developing public involvement.
King's Fund, 11–13 Cavendish Square, London W1M 0AN.
http://www.kingsfund.org.uk

NHS Centre for Reviews and Dissemination (CRD)
Providing the NHS with information on the effectiveness and cost effectiveness of treatments and the delivery and organisation of health care. Aiming to disseminate research to health professionals.
NHS Centre for Reviews and Dissemination, University of York, York, YO1 5DD.

Scottish Association of Health Councils
18 Alva Street, Edinburgh EH2 4QG

User participation in decision making

Chapter **Nine**

Patients' rights and responsibilities

Trevor Ride

- Patients' rights in Europe
- Patients' rights: an international review
- Health care consumerism
- Patients' rights: the principles of statutory involvement
- Analysing the issues
- Appropriate and accessible health care
- The media, information and communication
- The Patient's Charter
- The NHS Plan
- The professions
- Conclusion
- Endnotes

O V E RV I E W

Although the World Health Organization has continuously pushed for the raising of the rights of individuals to gain recognition in health care, there has been much reticence on the part of professionals and managers to take up this challenge. This chapter looks at the statutory rights of individuals and how these are supported and takes a stance on the ways in which consumers may choose to ignore their responsibilities.

'Consumerism' within the 'public services' in the UK made major advances in the early 1990s with the development of the Citizen's Charter. This was essentially a Prime Ministerial initiative by the then Prime Minister John Major leading a Conservative government.

In the 1980s, Prime Minister Margaret Thatcher instigated the internal market composed of purchasers and providers. This major policy drive became a regulator of rising costs in real terms and perceived inefficiency within the service. Whilst the doctrine of the market economy was a specific political intervention, the public perception eventually, in the late 1990s, became one dissociated with a philosophy that was out of touch with and inappropriate for the provision of public services. The philosophy of the population appeared to be essentially socialised rather than that of the Prime Minister of the time which was emancipated and capitalist.

In classic economic theory, consumerism leads the regulation of the marketplace and thus a market economy. The problem with the UK system was that the 'market' in health care was managed and therefore failed.*

At that time, again in the political context, John Major needed to demonstrate the relevance of contemporary consumerism to the political doctrine of the day. The mission, almost personally identified with the Prime Minister, was that the rights of consumers were raised, to function as the focus for leading innovation in several areas of public services. If anything, consumerism sought to soften the blow from a political ideology founded on principles of free enterprise and the market economy. The public perception of their rights and responsibilities and consumerism within public sector enterprises was not consistent with a market economy. As a result of the need to strengthen the public action of participants in the health care market, charters and statements of standards of services developed in public and private service sectors.

In the UK National Health Service, the Patient's Charter was published in 1991. This document set out for the first time the standards and levels of service that consumers of the NHS could expect. The Charter defined 10 rights and nine standards, setting a minimum standard throughout the country, with facilitation of local improvements (see Application 9.1). Subsequent charters were developed for primary care (1991) and mental health (1997).

PATIENTS' RIGHTS IN EUROPE

A study by Leenen et al (1993) commissioned by the WHO European Region on patients' rights in the region examined

---

* Several economic and academic points are raised in this argument, see further in Le Grand J, Bartlett W (eds) 1993 'Quasi-markets and social policy'. Macmillan, Basingstoke.

User participation in decision making

trends within the member states over the period 1970–1983 in relation to:

- health care consumers
- health care providers
- health care establishments
- regulation of healthcare systems
- financing.

From this and subsequent work emerged the *Principles of the rights of patients in Europe* (WHO 1994) which included:

- human rights and values in health care
- information
- consent
- confidentiality and privacy
- care and treatment
- application (implementation).

The study demonstrated that, whatever the health care system, increasingly countries shared the same principles for the rights of patients. Issues included:

- informed consent
- access to patients' medical records
- privacy and the confidentiality of data
- the rights of specific client groups (minors, people with mental health problems or learning difficulties)
- complaints procedures
- research, experimentation
- ethics.

Civil, penal, administrative and disciplinary law in health care, together with mechanisms for the protection and enforcement of these rights, were also examined. Overall it was found that legal frameworks and weak civil procedures did not always provide answers in what was seen as a balance between patients/clients and the 'system'.

The study identified the then present and future trends with responses such as 'the development of legislation on patients' rights'. This provided the overall context of health sector reform, emerging over that time, which became a platform for the common values of patients' rights internationally.

WHO Europe followed up with a consultation in 1994 to harness this growing movement and help countries develop clear policies, by defining the principles of patients' rights and placing them in a common European framework for action. From this, the

WHO EURO declaration was agreed which has become the basic framework for establishing and developing patients' rights and subsequent charters by the member states in the region.

The declaration was an attempt to formulate a set of patients' rights relevant to the way health care would be provided in the future and to improve the relationship between patient and health care provider. However, such developments cannot be taken in isolation from the social, economic and health sector to some degree or other within most countries across Europe. The extent to which such rights are emphasised depends on historic, cultural, economic, legal and other factors together with the organisation of health care in each country.

National situations vary in respect of legal frameworks, health care systems, economic conditions and social, cultural and ethical values. However, there are common approaches, which can be adapted to the needs of each country. The WHO *Principles* recognised these as:

- legislation or regulations, specifying the rights, entitlements and responsibilities of patients, health professionals and health care institutions
- medical and other professional codes, patients' charters and similar instruments, drawn up in the light of agreed common understandings between the representatives of citizens, patients, health professionals and policy makers and periodically revised in response to changing circumstances
- networking between and among patient and health care provider groups, recognising the distinction between citizen and user participation
- government support for the establishment and effective running of non-governmental organisations (NGOs) in the field of patients' rights
- national colloquia and conferences to bring the parties together to create and promote a shared sense of understanding
- involvement of the media in informing the public, stimulating constructive debate and sustaining awareness of the rights and responsibilities of patients and users and their representative organs
- better training in communication and advocacy skills for health professionals as well as for patient and other user groups, in order to further the development of a proper understanding of the perspective and role of all parties
- promotion of research to evaluate and document the effectiveness of legal and other provisions and the various initiatives taken in the diverse contexts of the different countries (WHO 1994).

User participation in decision making

Societal rights have become the province of government, determined by in-country conditions in many instances, whilst individual rights are the province of the patient/client.

WHO Europe has continued to advance this area of work with further resource documentation for member states produced in 1996. A network on patients' rights including 20 WHO members was established in 1997 and aimed by the end of year 2000 to include all 52 WHO member states (European Region). From 1998 this network has produced newsletters, including a report of the annual meeting and information from countries, together with reports of the annual network meetings. In addition, a WHO Collaborating Centre has been established on patients' and users' rights at the University of Canterbury, UK.

European comparisons

Fallberg et al (1996), together with the Nordic School of Public Health for WHO Europe, studied information on efforts to improve patients' rights and examine the role of patients and consumers in health care reform in 14 European countries. In addition to documenting the existence of laws, policy documents or patient charters, the conclusions show the future trends as follows.

- Individual rights will receive more emphasis.
- Patient-centred care focusing on consumer satisfaction will increase.
- Internal markets in health care will increase competition between hospitals and other health care providers.
- Quality will be a factor in competition.
- Patient power and organisation will increase.
- Health will be emphasised more as a basic need of people.

The study also documented the development of patients' rights in the 14 countries, showing the common themes and trends in establishing patients' rights, whether or not there was any basis in law. Some of the key issues to emerge in the comparison were as follows.

- Patients' rights have to be closely and continuously monitored and altered.
- Patients' rights are a combination of legislation and principles including ethical guidelines for different professional groups.
- There has been only limited specific legislation for patients' rights.
- Health insurance systems may in future develop in line with patients' rights legislation.

Patients' rights and responsibilities

- Patients' charters may emerge as minimum standards.
- Serious attempts in some countries to establish patients' rights are impeded not only by lack of funding but also by tradition and culture.

PATIENTS' RIGHTS: AN INTERNATIONAL REVIEW

In reviewing patients' charters internationally, the nature of the subject inevitably leads to the broader area of patients' rights in which charters may be seen as part of an enabling framework. There are 191 countries within the United Nations system. In response to the need to justify the support for consumer rights and enquire after the support that exists nationally, a survey by Consumers International (1996a) found over 30 countries with some form of framework for patients' rights. Together with the evidence from the study by Leenen et al (1993) and subsequent work within the WHO system, it is possible to see how patients' rights and charters have been developing in the regions of the world. Some are described here for their clarity and positive moves for change.

Asia and Pacific

Australia

The Australian Commonwealth government has a programme to improve the delivery of hospital services. At state level the charters include the basic rights for hospital care and health care in Australia, as part of the country's Medicare system. The Australian Private Health Insurance Council also has a patient's charter framework regulated by an ombudsman from within the Council structure.

South Australia

This charter sets out the rights and needs of individuals using the public health system. It is a commitment to services on the part of the public health system, to sensure that services are accessible and that they meet the needs of individual service levels under the Medicare system.

Hong Kong

A patient's charter describes both rights and responsibilities for the services of any of Hong Kong's public hospitals. It sets out the ways in which the community and the hospitals work as partners in a positive and open relationship with a view to enhancing the effectiveness of the health care process.

Indonesia

A Health Law, adopted in 1992, sets out provisions for patients' rights, including the rights to receive information; give informed consent; medical confidentiality; a second opinion; access to one's medical records; select one's physician and hospital.

New Zealand

A proposed draft code of rights for consumers of health and disability services, issued in 1995, has been criticised by consumer groups and patients' rights lawyers because of a let-out clause which allows the government to set aside any rights if 'resource constraints' make it impractical to give effect to them. The Consumer's Institute has also drawn attention to the fragmented nature of the public health system and the dangers this holds for consumers.

United States of America

Federal legislation has become embroiled in the political debate on health reform within the US. Various states have bills of rights for hospital patients. Any system of rights tends to be driven fiscally by a combination of health insurance and health maintenance organisations. The large number of disadvantaged people within the population and with no health insurance cover in practice would appear to have no rights other than those through civil and constitutional law and the ethical/professional codes of health workers.

Denmark

A National Board of Health circular from 1992 sets out the duties of physicians and the rights of patients. The rights include self-determination, information and consent.

Ireland

A charter for the rights of hospital patients was enacted in 1992. It includes access; courteous treatment; privacy; information; consent to treatment; confidentiality; right to refuse to participate in teaching sessions or research; complaints. The Irish Consumers' Association has been lobbying for a more comprehensive charter.

Patients' rights and responsibilities

Netherlands

A law on patients' rights came into effect in 1995. Consumentebond and the Patient/Consumer Federation have negotiated individual model agreements with specific groups of health workers.

San Marino

A 1989 charter sets out patients' rights and duties. The rights include access; prior consent; avoidance of research; information; an efficient and flexible system.

Sweden

Many rights are incorporated into existing legislation.

HEALTH CARE CONSUMERISM

Patient's charters do not stand alone in terms of patients' rights and responsibilities and are part of a much broader framework of consumerism and public awareness. Public participation in health care consumerism is a complex subject across a spectrum of socioeconomic, cultural, political and ethical issues.

Consumerism and strengthening the voice of the public as a user of services are not unique to health care but have developed as part of the general consumer movement. The whole concept of consumerism can be considered as 'the interaction that the consumers have with governments, business and other public, private and voluntary organisations'. However, the general focus is on the needs and preferences of the consumer who may then be viewed as the customer or client. In both public and private sector health care, this has given rise to a changed emphasis and a different way of looking at patients and clients.

Consumerism in health care is no different from consumerism in commercial businesses. This means:

- organisations being customer and consumer focused
- actively identifying who the consumer and customer is
- structuring services to meet the needs of consumers
- taking specific action to protect, educate and empower consumers
- stimulating need and awareness in users of services.

Over the past two decades in particular, organisations of all kinds have become more aware of the need to respond to the preferences and needs of the consumer. This is due in part to major demographic, economic, societal and technological developments. In addition, some of these relate to a wider access to education and information, changes in the nature and hours of work, changes in the economics and structure of the family unit, the consequences of increased life expectancy and the ageing population.

Emphasis on raising the rights of patients is, however, not a new phenomenon. It was first identified as the right to refuse in medical experimentation on human beings in the context of the Nuremberg Trials (1947). Over time and probably influenced by the Charter of the United Nations (1945), the adoptions of the Universal Declaration of Human Rights (1948) and the European Convention on Human Rights (1950), the rights of patients gradually acquired new meanings. This has resulted in the realisation that everyone is a stakeholder in the NHS and in their own health and as such should be responsible for outcomes of any intervention, as much as the professionals. This identification of a 'partnership in the decision-making process', especially in primary care, has led to greater participation of individuals in discussions about their health care with professionals and in decision making.

In terms of health care, interest has been affected by government in terms of:

- the role and duty of the state in guaranteeing the rights of citizens
- economic realities of scarce fiscal resources and equity of distribution
- ever-increasing cost of health care and the impact on national resources.

All these features of consumerist involvement and effective introduction of an ethical stance on defence of human and individual rights have been seen in other countries.

PATIENTS' RIGHTS: THE PRINCIPLES OF STATUTORY INVOLVEMENT

Whilst within Europe, the WHO has had a major role in advancing work on patients' charters and rights, globally, a range of organisations have also been developing similar work. Of particular significance and perhaps with the most potential impact has been the work developed globally through the consumer movement and particularly that of Consumers International (CI). A study by

Patients' rights and responsibilities

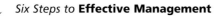

Six Steps to **Effective Management**

Consumers International (1996a) found 30 countries with some form of framework for patients' rights. In many cases, the protection was found to be weighted towards health care providers (particularly the medical profession) rather than consumers. Consumers International (1996b) developed a model framework for patients' rights which are described as:

- appropriate and accessible health care
- freedom from discrimination
- information and education
- choice of doctor or other health worker
- choice of health care establishment
- informed consent about treatment
- participation in an individual's own health care
- respect, privacy, confidentiality and dignity
- the right to complain
- redress in the event of injury.

ANALYSING THE ISSUES

Patients' rights are part of a movement that is gaining momentum globally. On the one hand their foundations can be traced to health being a human right and the developing awareness of human rights. This is not just a remote issue for developing countries but arises as a consequence of health care rationing and social exclusion. Of equal importance is the effect consumerism and individual decision making have on developed countries with issues such as whether children with Down's syndrome have a right to undergo cardiac surgery.

The development of the rights and charter concept is emerging not just in terms of setting out the obligations of the provider of health care (in many instances the state) but also reflecting the obligations that such rights place upon the consumer and recipient of health care. Whilst rights on the accessibility of health care to consumers may relate to issues of rationing, the right to health care that is clinically effective, evidence based and having a positive outcome and health gain as its orientation does not appear to feature.

APPROPRIATE AND ACCESSIBLE HEALTH CARE

Some of the terms used globally in relation to patients' rights are confusing in themselves, both in meaning and also interpretation.

Whilst health itself may be taken as a fundamental human right, such rights generally fall short of defining what 'health' actually is. The right to health care and service levels set out in many charters is more often set in the sociolegal framework and may relate to a right of access to a health care system, the emphasis of patient rights usually being on secondary (curative) as opposed to primary (preventive) care. There is a clear medical and legal domination in the majority of frameworks of patients' rights in various countries which may beg the question as to the actual nature of these rights, mainly because there is little appreciation by the medical professionals of the role that patients play in the success of each treatment intervention.

Many countries now emphasise freedom of choice within their health care frameworks but in practice this is not always possible. Whilst in the UK freedom of choice was assumed to exist, this has in practice been removed initially by the purchaser/provider contracting arrangements of the early 1990s and the arrangements that have subsequently replaced them. Many countries, including the UK, specify that services must be within available and affordable resources. Little connection is made between the importance of information and patient choice. Implicit in issues of the right of access to health care must also be the freedom from discrimination in that access.

Appropriate care is also about safe and effective care, i.e. the right person giving the right treatment at the right time and in the right place. This tends to be defined as curative, rather than preventive care.

The medical model and legal frameworks tend to dominate health care consumerism in many countries. Although there may be a notional freedom of choice, in practice this is not always the case. That freedom may also relate to freedom from discrimination in gaining access. Whilst in some countries this is explicit, issues may also relate to the nature of health care and services for ethnic minorities, transient populations and, in some settings, first-nation peoples. This gets to the 'nub' of the issues for individuals and collective empowerment of nations through major centralised decision making.

The lack of adequate or appropriate information is a frequent complaint by users of health care services. Although many countries have legal requirements for this, as in the UK, few users have the relevant opportunities and as such it is no guarantee of adequate or accurate information. Notional or actual consent to treatment is a problem of information as much as understanding. In many countries, this access to or sharing of knowledge remains weighted towards the benefit of health workers and facilities as

Patients' rights and responsibilities

opposed to the users of services. There are also tradition and cultural issues relating to communication of real and useful knowledge and the legal acquisition of knowledge, as in the databases containing information secured by the Data Protection Act (1998).

The right to choose a doctor, other health worker and health care establishment is a feature of patients' rights in many countries but again the practice in reality may be different. This is an issue also linked with patient information. Restrictions in choice of physician or GP may be as a result of available resources, the local responsibility of services, geographical and other local factors. There is an increasing trend for family physicians and general practitioners to be the gatekeepers for health services, thereby limiting the available choice or variety of care systems for patients. The general practitioners may be formally the primary contact between patients and health services but issues of patients' choice of other health workers are now emerging.

Patient choice may be limited by the specialist nature of treatment, limitations in its availability, resources and location. Whilst league tables show waiting list times for specific interventions, they may lack significant purpose if they are outside any frameworks for patient choice. Choice may also relate to the right to participate or not in treatment. This is controversial but requires patient involvement in decisions about their treatment, potential outcomes, options and choices available and is new territory to be embraced by health systems and health professionals.

The right to complain and receive redress covers more than issues of negligence, compensation and litigation. There are links with standards and quality service, professional regulation, malpractice and negligence that are related and need to be embraced within the overall frameworks of patients' rights. The issue of complaint and redress is not solely limited to malpractice and yet this is a key feature of the complaint systems of many countries. Complex processes as part of medical legislation exist in many countries but these do not always include basic issues of poor quality of service or overall breaches of patients' rights.

THE MEDIA, INFORMATION AND COMMUNICATION

The media have a significant role in raising public awareness on patients' rights and drawing attention to major health issues. These all form part of the process of public information which in turn informs the patient and is part of health care consumerism in the UK. Many consumer groups, health care agencies and providers publish vast amounts of information setting out standards of service and the rights and expectations for the public as consumers. Hospital league tables showing information on hospital performance have been controversial but they raise the public's expectations of their rights. Within UK public sector health care, this forms part of the government's 'open government' agenda.

The NHS is almost always cited in the media with failures and deficits being constantly reported on radio, television and in newspapers and followed up with commentary and reaction. In addition, there are health consumer watchdog programmes again highlighting patients' rights. These do little to promote faith in the NHS; in contrast, they frequently put the public off contacting the services and raise anxieties.

Information technology is increasing the pace of change in health care and is becoming an important medium for patient information. It gives access to decision-making processes and provides information amassed by government agencies, private foundations and academic institutions. Global accessibility to the Internet is increasing the potential awareness of patients not only in terms of rights but of all aspects of health and health care.

Within the UK, patients' charters of individual hospitals and other health facilities can be found on the World-Wide Web. Much information, including direct patient information, is available through the websites of many health consumer groups. The open availability of information plays a major role in health consumerism, giving patients an awareness of rights and raising expectations. It has produced the globally informed middle-class health consumer.

THE PATIENT'S CHARTER

The Patient's Charter launched in 1991 had a significant impact on the NHS. Following the implementation of the national charter, individual NHS trusts and public sector health care providers were required to develop their own individual charters and statements of service.

The concept of a health service charter, setting out the rights of patients/consumers, was attractive as part of quality frameworks for a health service in transition but the UK experience has been the subject of much criticism, public scepticism and, at times, political

Patients' rights and responsibilities

embarrassment. Research amongst NHS staff, patients and lay carers (King's Fund 1997) concluded that the charter concept had failed and was of limited usefulness.

Whilst the electoral pledges of the 1997 Labour government proposed a review of the charter, what emerged through the NHS Plan (2000) was a new framework of proposals to strengthen patient representation and public involvement in the NHS.

THE NHS PLAN

The NHS Plan (2000) contained a range of proposals to strengthen patient representation and public involvement in the NHS, to come into effect April 2002. These included the following.

For each NHS trust and primary care trust:

- patients' forum
- patient representation on trust boards
- patient advocacy and liaison service (PALS)
- annual patient survey.

For each health authority:

- independent local advisory forum.

For the whole local health community:

- local authority scrutiny committee.

Patients' forum and representation on boards

The new legislation provides an independent patients' forum in every NHS trust and primary care trust, giving direct input into the running of NHS services. Members are appointed by the NHS Appointment Commission, as representatives of their communities. Half are drawn from local patient groups and voluntary organisations and half from patients who have recently used the services of local NHS trusts.

There is cross-representation between forum and trust boards. Either patients' forums appoint one of their members as a non-executive director on each NHS trust/PCT board or each trust nominates one of its non-executive directors to join the forum.

Members of patients' forums have rights to:

- monitor and review every aspect of NHS services, including the PALS used by the patients whom the forum represents

- make inspections at hospitals, doctors' surgeries, nursing homes and other health care providers at all points of the patient pathway
- make reports and recommendations to NHS trust boards.

Patients' forums and their members are supported by a national patients' organisation to provide guidance, training and development to patient, carer and public representatives. Patients' forums and councils are funded at the NHS regional level but also with some local authority involvement.

Patient Advocacy and Liaison Service (PALS)

This service is provided as a conduit for complaints about the NHS Trust. Each Trust has to provide a PALS that:

- acts as a facilitator to resolve the concerns of patients, carers and families, with the power to negotiate immediate solutions or resolve issues quickly
- steers patients to advocacy services if this is requested or is appropriate
- provides accurate information on all aspects of the trust, including how to make a complaint
- acts as a gateway to people wishing to be involved in shaping the NHS.

Annual patient survey

NHS trusts conduct these by means of questionnaires or focus groups.

Patients' councils and local advisory forums

Patients' councils, an amendment to the original legislation, are aimed at strengthening the cohesion of the new system, by providing a mechanism to bring together the work of patients' forums across the entire local health community. Membership is drawn from local patients' forums. These will be separate from the local advisory forums, consisting of patient and voluntary agency representatives, which health authorities establish. Community Health Councils will continue until 2004, when they will be phased out.

Local authority scrutiny

As a result of the Local Government Act 2000, district and county councils can scrutinise local health services. Legislation gives Overview and

Scrutiny Committees (OSCs), with a lead role for county councils, an additional responsibility for scrutinising the local NHS.

All NHS bodies must provide OSCs with information about their services and operation. Chief executives of local NHS bodies are required to attend OSC meetings twice a year to answer questions about their organisations. OSCs report and recommend to the NHS bodies that they review. The NHS bodies have to provide clear justification for any recommendation which they do not accept. Health authorities have a specific duty to consult OSCs on any major changes to services in their areas.

Human Rights Act 1998

The origins of European human rights legislation can be traced back to the immediate post World War II era but successive UK governments were reluctant to encompass such laws into UK legislation until the Human Rights Act 1998. In terms of consumerism and users of health services, some of the important aspects include:

- the right to be heard and taken notice of
- the right to know who to talk to
- the right to explanations in plain English
- the right to advocacy
- the right to choices in having need met
- the right to promote human rights
- the right to access services.

Some of the key issues for health services are family life, discrimination of services and treatment against someone's will, accurate information, privacy and lack of respect. The impact of this major piece of legislation is now being realised in terms of major issues in the provision of mental health care, consent to treatment, the right to live and the right to die.

THE PROFESSIONS

With the continued modernisation of the NHS, there is now a clear recognition of the need for external reviews of the quality of NHS care. The Commission for Health Improvement has been established to inspect and monitor quality in all aspects of NHS hospital and primary care services.

In addition, there has also been recognition of the need to support clinicians and, in particular, poor clinical performance and

User participation in decision making

these proposals, 'Supporting doctors, protecting patients', whilst having a focus on the medical profession, have implications for all health care professionals in terms of frameworks for self-regulation, quality and performance monitoring.

Recently, the British Medical Association has endorsed the review of doctors' clinical practice through audit. Medical practitioners not fulfilling strict criteria have been enabled to retrain or retire, move their level of specialism or reduce their responsibilities. This is in line with evaluation of nursing competencies and Post Registration Education and Practice portfolios brought in by the UKCC during 1990–2000. Personal Learning Plans and Personal Learning Times have been provided as incentives for doctors, especially in primary care, to develop personal and professional practices. This also provides nurses with time out of practice for portfolio building, an improvement on previous experiences where no support was given.

Following the 2001 general election, as part of the continuing modernisation agenda for the NHS, the government has announced its intention to give patients stronger influence on the running of the health service and to strengthen regulation of the health professions.

CONCLUSION

There are early indications from government that consumer participation in the whole area of professional regulation will increase as a measure of increased openness and to secure public confidence in professional standards. Needless to say, this is a contentious issue.

The provision of public sector health services in the UK has been and continues to be a major political issue, irrespective of the particular government of the day. Whilst formal structures may not always exist, the fact that the state of the NHS becomes an electoral issue, even if limited to electoral cycles, gives the public and service consumers a key role as drivers of health consumerism within the political context of NHS policy.

Waiting lists, waiting times and even hospital cleanliness become important political issues, not just driven by the formal consumer movement but informally by the users of the service. Frequently, the public perceives failures in the service as a failure of government.

Consumer power was a developing concept in the later part of the last century but with the many changes in the service, may at times no longer seem to be part of the current political and

Patients' rights and responsibilities

managerial policy agenda. The work on citizens' charters laid particular emphasis on consumer participation in issues of organisational quality and standards. This has made minimal impact in health within a complex framework of many other formal and informal agencies entering the area of benchmarking and quality of service indices. The potential of health consumer power has been reduced by the planned abolition of Community Health Councils and no clear indication of any consumer-led alternative arrangements.

Health care professionals are under continued scrutiny as a result of publicised poor practice and national scandals, resulting in calls for greater public involvement in professional regulation but with national policy that may circumvent the key issues.

The challenge for health professionals together with health consumers is to embrace and understand the complexity of issues. Understanding these issues is not just about knowledge of rights but the complex structures and processes through which these rights can be exercised. All involved need to accept the reality of this participation. Policy makers, as solvers of user and consumer difficulties, themselves use problems and the subsequent processes of all formal and informal agencies to put outcome and health gain as the primary rights of patients. These are reviewed continuously to conserve the focus of users at the centre of health consumerism and the health consumer movement.

ENDNOTES

Rights under the Patient's Charter

- To receive health care on the basis of need, regardless of ability to pay.
- To be registered with a family doctor.
- To receive emergency medical care at any time, through your family doctor or the local ambulance service and hospital accident and emergency department.
- To be referred to a consultant, acceptable to you, when your family doctor thinks it necessary and to be referred for a second opinion, if you and your doctor agree this is desirable.
- To be given a clear explanation of any treatment proposed,

including any risks and alternatives, before you decide whether you will agree to treatment.

- To have access to your health records and to know that those working for the NHS are under a legal duty to keep their contents confidential.
- To choose whether or not you wish to take part in medical research or medical student training.
- To be given detailed information on local health services, including quality standards and maximum waiting times.
- To be guaranteed admission for treatment by a specific date no later than 2 years from the day when your consultant places you on a waiting list.
- To have any complaint about NHS services – whoever provides them – investigated and to receive a full and prompt written reply from the chief executive or general manager.

Rights under the Primary Care Charter

- To change your doctor easily and quickly.
- To be offered a health check on joining a doctor's list for the first time.
- To be entitled to request a health check if you have not seen a doctor in the previous 3 years and you are aged between 16 and 74.
- To be offered a yearly home visit and health check if you are 75 years or over.
- To have appropriate drugs and medicines prescribed.
- To be given detailed information about local family health services.
- To receive a copy of your GP's practice leaflet setting out the services the practice provides.

References

Consumers International 1996a The rights of patients. Consumers International, London

Consumers International 1996b Campaigning for patients' rights. Consumers International, London

Fallberg L et al 1996 Patients' rights in Europe: trends and prospects. *European Health Care Reforms – Citizens Choice & Patients Rights*. WHO Europe, Copenhagen

Patients' rights and responsibilities

Six Steps to **Effective Management**

King's Fund 1997 Review of Patient's Charter. King's Fund, London
Leenen H, Gevers S, Pinet G 1993 The rights of patients in Europe – A comparative study. Kluwer, The Hague
World Health Organization Regional Office for Europe 1994 Principles of the rights of patients in Europe. WHO, Copenhagen

User participation in decision making

Application **9:1**
Mary Cooke

Patients' rights and responsibilities and The NHS Plan

Labour spent much of its time in opposition developing propos-itions and plans for changing various public services. One of the services in need of more reform was the NHS. Although there was a series of shadow health secretaries up to the election in 1997, Alan Milburn is known to have engineered the ideas and preparation for the new NHS Plan published as a White Paper in July 2000.

There were several reasons for thinking about a new way of organising health care in the UK. First, the UK public was clearly not receiving a fair deal in health; neither were members of the public seen as using the health service fairly or equitably. There was inequality in health outcomes for people living in different areas of the UK that could not be explained. Second, funding in real terms was seen as being low, compared to European countries; the UK spent less than 7% of the Gross Domestic Product (GDP) on health services. Other countries spent up to 15% of their GDP on providing health care, support and social services for their popula-tions, in less densely populated countries, and where for some measures of health status, the people were rated as being more healthy than those in the UK. In the main, women's health in the UK was considered to be of higher risk compared with Europe (WHO 1997). The UK is placed 14th out of 29 countries in terms of infant mortality, 11th for male life expectancy and 18th for female life expectancy.

A third reason was that professionals generally did not see patients and the public as consumers or purchasers of the health care services, in spite of various challenges to the medical profes-sion such as media stories about unethical and illegal conduct by GPs and hospital doctors being challenged on their competence to practise. These problems were compounded by the General Medical Council and British Medical Association not acting sufficiently rapidly to protect some of their members from serious legal charges and costly litigation.

Some professionals were discontented with the service and their role. Resource figures for numbers of nurses, GPs and hospital doctors working in the NHS all showed difficulties with recruitment and retention of staff. The reasons were given as poor working conditions and low pay, especially in large city areas and some affluent areas of the country where staff could not afford housing on the national agreed pay.

There is a list of reading on these subjects at the end of the application.

THE NHS PLAN (DOH 2000)

The UK needs to show that its health system has been reformed to raise the health status of the population and that health policy objectives help define the concept of health for the country, to enable health to be treated as a social 'good'. Health also encompasses treatment and care and prevention of the causes of ill health in society so social and economic factors affect health. It is with this definition that The NHS Plan sets out its mission, the government's vision and the means by which change will occur. Many factors have an impact on whether the government's vision will be achieved.

- Increasing life expectancy to 77 for men and 82 for women by 2015.
- 15.8% of the population aged 60–74 and 7.8% aged 75+ by 2015.
- Dependency ratio increased to 308 per 1000 people by 2015.
- Dramatic increase $\times 3$ in cost of long-term care by 2030.
- Globalisation of health (problems and solutions) including space/time compression and industrial concentration that brings health threats and opportunities.
- The emergence of new health risks caused by increased trans-border flows of people, goods and services and capital.
- Increasing opportunities for enhancing health training and education via global information and communication systems.
- Increasing pressure for global systems of governance to deal with global issues.
- Trends in disease: shifting burden of disease from young to old and communicable to chronic, with continued threat of recurring infectious diseases.
- Increasing incidence of cancer due to age, health/lifestyle risks of population.

- Increasing trends in obesity in children and adults.
- Increasing proportion of children aged 11–15 smoking, from 10% in 1990 to 13% in 1996.
- Increasing poor mental health in children and young people.
- Public expectations: increasing individual access to health information that was previously dependent on professionals, particularly via electronic means.
- The rise of the empowered consumer, leading to increased challenges to professional and expert authority in health.
- Intensification of media role in assigning priority to certain issues and debates at the national and local level.
- Technology: influencing the setting in which health care takes place.
- Scientific advances and new knowledge: genetic developments, molecular genetics, bioengineering and biotechnology.
- The environment: improvements in air quality from major pollutants, increasing public concern with food safety, emergence of new diseases, increasing link between housing and health.
- Lifestyle: poverty and relative deprivation: smoking in children, obesity, rising trends in cancer diagnosis, more teenage pregnancies.

Possible interventions to deter the progression of determinants

- Devolution: in the UK to Scotland (25% more funding than NHS England), Wales (18% more funding than NHS England) and Northern Ireland (5% more funding than NHS England). Higher funding in these countries is not associated with better health outcomes.
- User involvement and empowerment: shift from individualist model of health to partnership model, professional autonomy challenged, more public decision making about health systems.
- EU institutions: EU treatises include health policy making. Reduction in boundary between EU countries (1998 European Court judgement). Increasing comparisons between EU countries on health outcomes.
- Service delivery: increasingly more managed and externally regulated system of health delivery, increasing desire to move to primary care setting, increasing influence of private sector management styles and organisation (PFI).
- Financing: rationing of services, low rate of expenditure in UK compared to EU on health, increasing pressure on financing

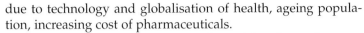

due to technology and globalisation of health, ageing population, increasing cost of pharmaceuticals.

- Priority setting: resource pressures from rising demands, costs,
  fixed budgets. Increasing scope of explicit rationing, including
  evidence-based medicine.
- Leadership and governance: increasing importance of networks, collaboration and interagency working in health,
  importance of leadership roles that involve responsibility
  beyond traditional roles based on hierarchy, position or professional occupation, shift to clinical standards and performance.
- Caring: diminution of caring in concepts of health care, nurses'
  increased responsibility, administrative and managerial roles.
  Most care remains informal and unpaid.
- Information and communications systems: increasing use of
  sophisticated technology for communication, comparison of
  NHS with other industries, IT for individual user rather than
  organisational system, marriage of clinical and financial data,
  relating individual to social data.
- Regulation: increasing level and scope of government regulation through public services, regulation within health concerned with performance, new regulatory bodies at national
  level concerned with health outcomes.
- Health professionals: erosion of professional autonomy, growth
  of management and increasing regulation of professional activities, motivational change in some professionals, problems with
  traditional workforce planning in health based on shortages,
  shifting roles and responsibilities.
- Location of care: increase in substitution of health care location,
  new technologies, mix of staff skills, achieving efficiency gains,
  shift from secondary to primary care, contraction of acute beds
  to medium and intermediate care, blurring of sectoral boundaries in care.

Outcomes that will be measured to test efficiency

- Burden of disease: disease burden shift from young to old, communicable to chronic disease, new infectious diseases. Increases
  in cancers, obesity, children smoking, mental illness including
  depression.
- Efficiency: decentralisation of management to local purchas-
  er/provider organisations, increasing focus on health outcome
  measures, for which location of care, treatment and management of human and financial resources are contributory factors

User participation in decision making

that require individual assessment and review. Efficiency measures drive increasing processes of substitution within health services.

- Effectiveness: use of alternative resource allocation mechanisms to hierarchical control such as service agreements in NHS, performance-related payment systems for providers leading to increased scope and diversity, reform of hospital payment methods tied to outcome measures and overall service objectives, innovation in mechanisms for allocating capital for health including PFI and a redistribution of capital through changing locations of care.
- Performance and benchmarking: increasing concern with organisational performance in health terms with clinical outcomes replacing traditional concerns with finance and administrative process, increasing use of national health targets, increasing desire to link health care funding to improved health outcomes.
- Quality: increasing concern with achieving consistently high standards of service across the NHS, increasing interest in outcomes rather than process measures of quality, increasing concern with measurement, comparisons and evaluation within health service.

The government's commitment to increased funding for the NHS from 2000 to 2004 follows the desire to move the organisation from its roots in welfare to new systems influenced by the needs of the population in the 21st century. The NHS will remain free at the point of delivery, for most interventions, but people are seen to have more disposable income, more people are in work and the government is ensuring that this pressure is continued in the disabled and single parent groups in society.

People's rights to health have not altered but their means of accessing health care have. More diverse methods of gaining information have been implemented: the NHS Direct service provided by nurses on-line and by telephone has influenced demand on health care. Information on the Internet has been improved and is formally designated to inform the public. Health and social service professionals in organisation bases (surgeries and clinics or drop-in centres) are the second level of contact for the public. Although many tasks once undertaken by doctors are now the remit of nurses, now unqualified nurses, physiotherapists and phlebotomists are doing the work, after initial training. These measures are designed to overcome numbers and skills shortages in qualified professionals.

Patients' rights and responsibilities and The NHS Plan

User participation in decision making

Consumers, for their part, are reliant upon the PHTs and commissioners of health and social care to determine local standards and levels of care intervention. However, the role and responsibilities of consumers are based on the NHS as a welfare system. The framework of the system ensures that most health care needs are met but the onus on the individual to participate as a member of collective society and manage their own health will become more apparent. The NHS is focusing on patients and this will eventually reduce demand on the services by devolving some responsibility to the public as partners in developing outcomes measurements for health interventions.

References

Department of Health 2000 The NHS Plan: a plan for investment, a plan for reform. Stationery Office, London

World Health Organization 1997 Highlights on health in the United Kingdom. WHO, Copenhagen

Further reading

Age Concern 1996 Not at my age: why the present breast screening system is failing women aged 65 and over. Age Concern, London

Age Concern 1997 Health care for older people: the ageism issue. Age Concern, London

Alderson P 1990 Choosing for children: parents' consent to surgery. Oxford University Press, Oxford

Allard A 1996 Involving young people – empowered or exploitation? Children and Society 10(2): 165–167

Allsop J, Mulcahy L 1996 Regulating medical work: formal and informal controls. Open University Press, Buckingham

Alzheimer's Disease Society 1997 Experiences of care in residential and nursing homes. Alzheimer's Disease Society, London

Audit Commission 1997 First class delivery: improving maternity services in England and Wales. HMSO, London

Bailar JC, Gornik HL 1997 Cancer undefeated. New England Journal of Medicine 336(22): 1569–1574

Barclay S 1996 Jaymee: the story of Child B. Viking, London

Barham B 1997 Closing the asylum: the mental patient in modern society. Penguin, London

Benzeval M, Judge K 1996 Access to health care in England: continuing inequalities in the distribution of GPs. Journal of Public Health Medicine 18(1): 33–40

Bynoe I 1997 Rights to fair treatment. Institute for Public Policy Research, London

Carr-Hill R 1992 The measurement of patient satisfaction. Journal of Public Health Medicine 14: 236–249

Consumers' Association 1996 The drug information gap. Health Which? October 167–170

Consumers International 1996 Campaigning for patients' rights: a consumer action kit. Consumers International, London

Council of Europe 1994 Participation by citizens-consumers in the management of local public services. Local and Regional Authorities in Europe No. 54. Council of Europe, Strasbourg

Dalziel M, Garrett C 1987 Intra-regional variation in treatment of end stage renal failure. British Medical Journal 294: 1382–1383

Dargie C 1999 Policy futures for UK health; pathfinder. Nuffield Trust and Judge Institute of Management Studies, University of Cambridge, Cambridge

Department of Health 1992 The health of the nation: a strategy for health in England. HMSO, London

Department of Health 1995 A policy framework for commissioning cancer services: a report of the expert advisory group on cancer to the Chief Medical Officers of England and Wales. Department of Health, London

Department of Health 1997 The patient's charter: mental health services. Department of Health, London

Department of Health 1997 The new NHS: modern, dependable. Stationery Office, London

Department of Health 1998 A first class service: quality in the new NHS. Department of Health, London

Department of Health 1998 Our healthier nation. Stationery Office, London

EC 1996 The state of health in the European Community: First Public Health Report. European Commission, Brussels

Fallowfield F, Hall A, Maguire G, Baum M 1990 Psychological outcomes of different treatment policies in women with early cancer outside a clinical trial. British Medical Journal 301: 575–580

Gillam S, Brooks F (eds) 2001 New beginnings: towards patient and public involvement in primary health care. King's Fund, London

Hogg C 1999 Patients, power and politics: from patients to citizens. Sage, London

McIver S 1998 Health debate? An independent evaluation of citizens' juries in a health setting. King's Fund, London

McPherson K 1990 International differences in medical care practices. In: Health care systems in transition: the search for efficiency. OECD, Paris

World Health Organization 1993 Health for All targets: the health policy for Europe. WHO, Copenhagen

Patients' rights and responsibilities and The NHS Plan

Section **Four**

THE IMPLEMENTATION OF STRATEGY AT LOCAL LEVEL

OVERVIEW

Man being . . . by nature all free, equal, and independent, no one can be put out of this estate, and subjected to the political power of another without his own consent. (John Locke 1690 *Second Treatise of Civil Government*, ch. 8, sect. 95)

This extract is one that is frequently used to demonstrate belief in the UK that democracy is a politically and socially accepted way of enabling organisations to generate consensus within their operative workforce and strength of purpose to move forward progressively and productively. Management of health care, the product of health services and methods of delivery combine together as a social exercise. That is, society requires its members to develop a system and ensure it works so that people receive what they need as health care. Management as a social exercise can only take place within a setting where consideration is shared with the people who receive the service and the individuals who shape the system that supports the service. This statement describes a complex social organism that changes perceptively in relation to the political definition of health and welfare at each election or during any reorganisation. It also takes account of the fact that people are different, have differing beliefs, yet can work together to a common purpose.

Public sector organisations are managed by statute and this broad approach to each public organisation's activity mostly coincides with public acceptance of the need for a health service. Policies that are directed at national strategies, such as the epidemiological problems raised by research into genetic manipulation of human chromosomes, may often seem far removed from day-to-day experience of clinical situations. But collectively, each interaction or experiential incident in an organisation, in a unit, ward or trust can be considered as a part of the choreographed movement of people in the system. They constitute variations in the character of organisations. The intraorganisational movements of beliefs, values and people have to be organised or there will be such inefficiency of action and lack of measurable outcomes that anarchy could prevail!

This section contains three main aspects of managing how decisions are made when the direction of the decision has already been formulated. First, the vision or philosophy of an organisation should be manifest in the way that the organisation is moving forward or progressing with its activity. Second, an overarching goal for the organisation should be clear, so that everyone who works in the organisation may be aware of what they are doing and why at an individual and collective level, yet be able to maintain each variation of character that enables change to occur positively. Each organisation interprets national and local policy through its strategies and will incorporate these in its aims so that the organisation flourishes as a whole. What is the reason for this method of enforced planning? Competitors may perish, the strongest organisation will survive:

What is our policy? . . . to wage war against a monstrous tyranny, never surpassed in the dark, lamentable catalogue of human crime. What is our aim? . . . Victory, victory at all costs, victory in spite of all terror; victory however long and hard the road may be; for without victory, there is no survival. (Sir Winston Churchill 1940 Speech. Hansard 13 May, col 1502)

In spite of internal reassurance and external gratification of success, the professionals in health services need more than rhetoric and philosophical words to work together, with patients and within the health system. The regard for change has to be positive for the sake of survival in an organisation. Expectations and needs of patients are incorporated into the planning of new services. These changes take place incrementally. Change and development of the organisation occurs in accordance with evidence for the need for change; efficiencies of costs and outputs, effectiveness and benefits of interventions are usually the drivers for change.

Chapter **Ten**

The practitioner and strategic decision making

Mary Cooke

- ● Introduction
- ● National policy and the influence on local strategy
- ● Promoting policies through strategic planning
- ● The private sector
- ● The role of health workers in developing strategies
- ● Conclusion

I shall be an autocrat; that's my trade. And the good Lord will forgive me; that's his. (Catherine the Great)

You don't manage people; you manage things. You lead people. (Admiral Grace Hoopern, USA)

OVERVIEW

The previous section provides opportunities to look at how government leads people to apply policy concerning the health services in the UK. Of course, various governments will lead in different ways and a view of how governments in other countries develop policies in different ways (Chapter Nine) gives an interesting insight into alternative ways of looking at problems.

Here, the ways in which national strategies can influence how we work 'at the coal face' are described. The methods of canvassing compliance among health professionals as well as users is interesting, using media and campaign initiatives to ensure the policies are implemented through effective strategies by enhanced incentives resulting from successful outcomes. You will have your own examples of how strategic actions can move change in organisations at all levels. Bring those examples with you when you read through this chapter.

INTRODUCTION

The philosophy of an organisation can be seen in its 'mission statement' which will provide the vision for the organisation's future within the context of its operative activities.

Policies are the aims of an organisation, giving direction for any decisions that are made to develop it in parts or as a whole.

Strategy comes from policy. Strategies are the ways in which the aims are enacted. They offer measurements of the success of the aims through benchmarks or milestones. The quality of the strategies and their intentions and the outcomes are all measured in different ways.

Decision making in clinical and managerial practice is guided by issues and standards of quality and also the level of risk contained in each decision for the participants. These points are dealt with in other parts of this book but are mentioned here in relation to the models of strategic planning described.

All parts of an organisation show that they comply with a policy by deciding on the strategy each will apply to fulfil the aims. It can be interesting to look at how a variety of different parts (trusts and health authorities) of a national organisation with a national policy and philosophy can interpret the framework to suit their own local aims for providing care. Interpretation is applied to each local strategy and each local group makes the best use of the resources available in following it through to the clinical level and each patient care package or pathway through the system (Etzioni 1967).

NATIONAL POLICY AND THE INFLUENCE ON LOCAL STRATEGY

So, we will look first at national policy and framework for strategy, then review how local trusts may interpret this and apply it to their mission statement, philosophy or local strategy. A strategy for

The implementation of strategy at local level

reducing teenage pregnancies is used here. Then, the nursing strategy in a trust will be reviewed in relation to the trust strategy and then we can begin to see how nursing decisions about local policy fit into the picture.

National strategy formation and reflexivity of policy development

We need to start with the aims of the NHS, because these lead the analysis of policy development. Other external features to be considered are the policies agreed by the government with the World Health Organization.

The now infamous policy change of the 1990s by Prime Minister Margaret Thatcher, supported by Roy Griffiths, developed the NHS into two sectors. The first sector (purchasers) comprised those organisations that planned and purchased health care as agents on behalf of the public. Secondly, there were providers – those who serviced the needs of the public by commissioning the purchasers. This change in emphasis in policy helped to refocus the NHS on the needs of the public rather than the needs of the professionals and staff who work in the service. This policy was introduced rapidly and without much discussion in Parliament. There were no pilot sites set up for testing the implementation so that all strategies to introduce and develop the policy were simultaneous across the UK. The government had decided that all providers were to become trusts. They were either primary care providers or acute trust providers or a combination of both, where care was provided for smaller populations. The main philosophy was that the health care demands of local people were to be better served by trusts that knew their population's needs. The purchasing authorities would develop profiles of the populations for which they would be contracting through GPs and local health authorities. The policy was developed into strategy from 'the top' down to the local areas and took about 15 years to be implemented. The changes had to be gradual and incremental. Many people lost their jobs as several tiers of management were removed to allow clarity of the decision-making process to occur and be seen to occur.

There needed to be a pathway of accountability so that the government could monitor how its policy was moving through the changes that were occurring. The changes needed to be measurable and clearly accountable. As a result health authorities and regions then became weaker. This was because the government needed to see clearly where decisions were being made, to ensure that government policy was being implemented, and which strategies were more effective. Trusts that used good ways of working were given extra funds and 'areas of best practice' were rewarded in other ways by government. Other confusing activities came from Region, where some strategies were being altered so that individual professional powerbases were being protected. So a tier of management at local level was removed. The trusts then reported directly to the Minister in the government about their strategic plans and activities for change incorporating the purchaser/provider split.

Local GPs began to purchase health care as independent fundholders (and business managers) in association with health authorities. The ways in which costs and budgets were calculated were based solely on past costings and levels of activity. Some contracting activity crossed boundaries with other trusts and confused 'local' with 'locality'. All trusts found it difficult to determine their boundaries. The trusts began to develop their own strategies and plans for building on their successes, where they could expand specific activity from the types of good practice they incorporated in their workforce speciality. The culture of each organisation began to alter to suit each executive team, the plans for each trust and their perceived needs to build up investment in designated areas that were defined by disease diagnosis. Secrecy about who was purchasing what from whom became the norm. Competition was rising but it was not clear whether costs were falling or whether the needs of people were being met. In fact, the costs of providing health care rose inexorably in line with the perceived value of the service by each provider trust, until the government capped activities in accordance with demands for quality and 'value for money' became the deciding feature of contracts. The government directly defined strategy for providers and purchasers at this point.

Health indices and self-assessment of health status by patients became a way of measuring the success of strategies. For some time there was no consideration of the differences between medical practices across the country or level of funding for each diagnostic group.

Health action zones were introduced and locality planning of health services was promoted. The health surveys for England and Wales (now separated) and Scotland began to show further widening gaps in the health status of populations (these publications can be accessed at the website www.opengov.org.uk and will change from time to time). Codes of practice, tax policies and Health & Safety at Work laws were introduced to prevent poor health and promote good health (Downie et al 1992). Other policies were developed to support the health agenda for change to health behaviour such as health promotion. This also includes disease prevention and age/gender-related screening programmes for specific illnesses and health checks for over 65-year-olds and immunisation for under-5s were introduced, coupled with financial incentives focused on the market-managed health system.

The government needed to see how the policy was shaping up in the accounts department – what extra costs was the policy involving? NHS managers found it difficult to decide how much each episode of care cost, how many staff were needed to work for the best effect and what long-term outcomes of each intervention were expected. It was easier to look at the short-term gains but these were not sufficiently positive in relation to the public and political expectations.

The government changed and the policy altered.

Local strategy formation

The managed market was abolished in 1998 by the new Labour government of 1997. GP fundholding practices and purchasing by health authorities were subsumed into primary care organisations, which then became trusts during 2001 and are working towards primary care collaborations for 2004. They were to take over the role of the health authority in purchasing health care for huge populations. The trusts had to publicise their activities, collate their audits and be measured against each other for efficiency and effectiveness. This was because the government, in its intention to become 'open and streamlined', needed to measure successful trusts against poorly performing trusts. Government assured implementation of its policy by publishing league tables of successful trusts that had worked together as a team to gain 'high' standards. This was designed to improve efficiency and effectiveness by using strategies that provided direction for the whole organisation rather than parts of each trust. Strategies of trusts have responded to this accordingly.

It becomes clear that there is a central plan for the NHS, based on focus group research into people's beliefs about health and health care that was defined as the Labour government took over in 1997. This forms the basis for the new policy. Evidence for making plans is available in the form of national (and local) statistics. Data are collected all the time about all aspects of our lives. The National Statistical Office (www.doh.gov.uk/nso) is the website for this. There have been several national surveys showing that

The practitioner and strategic decision making

237

strategies to implement policy affect people's health status and indeed their lifestyle. Planning as a result of this evidence is one way of demonstrating the impact of strategic thinking and developing of policies in an organisation.

Further national, local and internal audits and research described in the plan provide evidence for changes. Funding for the changes follows the more successful management outcomes of strategic development.

An example of developing strategy for local implementation of a national policy

One of the perceived requirements was that the public should take more responsibility for their health status. Into this was built a view that young people and the next generation of adults should become responsible for activities in association with reducing future health costs. One policy or aim is to reduce the high (the highest in Western Europe) rates of teenage pregnancies in the UK (to young women under 18) and the associated risks which include the following.

- Sixty percent of newborn babies are at risk of dying in the first year after birth and children aged 1–3 born to teenage mothers have the highest mortality.
- The sexual health of young women is reduced through rising rates of sexually transmitted infections.
- Only 40% of teenagers receive courses on relationships and sexuality.
- Four out of 10 teenage mothers experience postnatal depression.
- The costs to their primary families through low benefit payments for young people under 18.
- Young women are not encouraged to complete their potential via full or part-time education and are therefore more likely to be unemployed or unemployable.
- The short-term costs of offspring born to poverty and the reducing aspirations of young women in a stigmatising society.
- The government also recognised the need to reduce social exclusion that arises from teenage pregnancy (Payne 2001).

The policy demanded that from October 2000 to March 2001 the primary care organisations (while in the process of merging to become primary care trusts) had to plan their local strategies based on hard evidence of local need. More funds would be available for those trusts that provided full reports and detailed strategies. A government department was created – the Teenage Pregnancy Unit – to monitor and benchmark each health authority that would support the strategy at a local level, within each primary care organisation (DoH 1998).

1. Teams of Public Health Officers in health authorities were appointed.
2. Links within local areas were created between local organisations, voluntary groups, support agencies, social services, youth groups, family planning organisations, health visitors, midwives, health educationists, school nurses, headteachers, women's support centres and many other various groups, charities and professionals.
3. In some areas researchers from higher education were commissioned to review teenagers' ideas and the professionals' views of the issues associated with teenage pregnancy.
4. The local teams (point 2 above) defined the needs for their areas based on resources.
5. These were fed into the health authority strategy for implementation of the plans.
6. The Teenage Pregnancy Unit would decide on the funds allocated and monitor the stages and success of each health authority strategy at a national level.

This is one way of activating a national strategy, based on the guiding principles of reducing variations in health opportunities, that has four broad themes, one of which is the overview of the strategy as a report of 'joined-up local action'. The other three themes are 'the national campaign'; 'better prevention includes relationship education, contraceptive advice and services'; 'better support for teenage parents (including housing and childcare)'. Each theme requires corresponding local action (DoH 1998) which will include health workers, social services managers and head teachers, school governors and project leaders. The resources to support the strategy come from various sources for government funds and include mainstream funds and the Local Implementation Fund.

As a result a strategy is developed and published for understanding the problems of teenagers in a new way and with a different philosophical framework. Other intended outcomes from this initiative are closer working relationships between agencies that provide help and support to young people, the education services and housing authorities. This substantiates the government's

The practitioner and strategic decision making

239

philosophy, provides the framework for their policies and allows specific strategies to be monitored for success and good practice.

PROMOTING POLICIES THROUGH STRATEGIC PLANNING

Planning for health needs not only to involve all sectors of society but all levels of government, employers, workers and communities. Sometimes this is driven by world health policy or a need to provide health care that redetermines the outcomes of health for a given population so that the majority are not made less healthy by the minority. One example of this is the measles, mumps, rubella (MMR) vaccine that was almost compulsory for all babies and children of preschool age. The strategy was to reduce childhood death rates from these diseases and fetal abnormalities and disadvantage from poor opportunities created by loss of education. Fears of adverse events, resulting from research that showed a small percentage of children who developed asthma and breathing difficulties, reduced the number of children vaccinated. The total numbers of the childhood population covered by the immunology programme reduced so that the likelihood of the minority reducing the health of the majority was raised. The science of strategic planning arising from epidemiology has been demonstrated.

Any planning involves six steps.

1. Knowing where you are.
2. Deciding, quantitatively where this is possible, where you want to go and how to get there.
3. Deciding how far you can hope to get towards your target in a period of time (5 or 10 years).
4. Trying to get there in the time period.
5. Regular evaluation to see:
   - how far you have got
   - where you are in relation to the target
   - how you can do better in the future.
6. Amending the implementation plan.

This approach is used by the WHO at both global and regional level. Progress in the 12 global health targets of the Health For All programme (adopted in 1977 and agreed in 1981) is reported to the World Health Assembly every 3 years and an evaluation is made in

The implementation of strategy at local level

the following year. European targets feed into the WHO programme and national targets follow a similar pathway. Countries make their own definitions of the programme and determine their strategies accordingly.

The NHS Plan, published in August 2000, provoked a variety of responses. There are significant changes to structure, intentions and professional activity planned for the NHS and strategies to implement these will be the motivator for many local health links in the future.

These new plans are available at: http://www.doh.gov.uk/whatsnew/index.html

Strategy formation selects broad priorities in the light of the current situation and national development goals. These are then developed into strategies with, where possible, quantitative targets – broad programming. In detailed programming the resources needed to achieve the objective are estimated. Then the programmes are implemented and, finally, evaluated and the lessons learnt are used to revise the programme.

Evaluation is intended to be carried out by those providing the services, those using them and those responsible for managerial control at the different levels of the service. Sometimes this measurement process is called audit, as it is a means by which the quality of a service delivery is evaluated. It has several parts.

- First, it is necessary to reexamine the relevance and priority of the programme against the competing priorities and policies.
- Second, the actual progress has to be assessed against the planned benchmarks for success and criteria for outcomes.
- Third, the efficiency has to be evaluated by comparing the results achieved with the resources used.
- Fourth, the effectiveness of the outcome has to be considered.

Another system change that provides the background for strategies is clinical governance which determines a standard for the quality of the services. Some quality measures have an impact on the way in which services are purchased. If a service is of low quality then the purchasers will need to review their costs, to reduce them by reducing provision or raise funding of the service so that a higher quality can be achieved if the costs have not been calculated well. Øvretveit (1995) offers a succinct coverage of the features of purchasing for health and the measures to take to assure standards of care.

Commissioning for health care (planning and buying health care services according to the needs of a local population) incorporates features of both private and public purchasing (Fig. 10.1). In

The practitioner and strategic decision making

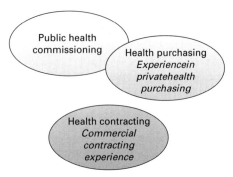

Figure 10.1   Health 'commissioning' is broader than 'purchasing' and 'contracting' and draws on experience from the commercial sector.

the past, it was largely concerned with contracting providers and mostly with acute hospitals. In the future, purchasing will be more strategic and less provider driven, with a greater understanding of the cost effectiveness of services and of other health-enhancing activities and with new types of services and treatments provided outside hospitals. Health-enhancing activities could mean further guidance for people when deciding on lifestyles and risks that are taken when, for example, we go skiing on holiday or take a car rather than a measurably safer rail journey or an air trip.

Risks related to strategies are mainly associated with costs and short-term outcomes rather than investments in long-term gains. In the UK, local strategies will be assessed through National Service Frameworks. Many new standards have been set and government measures introduced to assure they are upheld. The focus is on determining the expectations of the public and ensuring that the NHS and social services can meet these expectations.

THE PRIVATE SECTOR

The private health sector has been invited to work alongside the government to reduce waiting lists and to bid for work to be purchased by the commissioning agencies. Strategies for raising the health status of the public have to include all agencies, social services, local government and therefore not-for-profit and private for-profit organisations.

All these organisations relate to the NHS in many ways. It has taken nearly 50 years for the government to realise, though, that the major determinants of health lie outside the health care system and that inequities in health are only likely to be radically reduced through actions involving such sectors as income distribution, housing, agriculture, education and the environment (WHO 1986, p. 19).

The private sector is generally staffed by people who have been trained in the public health service, but often education facilities in private health care are open to trainees. The planning of health care as described above has to take account of housing, education and social policy sectors in order to make any progress. There are private and public agencies to contract for the supply of services and who also form a part of the method for evaluating the outcomes of the plans. The private sector has its own, often competing objectives and in some facilities, substantial power is exerted by external donors and international agencies which have their own agendas that may differ from those of the organisation. Some professional policy makers and strategists may favour the interests of their own groups (Walt & Vaughan 1986).

Strategies may also encounter opposition from powerful local interests. To be effective, planning and strategy implementation often becomes a process of negotiation and frequently develops into a tension between the desire of the centre to have its way and the need for local flexibility and discretion.

THE ROLE OF HEALTH WORKERS IN DEVELOPING STRATEGIES

Strategic documents from trusts are agreed for a time period of 3, 5 or 10 years. The government strategy for reducing teenage concep-

---

Box 10.1 Structures to support strategy decisions and resource use (adapted from Lee & Mills 1982, p. 89)

Target groups	Age, sex, income level, social class, ethnic group, geographical area
Function of services	Prevention, treatment, promotion, rehabilitation, support
Levels of care	Primary, secondary, tertiary
Broad disease problems	Malaria, diarrhoeal diseases, tuberculosis, AIDS, etc.
Client or diagnostic groups	Mentally ill, mentally handicapped, aged, children, pregnant mothers, etc.
Clinical specialities	Surgery, general medicine, etc.
Degree of dependence	Nursing and social support needed

The practitioner and strategic decision making

tion rates by 50% by 2010 described above is intended to be carried through over 10 years. Some strategies like this can be used to recruit, retrain and retain staff in health services. Other projects utilise people and their skills for short-term contractual periods or secondments. Usually, strategies are already agreed when people are recruited in this way and implementation of the strategy is all that is required. Some trusts accept the need to adopt a 'bottom-up' approach to planning, where staff involvement in the strategy and their 'ownership' of the project mean that it will be more successfully implemented and evaluated.

One such plan is the 'strategic direction document for nursing' that one trust drew up in response to its trust strategic direction statement. The stated aim of the trust is: 'to excel in treating patients' illnesses, promoting health and supporting health care education and research'. The objectives of the nursing strategy are therefore designed to complement the overall aims as far as possible.

A meeting of all senior nurses in the trust took place on an 'away' half day. The strategy was formulated through the various methods of 'forming', 'storming', 'norming' and 'performing' processes and thinking through the implications of how, where, when and who would be involved in the implementation of the strategy. First, the groups needed to define their rationale for the strategy.

We have attempted to keep our strategy succinct and our aims measurable in the belief that it will help to focus nursing activity in a world of constant change and pressure. We believe that it is flexible enough to adapt for the future, yet provide an anchor against the pressure of internal and external professional reviews yet to come.

Here, the group felt that an exercise such as this needed credence for the future, knowing that validity of practice as professionals was likely to be questioned.

Four themes were then identified from the trust's strategic direction statement and these were applied to practice.

1. The quality of nursing care
2. Clinical career pathways
3. Shaping the future of nursing practice
4. Research and development

These themes were then supported by statements of intent or goals that would be used to evaluate the level of success with which they were applied. Very clear targets were then identified that showed nurses on the units how they could contribute to the success of the strategy. The strategy was then circulated to all nurses in the trust attached to their pay slips and their return comments were collated for further circulation in each unit. In this way all nurses who wanted to be involved contributed to the strategy and were able to recognise

(continued)

(continued)

the part they played in its construction. A nursing and midwifery workforce of some 2500 people was contacted and communicated with in this way. The final strategic direction document was disseminated to all the managers in the trust and the nurses.

From this exercise, several role development needs were identified that were required to ensure the strategy would be applicable. These developments then created a clarification for career pathways for nurses at 'F' and 'G' grades. A programme was then devised and implemented to allow these nurses to gain management skills in support of changes in their roles. The result was a strongly supportive nursing workforce that could self-assess and understand how to discriminate between decisions concerning patients and those concerning the organisation. A further programme to identify and promote leadership was developed; however, it was found that this encouraged people to apply for posts in other trusts so in order to retain staff, the leadership programme became associated with the needs of the trust alone rather than management generally.

The strength of the exercise is that all the nurses who wanted to be involved could contribute. There were, of course, others who commented afterwards that they had not seen the papers and would have participated . . . this is inevitable in such a large organisation. Other outcomes of the exercise were that some nurses in particular specialities decided to apply the strategy to their role and clinical area in a more individual way. They created standards for practice and clinical guidelines for the education of staff. Some of these were then brought to the nursing Policy and Standards Committee. The work was not only disseminated across the trust but the pockets of good practice were used to raise the standards for other units. For example, venepuncture training booklets, guidelines and packages are now used to support internal training over all units. Nurses are expected to be responsible for their training and updating in line with Professional Education and Practice submissions and collation of material for portfolios.

CONCLUSION

Strategy formation cannot occur without sound policies with which to guide the focus for decision making in any organisation. The stakeholders in an organisation are all the workforce, not only professionals but also support staff and even external contractors who work on short-term projects in the organisation.

Strategies will only work if they can be applied to the roles of people and the consumers/users of services who carry them through

The practitioner and strategic decision making

within the culture of any organisation. Therefore everyone has to agree, either implicitly or explicitly, with the policies and strategies. To create strategies at the bottom of an organisation and have them taken to the top management is difficult but where a team of people work in a supportive manner, their roles and practices are seen as exemplary and their ideas can influence the organisation at all levels.

Theories of strategy formation are available and the main principles lie in planning. These principles have been used in this chapter to underpin examples of strategy formation and policy definition at world, national, local and individual level.

Acknowledgement

The author wishes to formally acknowledge and recognise the work done in 1997–98, in the Addenbrooke's NHS Trust Central Nursing Department, where she was privileged to participate in creating the Nursing Strategic Direction Document, published in 1999.

References

Department of Health, Social Exclusion Unit 1998 Teenage pregnancy. Department of Health, Social Exclusion Unit, London

Downie R, Fife C, Tannahill A 1992 Health promotion models and values. Oxford University Press, Oxford

Etzioni A 1967 Mixed scanning: a third approach to decision-making. Public Administration Review 4: 7–17

Lee K, Mills A 1982 Policy making and planning in the health sector. Croom Helm, London

Øvretveit J 1995 Purchasing for health. Open University Press, Buckingham

Payne D 2001 Babies of teen age mothers 60% more likely to die: news extra. British Medical Journal 322: 386

Walt G, Vaughan 1986 Politics of health planning. World Health Forum 7: 31–37

World Health Organization 1986 Intersectoral action for health. WHO, Geneva

Application **10:1**
Josephine Nwaelene

User involvement in strategic information planning in a chemical pathology unit:

extracts from a management project

This application looks at the problems experienced by a chemical pathology laboratory in producing quality output within the limitations of their information system. The officer who undertook this project decided that the most effective way to bring about change was to gather evidence of the current system's limitations as perceived by the workforce and, from this, suggest some practical changes that might be feasible within existing resource restrictions. She clearly appreciated the overall strategic drive of the NHS and that, unfortunately, this particular strategic area had been fraught with mistakes and inefficiencies. In working within existing strategic implementation in this way, she hoped to encourage a shift in a direction that would match the needs of the future rather than just of the present.

INTRODUCTION

Having always been enthusiastic about health care, I trained as a medical laboratory scientific officer and currently work in a busy chemical pathology laboratory in an NHS trust. This handles a workload of approximately 3 million tests per annum. I am involved in analysing patient and quality control samples. These require attention to accuracy and the ability to use the information systems for problem solving and to meet deadlines.

Generally, it is felt that the NHS has failed to use technology in an innovative way to support the improvement of the quality of health care and help deliver integrated services. In this NHS trust, there is the perception that the information technology infrastructure of the laboratory is inadequate and that this denies the lab's workforce the ability to meet the organisation's mission and goals. The chemical pathology department's information system is not flexible in terms of where to print patient reports, resulting in delay in GP patients receiving their test results. The ability to print locally and also to print at ward/outpatient locations would speed up the diagnostic process.

Because of these perceptions, it was decided to assess the current level of support given to the chemical pathology services by the existing information system, LMX. As a result, it was hoped to be able to make some recommendations to management.

THE RESEARCH

Data were gathered by means of a questionnaire containing nine questions. The first question asked for the respondent's grade. The following five questions asked the respondent to rate the current network information support system with respect to timeliness, adequacy, consistency, accuracy, cost savings.

Respondents were then asked if the current system increased production output and/or decreased staff workload. The final question concerned flexibility of the LMX and whether the current system would adapt to the changing needs of the pathology services.

RESULTS

Of the 200 questionnaires sent out, 185 were completed and returned. Of these, 22 were from clerical staff, 53 from medical lab assistants, 83 from medical lab scientific officers and 27 from managers. The answers can be summarised as follows.

- Timeliness – 69% poor, 31% average
- Adequacy – 98% inadequate, 2% adequate
- Consistency – 98% inconsistent, 2% no response
- Accuracy – 70% inaccurate, 21% not sure, 9% no response
- Cost effectiveness – 68% no savings, 32% no response
- Increased productivity – 52% no increase, 11% some increase, 37% not sure
- Increased workload – 71% increased, 29% no increase
- Flexibility – 76% inflexible, 22% flexible, 2% no response

These results were then considered alongside existing knowledge of operational practices.

The implementation of strategy at local level

EVALUATION AND DISCUSSION

The NHS is currently faced with a number of problems which include inadequate resource availability. For this reason, rationing and prioritising need to take place.

In order to assess and prioritise information systems activities, it seemed advisable to examine the current information system environment and attempt to predict the gap between current and future requirements. This assessment entailed obtaining a description of the functions performed by the current information system and its technical and functional effectiveness, as well as the opinions of the lab staff in terms of the usability of the system.

The analysis of the questionnaire confirmed that there were several problems with the current information system in the chemical pathology department. The problems included productivity of test results, the actual workload in the lab, flexibility, cost and quality issues.

The concept of productivity seeks to explore the quantitative relationship between the inputs and outputs of the current system. Productivity measurement is of interest to all members of staff in the lab, particularly the medical laboratory scientific officers as they are responsible for carrying out analytical assays on patient samples. It is also of particular interest to the operations managers as productivity measurement and forecasts are a crucial part of operational planning and control. Productivity is therefore intimately related to expectations of performance and quality.

The response to the questionnaire strongly suggested that the current information system did not reduce operation costs. Frequently, assays were rerun to ensure good precision. This resulted in a high level of expenditure on consumables. Also, the system encouraged excess use of paper. A new system needed to be designed whereby error messages were stored in the system for at least 24 hours.

To achieve cost leadership, chemical pathology must offer services which are fully acceptable to the consumer. These may be considered 'high quality' in the sense of conformity to specification. This may involve the organisation in some hard choices to be sure that its services exactly match consumer needs with no extra costly features.

CONCLUSION AND RECOMMENDATIONS

As with other business managers in the trust, pathology lab managers must always plan how they might achieve the objectives of the department. Strategies which are appropriate, feasible and desirable are most likely to help the department to achieve its mission and goals. However, the health care environment tends to be turbulent and unpredictable and strategic planning requires flexibility. New opportunities must be recognised and appropriate changes introduced continuously.

User involvement in strategic information planning

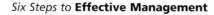

Six Steps to **Effective Management**

The analysis of the current information system must be used to make decisions on what would add best value to the pathology services. However, management has to consider the availability of internal resources (e.g. financial and human). It is important that serious functional weaknesses that might be preventing the lab from delivering a value service are minimised or eradicated. For this reason, management should be aware of technological opportunities which they could use to enhance the system's effectiveness.

It is suggested that improvements to the information system should focus on the following areas.

- Increased value to patients.
- Greater flexibility to accommodate future changes.
- Creation of a culture of high quality.

Proposed strategies for the near future could be as follows.

- Review the most cost-effective way to deliver specialised tests.
- Evaluate possible replacement of manual immunoassays.
- Introduce new chemistry analysers.
- Replace current HPLC equipment for assay of urine 5HIAA, HVA and plasma catecholamines.
- Link Behring BN2 and Immulite 2000 analysers to LMX lab computer.
- Improve dialogue with clinical groups, particularly paediatrics and oncology.
- Look for ways of improving the current networks and servers.
- Improve the quality of information entered into the PAS.
- Audit protocols against accepted best practice.

It is hoped that the evidence presented will facilitate the implementation of the above recommendations.

COMMENTS

The above extract, while omitting the additional work carried out by the scientific officer on examining the motivational and training requirements of the chemical laboratory staff, is still sufficient to demonstrate the potential for involvement at practitioner level with the modification of strategic issues. The officer was realistic in her suggestions for change, looking for improvements to the current system rather than, at this stage, the introduction of a totally new system that would carry a major cost implication. The involvement of such a large number of the staff, while potentially raising expectations that could not be fulfilled, could still be seen as an important tool for persuading senior management of the need for action and for gaining practitioner cooperation and ownership of future change.

Application **10:2**

Lenore Anderson

Reengineering: a case study

The NHS has been in a state of change over three decades. These changes have been in phases, usually as a result of a part of the system needing overhauling. Because so many of the changes were disjointed, they have not been coordinated to the needs of the organisation. Each organisation is responsible for its resource use, buildings, staff, expertise, capacity and capability. These assets are fluid. Some organisations have more, or 'better', assets than others and recruitment of staff from one place to another alters the range of assets of an organisation at any given time. There are times when an objective view of the organisation is required. Several trusts went through a process called 'reengineering' during the late 1990s, to try and reconstitute their management and systems structures so that they would be more efficient and therefore more effective. This case study offers an example of the process, from the personal perspective of a member of the reengineering team.

THE REENGINEERING PROCESS

Reengineering is a process by which a situation is examined in detail and a redesigned process is identified, implemented and evaluated to achieve an improved quality and/or financial outcome. The process involves the following stages.

1. Choose the reengineering team members.
2. Undertake a scoping study to identify projects that could lead to improved outcomes.
3. Identify and manage stakeholders; these people should then take ownership of the project and become the change agents that deliver a successful outcome.
4. Agree the projects that you will run with. Start with ideas that give you a quick win; this is known as 'cherry picking'. Success breeds success and later you can try more difficult problems, supported by your past success.

5. Test your project objectives in a pilot study.
6. Identify the benefits and risks associated with 'going live'.
7. Build a business case based on your pilot findings.
8. Manage your stakeholders to support your business case.
9. If your business case is rejected, find another route to success.
10. Monitor and evaluate the 'live project' to ensure that you are minimising the risks while maximising the benefits.
11. Celebrate success, but allow time for the change to become the norm and be embedded in the organisation's culture.

THE STUDY

The trust is an acute teaching hospital that has approximately 1300 beds and employs some 5000 staff with an annual turnover of £185 million. During the period 1998–99 over 82 000 patients were treated as either inpatients or day cases. Nearly 343 000 outpatient consultations took place. The trust embarked on a reengineering process to reduce the length of inpatient stay and improve the quality of patient care.

SCOPING

We held workshops and meetings with GPs, surrounding trusts and social services, resulting in the identification of a number of projects. Anecdotally, it emerged that patient discharges were delayed unnecessarily and in particular by external forces. The delayed discharges were defined as patients who required complex support from one or more agencies to facilitate a quality discharge from an acute trust. The scoping study indicated that complex discharge patients comprise 4% (3280 patients) of the total discharges from the trust.

A more detailed retrospective analysis of 120 medical, nursing, physiotherapy and occupational therapy case notes deemed as complex identified factors that contributed to delays in patient discharge.

- Discharge planning was fragmented with no clear accountability.
- Documentation was incomplete and varied from ward to ward.
- Referrals were late for 'needs-led' assessment.
- The causes of delayed discharge were 48% internal and 52% external to the trust. This exploded the hypothesis that the causes were outside the trust's own control.
- The highest cause of internal delay was referral to the occupational therapy (OT) service, at 32% of the total causes.
- The main origin of the delays in referral to OT were patients whose admission was via the accident service and medical admissions unit and patients outlying in wards not appropriate to their diagnostic grouping. These areas had no dedicated OT

service, as no funding had been made available. Patients had to wait until they transferred to their appropriate diagnostic ward.

A reengineering subgroup was formed to identify some solutions; this group included both internal and external trust stakeholders. It was important to find proactive members from all professions and agencies, so that ownership of the reengineering process was assured.

'CHERRY-PICKING' SOLUTIONS

Two projects were identified as likely to gain the most benefits for the trust: the introduction of a standard one-stop discharge document across the trust and the introduction of a rapid-response OT service. The second is described here.

A reengineering subgroup was formed and stakeholders identified to carry this project forward, enhanced by the creation of a rapid-response occupational therapist service.

PILOTING

A pilot study over a 13-week period was undertaken, its main aims being:

- proactive targeting of patients to avoid ward admission from attendees at the accident service and medical admissions unit
- to fast track patients in the admissions ward, to reduce the overall length of stay, preventing patients becoming dependent due to protracted hospital admission
- to respond to urgent requests for assessment during bed shortages
- to improve the quality of the care packages for individual patients.

Pilot findings

- The findings indicated that between 1100 and 1200 bed days could be saved per year.
- A new focus OT assessment tool identified the patients' needs and helped in the decision-making process that aided a safe patient discharge.
- The workload of the therapists was captured using the GRASP © Systems workload measurement tool (see Appendix) that quantified the resources required to achieve the pilot aims. The workload pilot and live studies were compared (see Table 10.2.1).

LIVE SERVICE

- A business case was presented to the trust board but failed to gain the required funding. It was agreed that the pilot study had

Table 10.2.1 GRASP © Systems workload data (age of patients 35–104 years)

Activity daily	Pilot data 13 weeks	Live data Jan–April 1999	Live data Jan–April 2000
No. of patients assessed	3.6 pts	5.35 pts	6.44 pts
No. of patients seen at assessment given a discharge on that day	0.65 pts	1.0 pt	0.9 pts
Contact time per patient	1.9 hours	1.3 hours	1.12 hours
Administration (including coordinating appropriate care packages)	1.0 hour	1.29 hours	2.2 hours
Meetings	0.75 hours	0.24 hours	0.59 hours
Proactive liaison	0.9 hours	0.8 hours	0.7 hours
Total required service hours	9.45 hours	9.28 hours	10.6 hours
Budgeted hours	7.2 hours	7.2 hours	7.2 hours
Provided hours	8.0 hours	8.35 hours	8.4 hours
Utilisation % (balance between workload and staff available)**	119%	111%	117%
WTEs required (5-day week)	1.5	1.5	1.68
Overtime worked	1.45 hours	0.93 hours	2.2 hours
Actual utilisation % (excluding overtime)	131%	129%	147%
Overall reduction in length of stay (days)	9.2	4.7	6.3*
Number of bed days saved per working year	1196	940	1191
Gross benefit pa @ £50 per day	59.8k	47.0k	57.5k
Staff costs pa	32.0k	21.0k #	32.0k
Nett cost savings pa[†]	27.8k	26.0k	27.5k

\# Staffing problems

* Other initiatives in A&E and community reduced the potential for this service to be the sole reason for a quality discharge

† Savings not realised as beds used for new emergencies or waiting list patients

** GRASP © Systems utilisation %:

    90–110% – creates a quality climate for both patients and staff
    111–125% – staff working to their maximum capacity
    126–150% – creating a quality gap
    > 150% – staff and patients potentially 'at risk'

The implementation of strategy at local level

proved that the changes were effective in that they improved the quality and timeliness of the care packages provided and that bed days could be released for emergencies and waiting list cases. The business case failed because it could not provide actual financial savings unless beds were closed and the project required £32 000 a year to fund.

- Following the failure to gain trust board support, we turned to major stakeholders, the chief nurse and medical consultants and presented our business case to the health authority. This bid was successful and the project went 'live' in January 1999.
- Two further 13-week studies were undertaken (see Table 10.2.1) to quantify the success of the reengineering process and the project outcomes.

CELEBRATION

Since the development of the rapid-response occupational therapist service, other teams of professionals such as A&E discharge planning nurses and discharge planning teams in the MAU have been developed and this service is at the heart of their success.

The project has been presented at local and national conferences and came second in the Eastern Region Danbury Quality Awards, Anglia Polytechnic University Business School 1999.

This case study indicates that, even if you have a good idea, that does not guarantee success as the reengineering process is fraught with problems. But if the change process is managed in a flexible way, good ideas will succeed.

APPENDIX: GRASP © SYSTEMS WORKLOAD TOOL

GRASP is an acronym for Grace Reynolds Application of the Study of PETO. The PETO study takes its name from the four researchers Poland, English, Thornton and Owens: three nurses and a medical director who developed a research methodology for measuring workload based on the individual needs of patients and staff.

Useful address

GRASP © Systems, Nurse Consultants International Ltd, 82 Deepwell Avenue, Halfway, Sheffield S20 5ST, UK

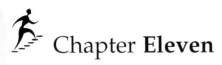

Chapter **Eleven**

Autonomy and initiative in implementing strategic decisions

Ann P Young

- **The implementation of strategic change**
- **Organisational control and managerial discretion**
- **The use of group processes**
- **Psychological reasons for individual variations**
- **Conclusion**

> The first step in change mastery is understanding how individuals can exert leverage in an organisation. (Kanter 1984, p. 209)

OVERVIEW

As must by now be very apparent, decision making is neither simple nor rational. It is with this in mind that this chapter explores the degree of autonomy and initiative that health care managers and practitioners have in the implementation of strategic decisions. For this, it will use a three-pronged approach of organisational style, group dynamics and personal preference.

The structure of the chapter is as follows.

- Variations in the implementation of strategic change.
- Techniques of organisational control, particularly looking at rules, targets and cultural norms and expectations.

The implementation of strategy et local level

- The use of group processes in implementing change with an examination of the use of power resources and preferred group roles.
- Personal responses to change with a focus on some psychological reasons for individual variations.

Throughout the chapter, the potential scope of the health care professional in the exercise of autonomy and initiative will be identified. Conclusions will be drawn on identifying and using personal space within the sometimes impersonal structures of the health care organisation.

THE IMPLEMENTATION OF STRATEGIC CHANGE

Health care practitioners work in a variety of settings but the majority in large organisations. Whether these are public or private, the usual pattern is for major change to be imposed by the chief executive on behalf of either government or shareholders. Even in the smaller concern, the owner often acts autocratically in making decisions.

However, this does not mean that health care professionals cannot have a marked influence on strategic outcomes. The initiation and implementation of change are very much a process of action and reaction and the following factors seem to be particularly important in health care.

- Degree of clarity of original strategic action.
- Detail contained in instructions for implementation of strategic decisions.
- Visibility of required outcomes.
- Follow-up on success or otherwise of implementation.
- Respective power relations of participants.

Degree of clarity of original strategic action

John Argenti (1993), in his book *Your Organization: What is it For?*, was particularly critical of the public sector's lack of clarity as to its aims and objectives. However, with multiple stakeholders it may be impossible to get agreement on a single-minded strategic direction. Health promotion versus illness treatment, emergency versus chronic care, high technology versus tender loving care all have a place but with limited resources, deciding priorities is difficult.

Detail contained in instructions for implementation

With the majority of health care under the umbrella of the NHS, the government sees it as politically important to direct strategy through the normal statutory processes of Parliament. Although statutes are supplemented by statutory rules and the NHS Executive supplies additional guidelines, the historical tradition in the UK has been for statute to lay only a fairly broad requirement on its public sector organisations. This does leave space for variations in the detail of interpretation at a more local level.

Visibility of required outcomes

Assuming that certain strategic outcomes are reasonably well defined, their visibility may be variable. An obvious required outcome of repeated strategic change over the last 15 years has been for costs to be contained. However, although the overall figures demonstrate a failure in achieving this, it is difficult to identify where there have been successes and where failures with accounting systems that have only gradually been reconstituted to reflect real costs and where the introduction of computer technology has been notorious for its failures.

More recently, government outcomes have been stated much more precisely (see section on Targets below) but their relationship to strategy must be questioned. Although highly visible, such as cutting waiting list times, they relate much more obviously to specific operational issues than more integrated strategic ones.

Follow-up on success or otherwise of implementation

The failure of changes to survive the immediate implementation stage has been the concern of a number of management researchers (Beer 1980, Kanter 1984). Several factors can be identified for this:

- change in leadership of the strategic change
- management systems not altered to support new strategy
- lack of support, understanding and commitment at practitioner level
- new strategy not made part of current organisational culture.

Such failures can occur in both public and private health care as the executive moves from one initiative to the next without adequate consolidation and evaluation of the first. For the public sector, the NHS has been a prime candidate for government interference due

The implementation of strategy at local level

to public sensitivity and political concern around the ballot box. In the private sector, increasing competition has encouraged a faster rate of change particularly associated with cost control and quality. In all sectors, as one change is implemented, it tends to get put to one side to make room for the next without proper follow-up.

Respective power relations of participants

There are many pressures for maintaining the status quo. One of the most important is that change may alter current power relations. Certainly, for the NHS, one of the aims of introducing general management in the 1980s was to curtail medical power. However, the implementation of government strategies has frequently had to be modified, even before being taken through Parliament, due to the power of the major stakeholders in health care. As Harrison & Pollitt (1994) pointed out, professionals can be challenged over or incorporated in any major changes. Evidence suggests that where incorporated, professionals will seek to reduce the managerialist implications of government strategy while, if challenged, some doctors will choose to ignore the changes and continue to work in their own way (Parker & Dent 1996).

ORGANISATIONAL CONTROL AND MANAGERIAL DISCRETION

With so much likely to lead to implementation failure, it is important that organisations do control their workforce in some way in order to avoid anarchy, although these controls may be both varied and unobtrusive.

Techniques of organisational control can be grouped into three main divisions (Child 1984):

- rules
- targets
- cultural norms.

These will be discussed in turn along with the scope for autonomy and initiative within their respective frameworks.

Rules

It is difficult to imagine any organisation without rules but some workplaces are more rule bound than others. The bureaucratic organisation typically uses rules to maintain clarity of purpose, roles and processes. Rules may have the status of law (for example, around employment legislation) or be decided locally (policies and procedures). The formal status of these will also vary but employees will normally have to have a sound reason for not following them or face disciplinary action.

In the implementation of major change, a number of dilemmas can arise. A situation is created where there is likely to be a lack of clarity. Old rules no longer seem to fit the new situations, new rules have to be constructed and communicated but this takes time. For the health care professional, several options are available:

- manipulate the old rules to fit the new situation
- create new rules to apply to local situations, even if this is done without going through the formal processes
- ignore the need for rules and base action on collaboration and consensus.

The need to still use the old rules seems to arise particularly around employment situations. How to define and pay jobs that are new or markedly changed and that no longer fit within the old hierarchy calls for some creativity. Managers are unwilling to risk jettisoning old rules in order to maintain cordial relationships with unions. Ways need to be found of maintaining the spirit of the old rule while making some modifications in its interpretation. For this to work, there needs to be respect and trust between the decision makers.

The usefulness of creating new rules means that the individual health care worker still feels that some control is being maintained. This may be important where the organisation is interfacing with external agencies where reliance on goodwill may be difficult to maintain. As collaborative ventures and external networks are seen as increasingly important in health care, systems of developing new rules rapidly and effectively should perhaps be developed. Bureaucratic processes are usually too slow and long-winded for current activities.

Health care professionals may decide to ignore the rules and work without them. This can arise in an emergency situation where others are left to worry about the rules while the professional gets on with the job in hand. To act alone may be justifiable but does carry a high risk. To act jointly with others adds support to the decision to ignore the rules and in the long run may encourage the organisation to reconsider the appropriateness of some of its rules in changing situations. It seems likely that such behaviour is usually enacted to support the overall aims of the organisation, rather than to undermine them (Brower & Abolafia 1995) and ideally should be viewed in a positive light.

Targets

Outcome and output measures are increasingly important in a competitive and resource-constrained environment. Although not new to the private sector, they have recently become much more explicit in the public arena and throughout both sectors are being applied more widely than just to financial measures.

Not surprisingly, one important system of organisational control is around the setting and meeting of measurable targets. One school of thought suggests that these can be motivational (Emmanuel et al 1990) but only if they stand a reasonable chance of being achieved. Some difficulties may arise in the public sector if financial and patient throughput targets in, for example, acute surgery are jeopardised by high numbers of emergency admissions.

As Young (1996a, p. 350) pointed out, 'Who chooses what measures is a question that should also be asked'. The government was largely instrumental in leading the move to output measures although professionals have not been averse to this in principle. However, initial measures chosen seemed to rely on what was most readily available and not on what was necessarily most useful and reliable (Spiers 1995).

Since then, nurses have adopted a range of output measures as part of quality initiatives with some success. Two drawbacks are that setting measurable targets for some aspects of quality care is difficult and often inconclusive while an emphasis on outputs may hide undesirable outcomes. For example, decreasing length of inpatient stay may place increased demands on carers and community services which have financial implications that should be offset against the hospital savings made.

For the practitioner, an involvement with targets seems unavoidable. Greater clarity and recognition of the purpose of care given by health care professionals other than doctors are on the whole positive to both the professional and the organisation. In most organisations, the professional standing of the practitioner is respected and decisions on clinical targets are negotiated and agreed, with the professional having a major voice in this process. For other targets, the picture is more mixed. Where finance and staff numbers are concerned, the professional is likely to have less authority but may still be able to negotiate targets on the basis of

Autonomy and initiative in implementing strategic decisions

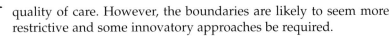

quality of care. However, the boundaries are likely to seem more restrictive and some innovatory approaches be required.

Cultural norms

The strongest type of organisational control is through the use of culture. If an organisation has a very strong and cohesive culture, without consciously realising it, workers are likely to see the same things as important, be aiming for targets that achieve and maintain these things and tend to behave in ways very similar to each other. The need for formal rules and explicit targets is minimal. In fact, if rules and targets are proposed that fail to match with the culture, they will simply be ignored. In such an organisation, there seems to be plenty of freedom and scope for initiative as, by choice, the employee will only choose to behave in ways that match the culture.

However, very few organisations have such pervasive control although elements of it may be recognised amongst certain professional-led concerns. This may include health care but, on the whole, the bureaucratic pattern of behaviour is as strong, if not stronger, than the professional one although the latter cannot be ignored as it has implications for the implementation of strategy.

Cultural norms are slow to change. Therefore, the implementation of imposed strategy in these circumstances is likely to be uncertain or unsuccessful. Certainly the imposition of markets, 'managed' or 'quasi' though they were, was only partially successful as a competitive market approach was so alien to the health care professional culture. Beliefs in equality, collaboration and the public good seemed at odds with contracts, business plans and a secretive environment (Young 1996b).

For health care professionals, their view of autonomy hinges largely on this professional culture. Health care organisations are very much multicultural concerns, with a number of professional, business and managerial perspectives. Such a plurality of groups, while potentially leading to conflict, does avoid the almost unseen straitjacket of one strong unitary culture that is almost impossible to resist. Practitioners and middle managers have become adept at moving between these different cultures. In the implementation of strategy, they will use different arguments with different superiors in order to facilitate the choices that they want to make. For example, cost–benefit analysis will be heard by the finance manager, quality initiatives will be supported by the director of nursing and the use of clinical knowledge will be respected by medical colleagues.

The implementation of strategy at local level

The discussion so far has focused on the possibilities for autonomy and initiative within the organisation as a whole. However, although strategy is usually imposed via the executive and filtered through the hierarchy, health care structures have become less bureaucratic. Increasingly health care professionals are being expected to participate in strategic implementation within project groups. Even within the hierarchy, there is usually an expectation of some shared decision making with immediate peers and subordinates. An understanding of group processes and the possible scope for autonomy and initiative in these settings is therefore important.

It seems likely that the main sources of scope for the health care professional are through the use of:

- power resources
- preferred group roles
- group processes.

Power resources

Most individuals have access to certain power resources. Dahl (1961) suggested that no individual as a member of a group is entirely lacking in access to some influence resources although these are unequally distributed. In an organisational setting, an important point to emphasise is that the individual is a member of at least one group, probably more than one, that can call on particular resources. The health care professional is part of a particular professional group, an employee of a multiprofessional directorate, a member of a project team, a participant in a staff development exercise, and so on. People are often surprised at how, by extending the number of groups within which they operate, they can markedly increase their sphere of effective action.

In a community setting, Dahl identified the power of social standing, access to wealth, access to legal powers of office, popularity and control over information. For the health care professional, these need to be reinterpreted. Popularity and control over information are potentially interesting to the practitioner who may feel low status and poorly paid compared to a number of other professional and managerial colleagues. Popularity is a difficult concept but the popular individual is someone who is well known in the organisation. Length of time in the organisation seems to be important here as well as approachability. The deputy who satisfies these criteria may well have more influence on the implementation of strategy than his or her boss who has only recently taken up post. The porter or receptionist who is in contact with a large number of individuals every day can choose to facilitate or sabotage change through control of the informal grapevine. This may seem rather an extreme example but professionals who undertake roles that frequently bring them in touch with a large number of strategically key individuals can use this as a source of power.

Morgan (1997) listed some important sources of organisational power (p. 171). In addition to those already mentioned, there are:

- control of scarce resources
- control of boundaries
- control of technology
- control of counterorganisations.

These resources are only sources of power in a group if they are not found in other members of that group. Control over a budget equal in size to those held by others in the group will not give power; sole control of specific external alliances needed to develop particular strategic collaborations may well do so.

As Dahl discovered, a resource is only ever a potential source of influence. For some reason, individuals may choose not to use an available resource. This chapter now moves on to discuss some individual differences displayed by members of a group.

Preferred group roles

Belbin's team roles are widely known and used but he extended his ideas to identify which of these seem to match with clearly prescribed work and which roles facilitated a greater degree of scope and freedom (Belbin 1997).

Those individuals least willing to make use of any scope for initiative would be 'completers' and 'implementers' where their greatest satisfaction is gained from painstaking application. 'Specialists' may also be content to follow prescribed work instructions if they relate to their specialisms.

Those that prefer some room to manoeuvre and to be involved in actual decision making are 'shapers' and, to some extent, 'coordinators' and 'specialists' (where their interest is engaged). Greater amounts of scope with plenty of space for creative work are particularly attractive to 'plants' but 'shapers' also respond well.

Where initiatives involve the need to seek out others for joint work and new contributions, the 'resource investigator' is particu-

The implementation of strategy at local level

larly able, supported by the 'team worker'. For the 'monitor-evaluator', the chance to stand back and evaluate the usefulness of various activities is important and will enable the organisation to make more constructive use of potentially unproductive time. Thus, giving the 'monitor-evaluator' sufficient autonomy can lead to valuable strategic outcomes.

Employees have a spectrum of team roles with which they can function although two or three are likely to be preferred. For the professionals, knowing what these are, as well as which roles they are not suited to, is an important component in making the best use of any potential lack of clarity in implementing strategic change.

Group processes

As well as power relations, certain actions arise in groups due to subtle pressures to conform to group norms and expectations. Although at the start of the implementation of some strategic change, the group as a whole may be against the change, if one influential member of the group supports it, others may start to follow. Rogers & Schumacher's categories (1971) are still useful. They envisaged a continuum from change to status quo as follows.

Change
- The innovator – proactive during the process of change
- The early adopter – readily accepts the change
- Early majority – the first group to follow the early adopter
- Later majority – other groups follow suit
- Laggards – a reticent group who tend to remain sceptical although not openly hostile to change
- Rejecters – openly oppose change

Status quo

Imposed change, directed from above, needs a somewhat different strategy from participative change (Hersey & Blanchard 1988). With less choice being available to the practitioners over the style of change, certain responses may seem to be required from the group as a whole. Group behaviour will tend to influence individual behaviour which in turn affects individual attitudes towards the change through a process of dissonance and compliance. The ability of some to resist these pressures, even sufficiently strongly to take others with them, is what makes the implementation of strategy forever uncertain. The reasons for this are now explored.

Autonomy and initiative in implementing strategic decisions

PSYCHOLOGICAL REASONS FOR INDIVIDUAL VARIATIONS

So far, this chapter has examined the effect of different types of organisational control and group functioning on individual ability to demonstrate autonomy and initiative. However, 'the problem of control exists, so to speak, inside the skin of the person' (Zaleznick 1966, p. 58). A more overtly psychological approach to the topic can give some insights not found elsewhere.

McKenna (1987) suggested that there are two fundamental psychological approaches. The first, the ideographic approach, views the individual as a well-integrated organism which reacts as a whole to various situations with past experience and future intentions contributing to present behaviour. An example of this approach is psychoanalysis. At the other extreme, the nomothetic objective is to isolate various personality variables that can be scientifically measured under controlled conditions (for example, the work of Eysenck 1967). The former can be criticised as being inaccessible and not easily lending itself to scientific measurement; the latter because in reducing the personality to certain types or traits, the richness of individual experience and learning is lost. Modifications exist which compensate for some of the disadvantages but the divide still remains.

This chapter suggests that an ideographic approach, more particularly a psychoanalytic perspective, can:

- open up ways of dealing with issues that can barely be approached from other directions
- allow work to be done on the complexity, conflicts and ambiguities of motivation and meaning of people's emotional lives
- respect the integrity of individual experience (Craib 1989).

A number of writers have identified the usefulness of a psychoanalytic contribution to understanding in this arena. A link was made by Rustin (1991) between individual power and change. Responding to the need for change requires giving up a sense of omnipotence as the resultant 'not knowing' may be a source of fear or threat. For this reason, the individual may resist, sometimes unconsciously, and when this is multiplied, the wider picture emerging may be one of institutional resistance.

Psychoanalytic theory is implicitly about power. Without tracing Freud's developmental theory in detail, his emphasis on parental power and infant powerlessness once it realises its own separate identity underpins the love/hate ambivalence towards parental figures and the ways that are learnt of dealing with the anger and frustration resulting from imposed authority and the prevention of immediate gratification (Freud 1994). This early learning can be seen to have a major influence on later relationships, including those that are work related, around subordinacy and responses to authority.

Compliance, aggression or detachment

Of Freud's work, his description of defence mechanisms, the ways that the ego protects itself against instinctual demands of the unconscious, is apt. Defence mechanisms are potentially observable and recognisable and many remain within the limits of the normal (Freud 1966). Karen Horney, spending most of her adult life in the USA, related the feelings of helplessness found in the child to the highly competitive culture in which its development took place (McKenna 1987). These feelings would continue into adult life as a compulsive striving for love and power, based on the conflicting need for parental love and fear of parental mistreatment (Sayers 1991). The inevitable base anxiety caused is dealt with through four defence methods: search for affection, submission, power or withdrawal. These defences are based on the assumption that:

- if you love me, you will not hurt me
- if I give in, I shall not be hurt
- if I have power, no-one can hurt me
- if I withdraw, nothing can hurt me. (Horney 1937)

The individual seeks affection through love, pity or sex and power through competition, wanting to be right and have one's own way and controlling others. Although Horney saw these defences as initiated in early development, she accepted cultural reinforcement of certain characteristics and described three distinct types:

- the compliant type – moving towards others
- the aggressive type – moving against others
- the detached type – moving away from others.

However, it is unlikely that an individual will only adopt one of the above although being more at ease with one style than another. Instead, it seems reasonable that the unconscious will adopt different defences at different times depending on circumstances and its internal learnt repertoire.

Recognition of the three character types relies on teasing out the most likely manifestations experienced in the workplace. Some suggestions are as follows.

Autonomy and initiative in implementing strategic decisions

The compliant type – moving towards others and therefore seeking affection and submission

- Obeys rules
- Follows instructions and procedures
- Does not question instructions
- Seeks approval from others
- Is comfortable with circumscribed work relationships
- Values clear roles and clarity of work requirements
- Avoids uncertainty, does not put her/himself forward for new projects

The aggressive type – moving against others and therefore seeking power

- Wants own way
- Wants to do what is right (in her/his view)
- Sees others as competitive
- Builds coalitions through networks, horizontal and vertical
- Sees resources as a source of power
- Has an instrumental approach to work and to others

The detached type – moving away from others and therefore seeking withdrawal

- Refuses to face reality, stays fixated to past role behaviour
- Postpones or opts out of decision making
- Worries about trivia
- Voices criticism of work and work colleagues
- Welcomes isolation
- Appears depressed or manic

The aggressive response seems to be the one most closely associated with initiative while the detached type will welcome autonomy. However, if the culture of the organisation rewards independence, even the compliant type may show initiative to gain approval.

Implications for the organisation

'It is easier to beg forgiveness than to ask permission' (an old Jesuit saying) was quoted by Kanter (1990) in order to bring home to her audience this very point. The importance of having an organisational culture that is supportive of individual initiative is all about survival in a competitive environment. The above discussion suggests that whether the individual 'begs forgiveness' or 'asks permission' will depend on some deep-seated psychological factors. If the professional's defence mechanisms move him or her towards a compliant style, then the individual is more likely to seek permission; if his or her preferred style is aggressive, or even detached, the fear of losing affection will not be the prime motivator. In this case, doing what the individual wants to do without too much regard for the consequences does display a possible manipulative or unbothered approach. It also indicates a somewhat cynical view of 'begging forgiveness' but perhaps it would be wise not to pursue this line of thought!

The value of bringing together the above strands is not to provide a quick fix for those in charge of organisations. Zaleznik & Kets de Vries (1985) suggested that in presenting psychoanalytic knowledge to the modern manager, the outcome needs to be a journey where:

> Reflection . . . and paying heed to one's own experience will be infinitely more valuable than grasping for answers. Such reflection will hopefully tame the urges of power and aggression and discover and utilise talents.

CONCLUSION

The final step of this chapter is to bring the previous conclusions together. Melucci (1989) suggested that collective (and individual) action must be understood in terms of processes through which individuals communicate, negotiate, produce meanings and make decisions within a particular environment. Although researching social movements, some of his conclusions could usefully be transposed to the issue of power and change in the workplace. For example, the loci of power are no longer exclusively at executive level, with the existence of 'subterranean' dimensions in contemporary social life. He also worked on the notion of 'public' or 'open' spaces where the plurality of individuals and groups can interact and the existence of networks that are submerged or private, as well as those that are visible. He avoided the conclusions of other social movement theorists that groups not achieving political change have failed. Although visible change is one outcome of successful power relations, the individual who self-consciously practises in the present new ways of behaving that will enable future change is exerting power in a successful way.

Autonomy and initiative in implementing strategic decisions

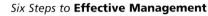

It seems possible, therefore, that the very complexity of health care organisations lends itself to the development of a heterogeneous model that can support autonomy and initiative in implementing strategic change. The following list attempts to pinpoint the potential actions that individual health care professionals can take to enhance their ability to influence strategic outcomes.

- Consciously recognise personal use of defences.
- Recognise and respond constructively to authority issues of subordinates and superiors.
- Develop and utilise constructive change tactics that match preferred psychoanalytic style.
- Work on strengthening secondary team roles where this will enhance initiative.
- Recognise group pressures and consciously accept/reject them.
- Identify personal power resources and work on enhancing and enlarging these.
- Network via individuals/groups to influence key decision makers.
- Develop arguments for professional autonomy that work at both rational and emotional levels.
- Identify desired targets and include these in annual plans.
- Embrace more flexible roles with enthusiasm.

Although this list may seem overpositive, as long as the individual professional does not fall into the trap of believing all things are possible, then it does identify areas where influence on strategic decisions might occur. However, woe betide that professional if she or he forgets that both the wider context as well as other individuals in the organisation will also be actively attempting to shape the future and in so doing will modify or restrict the professional's scope. It is indeed a pattern of action and reaction but by placing the individual's potential learning about personal choices at the centre it does hopefully encourage a more contented and forward-looking participant of any health care organisation.

References

Argenti J 1993 Your organization: what is it for? McGraw Hill, London
Beer M 1980 Organization change and development: a systems view. Goodyear, Santa Monica, California
Belbin M 1997 Changing the way we work. Butterworth-Heinemann, Oxford
Brower R, Abolafia M 1995 The structured embeddedness of resistance among public managers. Group and Organization Management 20(2): 149–166
Child J 1984 Organization: a guide to practice and problems. Harper and Row, London

Craib I 1989 Psychoanalysis and social theory. Harvester Wheatsheaf, Hemel Hempstead

Dahl P 1961 Who governs? Democracy and power in an American city. Yale University Press, New Haven

Emmanuel C, Otley D, Merchant K 1990 Accounting for management control, 2nd edn. Chapman and Hall, London

Eysenck H 1967 The biological basis of personality. Thomas, Springfield

Freud A 1966 The ego and the mechanisms of defence, revised edition. Hogarth Press, London

Freud S 1994 The dissection of the psychical personality. In: Clark H, Chandler J, Barry J (eds) Organisation and identities. Chapman and Hall, London

Harrison S, Pollitt C 1994 Controlling health professionals: the future of work and organization in the NHS. Open University Press, Buckingham

Hersey P, Blanchard K 1988 Management of organizational behaviour, 5th edn. Prentice Hall, London

Horney K 1937 The neurotic personality of our time. Routledge and Kegan Paul, London

Kanter RM 1984 The change masters. George Allen and Unwin, London

Kanter RM 1990 The human factor. BBC TV

McKenna E 1987 Psychology in business. Lawrence Erlbaum Associates, Hove

Melucci A 1989 Nomads of the present. Hutchinson Radius, London

Morgan G 1997 Images of organization, 2nd edn. Sage, London

Parker M, Dent M 1996 Managers, doctors and culture: changing an English health district. Administration and Society 28(3): 335–361

Rogers E, Schumacher F 1971 Communication of innovation: a cross cultural report, 2nd edn. Free Press, New York

Rustin M 1991 The good society and the inner world – psychoanalysis, politics and culture. Verso, London

Sayers J 1991 Mothering psychoanalysis – Helene Deutsch, Karen Horney, Anna Freud and Melanie Klein. Penguin Books, Harmondsworth

Spiers J 1995 The invisible hospital and the secret garden: an insider's commentary on the NHS reforms. Radcliffe Medical Press, Oxford

Young AP 1996a Who sets the business agenda? Journal of Nursing Management 4: 347–352

Young AP 1996b Marketing: a flawed concept when applied to health care? British Journal of Nursing 5(15): 937–940

Zaleznik A 1966 Human dilemmas of leadership. Harper and Row, New York

Zaleznik A, Kets de Vries M 1985 Power and the corporate mind, 2nd edn. Bonus Books, Chicago

Autonomy and initiative in implementing strategic decisions

Application **11:1**

Ann P Young

Managerial perceptions of initiative

This application gathers some opinions on initiative in the workplace from interviews with a selection of middle managers in a number of hospital settings (both NHS and private). They were asked for their views on how much initiative they thought they had, what blocks to initiative they had experienced and what ways around these restrictions they had found. Selections of their responses are presented below.

QUESTION 1: HOW MUCH SCOPE FOR INITIATIVE DO YOU HAVE?

Initiative? Yes, definitely encouraged in my workplace. I think I'm actually very fortunate as my post was new and I very much direct what I do.

We are definitely innovative, not 100% encouraged but if they see it working, you're not going to be stopped.

Yes, the lot. You pick up things out there that aren't going right or the nurses aren't happy with them. Let's take it, let's investigate it, let's move things forward, let's see if it's happening in other places, let's pick up things and go with them.

We have our problems here, particularly in the community. But one thing we've all felt is that the trust board have let us try and sort the problems out ourselves.

Absolutely tons, yes. I think it's partly this particular trust. For example, my bosses do give a lot of latitude because they have been happy with how things have gone in the past. They tend to trust you and let you go off on your own. Obviously you report back to them. Part of it is again the department we're in and the fact that everything is changing all the time, so we're always entering new territory. It's new stuff all the time.

It's very difficult to say where the boundary is because they have never ever said no. I'm sure they will. But I'm not going to do anything that's going to cause problems. At the end of the day, I want to make things run more efficiently and make my job easier. I've been here long enough to know what is possible.

Comments

All the managers saw themselves as having some initiative, even if it was within fairly circumscribed boundaries. Many saw themselves as having considerable freedom as long as they were working to the broad requirements of the service.

QUESTION 2: WHAT BLOCKS TO INITIATIVE HAVE YOU EXPERIENCED?

Biggest thing is time.

A large chunk of my working week I was in bed bureau and in the hospital, sorting out, troubleshooting, working through the problems of the day. This then means the stuff on your desk that you want to move forward, a good example then was of clinical supervision, actually begin to fragment and you can't build up the impetus again. Because I have such a wide remit, I seem to have a lot on the go at once, a lot of balls in the air at any one time. But then when the operational stuff starts to go a bit pear-shaped, I find that they all have to be thrown aside to get on with that. And then we have to learn to wait till we have the time. So I would say that I am limited by time.

Within limitations, because . . . my problem is time, basically.

I think a lot of people win initiative and this is one of the areas where we don't publicise what we do. You know, if we do something good, we just get on with it, we don't share it with people.

New work creates initiative up to a certain level which is very good. But once you go beyond a certain saturation point, I guess, where people become frustrated where they have no guidance or leadership, then it turns into frustration or animosity or lack of morale, and we have to go back and build it up again with the shirtsleeves approach. So I think there has been quite a lot of freedom which translates itself sometimes into worries about where you should be going, what you should be doing. So you think, I don't really know what I should be doing!

It was not managers or other people that seemed to be the major restrictions on the use of initiative but the problem of heavy and uneven workloads, with insufficient time to give to the more strategic initiatives that the managers wanted to implement as compared with the urgent operational issues that demanded their immediate attention. Some problems were compounded by poor communication and a lack of any direction which one manager experienced as seriously debilitating.

QUESTION 3: HOW DO YOU DEAL WITH RESTRICTIONS ON YOUR EXERCISE OF INITIATIVE?

I have lot of scope if I have the energy. I've moved around a lot and I believe that this gives a lot of ideas, gives energy.

Sometimes I do it and they know about it after the event.

I do find ways around restrictions but sometimes it's not easy, but once I get my teeth into something, I don't let go. I go round the walls. I think. Often we have to negotiate things.

I do feel that we have the support of nurse initiatives. But whether it's clinical support, I don't know. I don't know whether the pressure of the audit committee on these places drives us. We don't audit as good as we should audit and we can use this to support arguments for change.

There are times when I see what the board wants and it's not popular, but it's not popular throughout the trust. It's something, or may be something, the trust has no power over. And I think my job then is to intercede for the board. And to try to debate it, explain it, so that it's not just a blanket thing, a thrown down thing. Sometimes, for example, a policy comes out and some people feel strongly that that's not quite right. And yeah, I can see that. So then it's up to me to say, hang on, the view I am getting from some of my colleagues is that perhaps you should rethink that. Sometimes the board will say there's nothing we can do about it. And sometimes they may say, and do say, oh, we hadn't thought of that. Let's just think about it a little, and they modify something slightly to accommodate views.

There have often been compromises along the way. I can't think of one particular thing where I've come out thinking, I didn't win. I may not have won but I've reached a compromise that I am happy to go forward with. But you always go in to win whatever battle, don't you? But I think I recognise that it isn't always possible to go in and win the battle totally. You have to accept a halfway house sometimes.

It's about making sure that policies and procedures actually work for the people at the coal face, using these to help them, interpreting things in the broadest and most flexible manner.

Comments

Determination and risk taking were noticeable characteristics here for the managers who experienced the greatest level of personal initiative. However, experience had enabled them to judge levels of risk. Success was seen to reinforce others' faith in their abilities and increased levels of trust enhanced more freedom. There was also the realisation that the ability to negotiate, compromise and be flexible was an important component of success in developing new ideas and ways of working. Change does not happen overnight.

Managerial perceptions of initiative

Application 11:2

Ann P Young

Assertiveness and leadership skills

Although an ability to respond to changing circumstances varies with our particular personality characteristics, it is possible to learn new skills or develop ones in which we are weak. The ability to be assertive and the willingness to adopt leadership roles will predispose the individual to participate positively in change. However, if the person is naturally passive or lacking in confidence, conscious work needs to be done on developing these more outward orientated skills.

The two exercises below are not intended to be any more than a taster of what can be done to recognise and act in these areas of self-development. There are numerous texts that will give a comprehensive programme for those interested.

Exercise 1

Being assertive does not mean being aggressive but it is still very different from the passive, rather apologetic style so often seen. The grid in Table 11.2.1 (adapted from O'Reilly 1993, p. 45) presents some difficult situations and suggests what might differentiate the passive, aggressive and assertive responses.

The grid is left unfinished for you to fill in some difficult situations in which you have found yourself. Try to identify a range of recognisable responses and fit them into the appropriate spaces. Then revisit the whole grid to see how your preferred or actual responses matched. Finally, although assertive responses are usually successful in supporting a positive work climate, identify some situations when an aggressive or passive response would be more appropriate.

Table 11.2.1 Assertiveness exercise

Situation	Passive response	Aggressive response	Assertive response
1. You are making a request for help	Mary, I don't suppose there's any chance that you could	Mary, get this done now.....	Mary, would you please...
2. You are refusing a request from someone else because you can't spare the time.	Oh dear, I do hope you don't mind but it's not easy to fit that in right now.... Oh, OK	You must be joking! I've got so much on my plate I'm snowed under.	I can't help right now as I've got a meeting in 5 minutes.
3. Someone interrupts you while you are in the middle of explaining something.	I'm sorry... I hope I haven't confused you.	Angry stare and then ignore the person.	I want to explain the whole process and then I'll be pleased to deal with questions.
4. You attend a meeting at which the chairperson ignores your attempts to contribute.	Ignore her and surreptitiously catch up on some paperwork.	Butt in when someone else is speaking.	Raise your hand and say 'Please may I contribute at this point, John?'
5. Someone makes a sexist remark, calling you 'dearie'.	Make no comment but feel resentful.	Back off .... I'm not your dearie.	Smile and say firmly, 'My name is Ann. Now what can I do for you?'
6. Your manager is angry because you have made a mistake through not checking your work carefully.	Oh dear, I am sorry. I feel dreadful. Please forgive me.	Nobody's perfect. Anyway, you make just as many mistakes as I do. Perhaps more!	I'm sorry. I was wrong. I'll be more careful in the future.
7.			
8.			
9.			
10.			

The implementation of strategy at local level

Exercise 2

Successful leaders combine a number of different skills. Gaining an awareness of these, along with conscious practice, will assist professionals to move into and/or strengthen their leadership roles. It is suggested that a leadership action plan is developed. Activities might include the following.

1. Identify some national and international leaders in a variety of fields. Why did you choose them? What do you admire and/or dislike about them?
2. Whom do you consider to be successful leaders in your workplace? Ask to shadow one for a day.
3. If this works well, you might want to suggest the development of a mentoring relationship with this person.
4. Look at your achievements over the last year. Which of these involved some aspects of leadership? Even in informal settings and one-to-one relationships, you should be able to recognise some relevant skills. Note them and praise yourself for your success.
5. Look for opportunities to use your initiative, raise your profile and enhance leadership skills that are still 'embryonic'. For example:

   ● set up a small-scale project that will help illuminate or solve a problem that affects more people than yourself
   ● offer to chair meetings, initially the smaller and less formal variety if you are new to this
   ● discuss with your boss the opportunities for 'acting up' that could be offered you.

6. Identify some courses that would be useful to you in developing leadership skills.

This is by no means an exhaustive list. Look at some of the large range of practical management and leadership books in bookshops and libraries. The applications in this book should also give you plenty of ideas.

However, reflection must be turned into action. The following is a suggested format for a leadership development action plan in which to insert the specific activities you have decided to pursue.

Objectives	Review date
Short term – tomorrow to 3 months	
1.	
2.	
3.	

(continued)

(continued)

Middle term – 4 to 12 months

1.

2.

3.

Long term – 1 to 3 years

1.

2.

3.

Ideally your action plan should be part of a wider development programme which is discussed with your manager and/or mentor on a regular basis.

Reference

O'Reilly P 1993 The skills development handbook for busy managers. McGraw Hill, London

Assertiveness and leadership skills

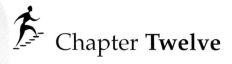

Chapter **Twelve**

Using clinical research to underpin decision making in health care: a case study approach

Christopher Loughlan

● Background

● Methods

● Results

● Involvement in clinical practice

● Influences in changing practice

● Negative influences

● Implementation

● Department/ward level

● Trust level

● Conclusions

● Discussion

OVERVIEW

Since the early 1990s there has been growing interest in using the results of research to improve both the health of the population and the provision of health services. This work comes under a number of headings such as 'evidence-based practice, clinical effectiveness and implementation of research findings'. At the root of these activities is a concern that there is considerable scope for improvement in clinical decision making (Dunning et al 1998). Such work has been stimulated by improved access to research findings, the quality of the evidence, variations in the level and quality of service provision and, as huge resources currently underpin service

The implementation of strategy at local level

provision, a general concern for greater accountability (Gray 1998).

Clinical governance has been defined as:

> A framework through which NHS organisations are accountable for continuously improving the quality of their services and safeguarding high standards of care by creating an environment in which excellence in clinical care will flourish. (NHS Executive 1999)

Within the new NHS clinical governance framework, more emphasis will be placed on demonstrating clinical effectiveness in treating patients. This will have direct implications for health care professionals and the way in which clinical practice develops. At the root of these changes is a determination to continually enhance the quality of patient care (DoH 1998). In short, does current practice match 'best practice'?

Ongoing professional development will have three dimensions: what an individual does, how a ward/department (the operational entity) is organised and what a trust (the organisation) provides in terms of commitment and infrastructure (Sewell 1997).

BACKGROUND

Addenbrooke's is a major teaching hospital and a local district hospital for the 300 000 people who live in Cambridge and the surrounding area. It has 5000 staff, over 1000 beds and a budget in the region of £185 million. The Department of Health, University of Cambridge, Medical Research Council, Cancer Research Campaign, British Heart Foundation and Wellcome Trust are some of the bodies who directly support research at Addenbrooke's. In 1998–99, in excess of £30 million of dedicated research facilities opened, providing state-of-the-art facilities for over 1400 research projects – the largest figure for any provincial UK hospital.

The Trust Research and Development department joined forces with the Judge Institute of Management Studies, University of Cambridge, to assess the needs of nursing and professions allied to medicine (PAM) staff in relation to the theme of clinical practice development. The study 'Improving your practice' set out to undertake a survey of understanding and needs in relation to clinical practice development. In particular, it sought views at individual, departmental and organisational level.

The study used the following working definition:

> Clinical practice development (CPD) relates to the changing nature of your clinical care for patients – it is concerned with action, what

Using clinical research to underpin decision making in health care

281

Six Steps to **Effective Management**

you do to and with patients, and the way in which at a practical level you systematically advance your care.*

It sought to differentiate between development that was patient (clinical) based and that which was generic (e.g. lifting and handling, dealing with abusive patients, HIV risk). This definition, however, was 'challenged' in the study: 'Staff have different perspectives on CPD – different training (diplomas, degrees), all having different emphasis on research/clinical development' and 'CPD is used as if it is something set up and agreed and known, but not to me!'

METHODS

A project team was established to take responsibility for the organisation of the operational arm of the study. Two field workers were seconded from the Trust – one nurse and one physiotherapist. A condensed, informal, semi-structured course on research methodology was provided by the Judge Institute of Management Studies. The general approach was informed by good practice guidelines for small-scale social research projects (Denscombe 1998). The provision of this (unique) course enabled the two field workers to gain a fuller understanding of the theoretical basis for and approaches undertaken in the study.

Four areas/departments and one specialist professional group were chosen in consultation with the chief nurse. These 'areas' were to reflect a broad cross-section of current level, expectation and needs within the Trust. The five areas were:

- Specialist Nurse (SpN)
- Department of Medicine for the Elderly (DME)
- Oncology (Onc)
- Theatres (Thea)
- Physiotherapy (Phys).

Project team members met with a general manager who represented each of these areas. The purpose of this meeting was to inform them of the study, gain an insight into the 'local history' and ultimately attune them to further participation in future developments as a result of the study. The study used a dual method of questionnaire and focus group discussion. The questionnaire gave an

---

* This definition came out of a number of discussions in the project team who were in consultation with health professional staff within the Trust.

The implementation of strategy at local level

282

opportunity for all staff within an area to comment. The focus group provided an opportunity to gain more insight into particular themes and enabled participants to raise their own concerns and questions. The general approach to and conduct within a focus group was informed and guided by good practice guidelines for applied research (Krueger 1994).

A questionnaire was devised by the project team and then piloted in other areas within the Trust. The questionnaire was distributed using the internal mail system to all staff (n = 401) in the five areas with the exception of those staff who were invited to the focus group discussion. Service centre managers were asked to nominate up to 12 staff to attend the focus group. One follow-up letter was sent to all non-respondents.

No incentives were used to increase the response rate. The study was undertaken in the period September–December 1998.

RESULTS

Questionnaires used in the analysis equated to a response rate of 45% (the true response rate = 49%*). The low response was particularly noticeable in the larger departments, namely Oncology and Theatres. Figure 12.1 shows the return rate by sector to the questionnaire. There was good participation (n = 53) in the focus groups by all departments.

In relation to employment status we found that large numbers of participants were part time: in Oncology 21%, in DME 40%. Participant details reflected a broad section of junior to senior mix with two exceptions: Oncology was at a more senior level whereas DME and Theatres were at the lower end of the spectrum. Most staff were in the 20–39 years bracket with the exception of Specialist Nursing which had 27% of their numbers in the 50+ years group.

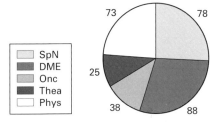

SpN
DME
Onc
Thea
Phys

73   78   25   38   88

Figure 12.1   Response by sector.

* A number of questionnaires were returned unopened and others were returned blank; some were returned after the cut-off point for analysis.

The implementation of strategy at local level

INVOLVEMENT IN CLINICAL PRACTICE

Figure 12.2 shows that a large number of nursing and PAM staff thought their practice had changed. Thus clinical practice development had been occurring through existing processes within the organisation.

Two groups had larger numbers of staff who thought that their practice had not changed over the last year: Theatres (28%) and Physiotherapy (20%). Because participants in both these groups contained relatively larger numbers of auxiliary and health care assistant staff, it is possible that the question was inappropriate.

INFLUENCES IN CHANGING PRACTICE

Participants were asked what had been the major influences in clinical practice development. Figure 12.3 depicts the range of positive influences. In addition to the four categories above, 'self-

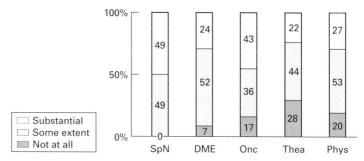

Figure 12.2 Involvement in clinical practice development.

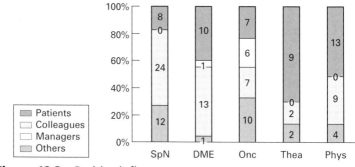

Figure 12.3 Positive influences.

motivation' was seen as a positive influence in all areas except physiotherapy.

NEGATIVE INFLUENCES

What held back or prevented development? There were three clear
factors: time, workload and staffing levels. This was summed by
one respondent:

> I am motivated and have sufficient education and skills to assess
> and implement developments in clinical practice both personally
> and throughout the Trust. However, this is not possible … the
> emphasis is on survival.

Staff were asked whether they would be prepared to initiate clinical practice development. The study found that they were and this
willingness was strongly confirmed in the focus groups. There was
a marked degree of unwillingness, however, in DME (33%),
Theatres (28%) and Physiotherapy (27%).

IMPLEMENTATION

With respect to planning the implementation of practice development, a polarisation of viewpoints emerged. This polarisation was
expressed in the following quotes:

> This type of work has to be done in people's off-duty time; it is hard
> to get people to give that up after hard long shifts on the ward.

> Clinical practice development is an integral part of working ethos
> and attitude.

Staff were asked what form of support they would like to see for
practice improvement and the answers fell into three dimensions:
colleagues and management, adequate time and resources (educational, academic and IT).

In relation to method of working, staff expressed a clear preference for working in small groups (Fig. 12.4*). The preference for
working in small groups was found across all areas (Fig. 12.5).

Are you familiar with team plans?

Whilst there was general familarity with plans for clinical practice
development, large numbers reported lack of knowledge: Theatres

---

* Percentages do not tally to 100 due to non-response.

Using clinical research to underpin decision making in health care

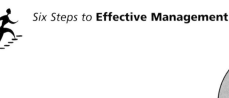

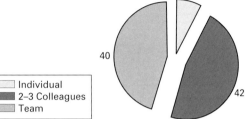

Figure 12.4   Preferred method of working.

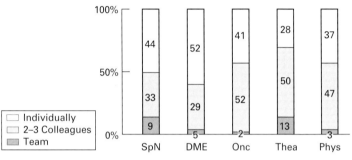

Figure 12.5   Method of working by group.

(78%), Physiotherapy (43%) and Oncology (38%). As the sample contained a broad section of health care workers, familiarity of actual plans may not have been entirely appropriate.

Time and value of practice development

As to whether time was 'set aside' for development, the survey found considerable variation across departments (Fig. 12.6).

Though time was apparently not made available, staff still placed a high value on this resource. Many participants expressed concern that apparently there was no practice development whatsoever.

DEPARTMENT/WARD LEVEL

Participants were asked to grade (low–medium–high) a range of factors that contribute to practice development at departmen-

The implementation of strategy at local level

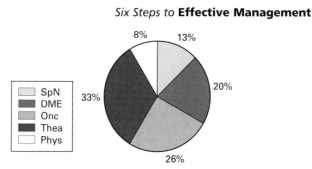

Figure 12.6   Time not made available.

tal/ward level. Priority need was where 50% of responses classed the topic as 'high'. Priorities at departmental/ward level are expressed in Table 12.1.

Within the criteria outlined above, the following needs were *not* viewed as a high priority: finding the evidence, appraising the evidence, educational manual on clinical effectiveness.

TRUST LEVEL

Participants were asked to grade (low–medium–high) a range of factors that contribute to practice development at Trust level. There was consensus over the following topics:

- agreed protocols for multidisciplinary team working
- local protocols/guidelines
- dedicated time.

Table 12.1 Priorities at departmental/ward level

Department	Priority
SpN	Maintaining or improving understanding of 'best practice'
DME	Applying the evidence: 'best practice'
Onc	'Best practice': journal discussion; meetings with colleagues
Thea	No clear priorities from questionnaire*
Phys	'Best practice': meetings with colleagues

* Theatre staff focus group participants expressed all of the above as a priority.

Using clinical research to underpin decision making in health care

CONCLUSIONS

The major conclusions with respect to training needs are twofold. At department/ward level: maintaining or improving understanding of 'best practice', applying the evidence and, to a lesser extent, formalising meetings with colleagues were viewed as a high priority. At Trust level, agreed protocols for multidisciplinary team working, local protocols/guidelines and dedicated time were viewed as a high priority. However, one of the main findings in this study reinforced the principle that the organisation infrastructure, e.g. the basics of staffing, time allocation and management support, has to be in place before clinical practice development can be comprehensively tackled.

Three linked factors, namely time, workload and staffing, have an immense bearing on both the potential and likelihood of successful clinical practice development. The context in which current clinical practice takes place is so varied that any practice development must take account of 'local' factors. There are, of course, a number of factors at play here: management lead, staff motivation, resource capacity and application, 'baseline' starting point, to name but a few. Specialist nurses were highly motivated who found their method of working (in addition to their specialist area) stimulating. The scale and scope of change and clarity of management support in one nurse area were seen as major contributing factors to lower morale in the staff surveyed.

The desire to work in small groups came out strongly. One of the most difficult issues centred on the application of practice development; the notion of 'time out' or 'time away' from the clinical interface still surfaced. There was an apparent polarisation of views in this respect. A large number of staff work on a part-time basis which makes it extremely difficult for them to catch up on practice development. From an organisational perspective, two positive features were noted: the notion of 'best practice' seemed to have wide currency and there was strong support for initiating practice development.

DISCUSSION

This study was found to be a useful and valuable exercise. It provided a snapshot of views on clinical practice development and a body of knowledge from which management can plan and take action. The question of the 'low' response rate and related bias has to be addressed. That nearly half of the sample chose to return the questionnaire can itself be viewed (positively or negatively!) as an indicator of interest in and commitment to clinical practice development (Loughlan & McAlpine 1998). It is clear that a positive bias was not reflected in the participants' views, e.g. see responses in 'change in clinical practice over the last year', 'negative influences in changing clinical practice'. These findings lend weight to the view that the study did indeed reflect a wider, more generalisable picture.

The implementation of a Trust-wide strategy on clinical practice development has to be placed in the local context. This would entail having a good grasp of the contextual factors outlined above in the conclusions. It is not clear how practice development and the pressures of clinical workload can be integrated. Whatever form practice development takes, there is a growing realisation that there needs to be a mechanism by which development occurs 'within practice'. The role of a respected, autonomous 'local facilitator' might be a useful catalyst in helping to implement practice development. Specialist nurses were in an advantageous position and would be extremely well placed (workload permitting!) to take on such a developmental role.

Recognition of the preferred form of working (i.e. working with 2–3 colleagues in teams) will have important knock-on effects. There are important implications here for management in terms of networking, communication, coordination and monitoring. There would be a significant increase in administrative workload but the assumption is that clinical practice development and staff working practices would be greatly improved.

How can part-time staff be more efficiently included the 'normal' process of clinical practice development? Exceptional and innovative methods may be needed to help ensure that such staff do not 'lose out'. Recent developments in 'clinical supervision' may address these concerns. As clinical practice development will involve a continual cycle of work, thought should be given to how management, in liaison with clinical staff, can sustain and support this process.

Interest in 'best practice' coupled with a willingness to initiate practice development came out strongly. This could provide a basis for substantial progress in future years and shape direction in the light of new responsibilities within the clinical governance framework.

Acknowledgement

The author would like to thank the Cambridge Education and Training Consortium for their financial support in the project. In

Using clinical research to underpin decision making in health care particular, Freya Adams and Helen Phoenix of Addenbrooke's NHS Trust, as field workers in the project team, contributed greatly to the study. Jonathan Ford, Research Associate, Judge Institute of Management Studies, University of Cambridge, created a learning environment within which the study was conducted, commented on earlier scripts and provided guidance throughout the period of the study.

References

Denscombe M 1998 The good research guide. Open University Press, London

Department of Health 1998 A first class service. Quality in the NHS. Stationery Office, London

Dunning M, Abi-Aad G, Gilbert D, Gillam S, Livett H 1998 Turning evidence into everyday practice. King's Fund Publishing, London

Gray MJA 1998 Evidence-based health care. How to make health policy and management decisions. Churchill Livingstone, London

Krueger RA 1994 Focus groups. A practical guide for applied research. Sage Publications, London

Loughlan C, McAlpine CA 1998 Skills and support in the application of research to health care in an NHS trust. Health Bulletin 56: 725–732

NHS Executive 1999 Clinical governance: quality in the new NHS. Department of Health, London

Sewell N 1997 Do you work in a learning or improving organisation? British Journal of Health Care Management 3: 315–317

Application 12:1

Christopher Loughlan

Findings and methodology

DEFINING THE TERM 'CLINICAL PRACTICE DEVELOPMENT' (CPD)

One of the initial unexpected findings of the study described in Chapter 12 related to the broad definition of the term 'clinical practice development'. Diversity in many contexts is a sign of health but the study team came to the conclusion that such diversity in meaning and definition was counterproductive. If a clinical unit (the physically and professionally bounded area of work) is critically assessing how to improve CPD then there has to be agreement by all professions within the unit as to what constitutes CPD. With the move towards multidisciplinary health care in practice, the survey tool could be used to debate and critique current definitions of the term.

THE CPD PARADOX

The survey revealed that there was not so much a broad spectrum but a polarisation of view as to how activities could best contribute to CPD. The much-used conference attendance was cited but there was a strong criticism that broader dissemination to the unit was minimal, if not non-existent.

Within this debate there was a tangential but related theme: 'practice as dynamic'. Practitioners viewed their practice not simply as habitual or routine but constantly evolving through time. Thus CPD was viewed as a 'product of time'.

Within a clinical governance framework, it is clear that CPD cannot be left to haphazard, unintended, unplanned activities but will require a systematic, structured and resourced plan which can be evaluated. Thus each clinical unit needs some sort of datum line from which to plan, implement and assess progress. The survey tool could be part of the baseline activity for such an objective.

PRACTICE DEVELOPMENT LEADERSHIP BY MANAGERS

In keeping with other research findings, this study confirmed that practitioners looked towards their professional colleagues as a positive source of influence in CPD. What role should unit managers play in this important area? Clearly lessons from change management suggest that one indicator of success centres on who sets the agenda. How will a manager succeed, then, if faced with external drivers (best practice, evidence-based practice and broader clinical governance responsibilities) against a backdrop of local clinical concerns and the immediacy of day-to-day routine practice?

Senior managers might usefully review how they understand, facilitate and resource CPD. This might include being clear in development priorities, communicating and pursuing innovations in a more focused way and techniques for winning the support of staff. Another area where senior managers might make an important contribution relates to multidisciplinary working. Increasing emphasis could usefully be placed on practice development projects as multidisciplinary developments and project management techniques could be used to help integrate and support staff.

Management would be viewed more positively if they took responsibility for the management and production of multidisciplinary protocols, leaving content to clinical staff. These protocols may help structure the shape and nature of involvement of nurses and PAM staff and help to balance and facilitate their contribution when working alongside medical staff, service managers and others. Such protocols may be viewed as restrictive by some staff but should be promoted as an enabling agreement or way of working which provides an outline of how teams might work together on development projects or programmes.

Section Five

MANAGING RISK AND CRISIS

OVERVIEW

'Lack of control may produce the basic cause for a potential incident. This potential incident leads to a substantial condition and an actual incident occurring.' This explanation of the domino theory by Anderson in Chapter Fourteen underpins the relationship between risk and crisis, one deficit leading to another and hence the fall of the dominoes.

The management of decisions in situations of uncertainty, lack of clarity about the real issues and potential or actual conflict have been features of a number of the examples and applications in previous sections of this volume. Practitioners and managers will appreciate the reality of this setting and will have sought ways of dealing with these 'sticky' problems. Section Five draws many of these threads together and puts them in a context that provides not only some frameworks with which to understand these issues but also some strong practical advice on dealing with the immediate and longer term features of risk and crisis. The overall emphasis, although managers have to take short-term remedial action, is on working towards more permanent solutions at both organisational and personal level.

Hunt sets the scene with a critical account of the ethical and legal implications of practitioner and managerial actions in situations of risk and crisis. Chapter Fourteen builds on this to present a very practical view of managing risk. The importance of a strategy that involves the whole organisation is seen as essential. The final chapter concentrates on the management of crisis. Dolan tackles the integration of theory and practice by taking the personal perspective although setting this within the current context of health care changes and organisational culture. He emphasises the importance of types of reflective practice and the development of an attitude that sees crisis as a learning tool.

The overall conclusion has to be that there are no easy solutions. Decision making will always be an activity that challenges, surprises and frustrates, particularly on a day-to-day basis, but it can also be creative and rewarding if the big picture is kept in mind.

Managing risk and crisis

Chapter **Thirteen**

Managing risk and crisis: legal and ethical implications

Beverley Hunt

- ● Policy directives or a prescription for risk management?
- ● A cultural dilemma?
- ● What are the values inherent in risk management?
- ● What are our motives and intentions for implementing risk management?
- ● Can we eliminate health care risks?
- ● What are the consequences of taking risks?
- ● What standard of care or level of risk should the public expect?
- ● Should organisational goals come before professional duties?
- ● Conclusion

OVERVIEW

Conceptually, risk management, ethics and law are connected by the principle of non-maleficence: *doing no harm*. In relation to risk management, this principle may be understood in various ways: as harm as an unintended outcome, harm as future outcome, harm as a consequence of an action or an omission, harm through inexperience, harm through ignorance, harm through resistance to change as well as psychological, physical or environmental harm. Therefore, the concept of risk management as protecting patients from harm merits consideration of the implicit relationship between the intentions of health care, concepts of harms within the confines of health care delivery and the expectations of society.

In this chapter, my argument is based on four broad factors.

1. The government will have failed to exercise the level of moral responsibility expected by society if risk management is seen only as a set of procedures and policy directives to be implemented in the NHS.
2. Successful implementation of risk management in the NHS will depend on the values, motives and intentions of individuals working within the health care system.
3. Organisational goals can sometimes take precedence over professional duties, thereby limiting the manager's ability to take the course of action that will reduce risks in the care environment.
4. Change can only be achieved if attention is paid to the underlying culture of the organisation and the values, motives and intentions of those who work within it.

These factors will be considered in the form of the following six questions.

- Are the government's policy initiatives a prescription for risk management?
- What are the values, motives and intentions of risk management?
- Should we try to eliminate risk in health care delivery?
- If not, what are the consequences of taking such risk?
- What standards of care should the public expect?
- Can organisational goals take precedence over professional duty?

POLICY DIRECTIVES OR A PRESCRIPTION FOR RISK MANAGEMENT?

Over four decades ago, Drucker (1957) stated that managers of the future will have to take more risks for a longer period of time and that risk-taking decisions will have to be made at the lower ends of the organisation. This statement resounds throughout the NHS today, as responsibility for standards of care are devolved to individuals at all levels of the organisation. Now, more than ever before, managers are required to think beyond their organisation silos to seeing the NHS as a collective whole.

Governing both the provision and delivery of health care today is an ethos that equates protecting patients from harm with a state-imposed prescription for NHS trusts and primary care trusts (PCTs) to implement clinical risk management. This is to deal with the public's reaction to the preventable serious failures in the treatment and care of patients. The prescription for risk management is evidenced in initiatives developed from the quality assurance agenda of the 1980s. For example, the World Health Organization (WHO) (1989) stated that 'to ensure quality is to ensure that patients receive such care as is most likely to produce the optimal achievable outcome . . . consistent with biological circumstances . . . concomitant pathology . . . [and the] *lowest achievable risk to the patient'.*

More recently, the quality agenda has been taken further in the White Paper entitled *A First Class Service* (DoH 1998), which outlines the framework for clinical governance and the requirements for a leaner, stronger health service with statutory accountability across various offices and professional groups. The underlying principle of clinical governance is to ensure that a high quality of care is provided to patients, that standards continually improve, that there are clear lines of accountability, risk management plans are implemented and adverse incidents are reported.

This national framework will bring together a number of initiatives to oversee and evaluate the types of clinical care that patients receive and, make recommendations on the best outcome-based treatments available, thereby removing the need for individuals to define their own type of treatment. For example:

- the National Service Frameworks (NSFs) outline the process of treatment for specific disorders including mental health, coronary heart disease, cancer care and older people's services, to address problems relating to fair access, efficiency and effective delivery and user involvement
- the National Institute of Clinical Excellence (NICE) appraises 'best' interventions and treatments and offers authoritative guidance on the highest standards of care
- the Performance Assessment Framework (PAF) focuses on the delivery of timely, appropriate, clinically and cost-effective health care that meets the needs of the local population
- the Commission for Health Improvement (CHI) is a patient-focused, rather than cost-focused, framework for ensuring that NHS institutions are accountable for their actions.

Several other changes, including the initial framework of clinical risk management that was set up in 1995 to enable NHS trusts to

Managing risk and crisis: legal and ethical implications

settle claims quickly, have been adopted. For example, the Existing Liabilities Scheme (ELS) provides financial assistance for cases costing over £10 000 where the incident occurred before 1 April 1995. Claims after this period are settled, subject to excess, by the Clinical Negligence Scheme for Trusts (CNST). This scheme allows NHS trusts and health authorities to pool the cost of clinical negligence by paying into the scheme in advance of any claims arising. The National Health Service Litigation Authority (NHSLA) administers the CNST and members of the scheme who operate an acceptable risk management system also benefit from financial remuneration. In relation to this scheme, four objectives of risk management are prevention, identification, assessment and correction of health care-related injuries.

The Health Act 1999 Section 18 states: 'It is the duty of each Health Authority, Primary Care Trust and NHS Trust to put and keep in place arrangements for the purpose of monitoring and improving the quality of health care which it provides'. This Act has introduced a number of changes to the structure and management of the NHS in the UK. For example, the quality assurance and partnership provisions outlined in the Act include a statutory duty of quality in health care and affects all health service members, including non-executive directors (NEDs) and chairs. Taken together, these initiatives send a clear message that while practitioners are responsible for the domain of treatment and care, the quality of that care and treatment is monitored and measured not only by the practitioners concerned but also the law, the state and society at large.

A CULTURAL DILEMMA?

An increasing number of recent high-profile medical and nursing wrongs to patients are thought to be due to a culture where service developments alongside recruitment and retention issues have led to sustained internal pressures on managers and affected their capacity to be effective. Simons (1999) identified three types of internal pressures which can affect the level of risk exposure in organisations. References will be made to these throughout the chapter.

- Risks due to culture.
- Risks due to growth.
- Risks due to information management.

Managing risk and crisis

However, Smith et al (1957), in an analysis of the term 'culture' in relation to education curriculum analysis, identified three components of culture, which may be helpful when thinking about the culture of the NHS. *Universal* components of culture accepted by all of society include conventions about, for example, what conduct and work everyone expects. *Special* components of culture are concerned with vocational skills, customs or expertise of social groups, for example, medicine or nursing. And thirdly, *alternative* or 'counterculture' components for those who are dissatisfied with the specialist or universal ways of thinking and doing.

The prescription for risk management in the NHS reflects the need for managers to bring about sustainable change in its universal and special cultural components. But sustainable change in NHS culture cannot be achieved simply by transmitting the values and beliefs as portrayed in the risk management agenda onto the existing NHS culture. It is also not possible to do so by reproducing the ways in which the specialist professional groups work.

Moreover, it could be argued that while the prescription for risk management is intended to help professionals, managers and the general public to reinterpret the current NHS culture, it does so in ways that reflect patients' health care problems, patients' and professionals' experiences of and within the health care system as well as the requirements for public protection and dissatisfaction with the dominant health care culture.

Clinical risk management is thus a framework for patient safety that will continue to impact on practitioners and managers alike. The multifunctional role of managers includes leading and managing human, financial and clinical resources for effective day-to-day care of patients as well as a delegated responsibility for managing the strategically improving health care delivery. Translated into operational functions, the role includes:

- empowering individuals to take responsibility for their practice
- creating an inclusive participatory approach that inspires ultimate ownership by patients and practitioners working together to develop a culture of openness, trust, respect and integrity
- adopting a whole-systems approach to risk management that takes account of the complexities of organisational life and ensures that ideas on ethical management are connected to the day-to-day overall management of patient care
- managing information flow across different health and social care organisations, particularly in relation to patient-related data.

For example, taking a nursing perspective, the cultural norm in the UK lacks a critical, nurse-centred approach to uncovering the real

Managing risk and crisis

costs – human, financial or emotional – of nursing negligence or nursing malpractice. This has far-reaching implications for managers because although the base figure for general malpractice claims has doubled since 1997, what is not known is how much of this is caused by nursing negligence as a contributory factor. Knowledge of the actual harm to patients and/or benefits of care with which nurses are directly involved should be made known as part of the culture of openness.

One way to explore this further is to examine the substance of cases brought before the professional regulatory body for nursing, the Nursing and Midwifery Council (until 2001, the UKCC), and the reports of the Health Service Commissioner (HSC). This would clarify the extent of reported nursing negligence and the lessons that can be learned from these cases to enhance nursing practice. To do otherwise would be to support, albeit unintentionally, practices that dominate and stultify nursing itself, with resultant harm to patients.

There is also a pressing need to ensure that there is interaction between the NHS complaints procedure and the regulatory bodies. For example, in evidence provided by the UKCC to the Parliamentary Health Select Committee, the UKCC stated:

> Consideration should be given to how the NHS complaints procedure can be more effectively interfaced with the jurisdiction of regulatory bodies and to making more explicit to the public the respective roles of the Health Service Commissioner and the regulatory bodies.

Professional regulation forms an indirect but important part of risk management because it has the authority to regulate the behaviours and practice of practitioners that can destroy public trust as well as the organisation's energy and performance.

The foregoing factors raise value-based issues concerning, at one level, a state interventionist approach to the values inherent in providing and delivering health care and, at another level, an organisation- or person-centred approach.

WHAT ARE THE VALUES INHERENT IN RISK MANAGEMENT?

Health care is a complex values-centred political process in which value judgements of the state, individual health care providers, professionals, patients and the public at large impinge on each other and on the structure, process and outcomes of the health service, with resultant value conflicts. Values are not absolute and difficulties may arise from trying to prioritise competing values. One implication arising from this position is that it is impossible to satisfy or uphold the values of everyone in the environment of care. New (1999, p.58) takes the view that the 'DoH should produce a statement of NHS values, [together] with an explicit acceptance of the need to trade off values against each other'.

However, the values underlying the objectives of the NHS when it was first set up in 1944 emphasised equal opportunity to benefit, a comprehensive service and free access at the point of delivery. Alongside these objectives were certain freedoms including the 'freedom of the doctor to pursue his own professional methods in his own way . . .' (HMSO 1944, cited in New 1999, p.22). During the prevailing political ideology of the 1980s, the values underlying the NHS emphasised an economically driven cost-effective and value-for-money approach to health care.

More recently, emphasis has shifted from the economic, values-based approach to health care, with taken-for-granted freedoms, to a more patient-centred participatory approach to care, thereby trading off professional freedoms for professional accountability and integrity. The shift in emphasis has come about in an attempt to address the loss of public confidence in the health service and the need to make more explicit the moral values inherent in the NHS. It seems that the foregoing prescriptive framework includes moral values such as honesty, universality, choice, respect for persons, caring, professional accountability and professional integrity, all of which may be ranked differently by the different stakeholders mentioned above and which could potentially be in conflict with each other.

For example, a patient's biologically determined first-order value may, at the point of care delivery, be in conflict with his or her choice, freedom and autonomy. Similarly, the term 'accountability' will mean different things to different people, depending on the grade of staff and the professional, organisational and legal expectations of those to whom that member of staff is accountable. Therefore, as it is impossible for managers or indeed the NHS to uphold everyone's values, managers must have the capacity to trade off or balance the different values without subjecting themselves, their staff or patients to danger or harm.

There are less obvious differences affecting the public at large. In this regard, public values may be defined as 'conceptions of the morally desirable in the realm of state activity' (New 1999, p.ii). This definition is consistent with the view that the provision of a health service and health care is a state activity. Furthermore, it would seem that risk management in the NHS is also a state activity. If this is so, what then is the role of the manager in managing risk and values to overcome possible harm to staff and patients?

Many managers are aware that the health care decisions they take or have made for them raise fundamental issues about their beliefs about the provision and delivery of health care. Additionally, this raises concerns about their cultural roles as managers within health care organisations, the role of politics in health care and their accountability, including the authority and responsibility that are vested in them as managers.

Several implications flow from this. First, while it is important to question why politics is involved in health care reform, it is also worth noting that the role of politics in health care is about the distribution of justice and justification of its power in society. In this respect, power is about the means to destabilise, pursue and achieve ends held, in this case, by specialist professional groups and to prevent other groups pursuing ends that are counter to those being claimed by the politicians.

Second, there is a need for managers to have a critical awareness of the values against which they make their day-to-day professional judgements. Third, having made known the values base from which they operate, managers need to challenge the status quo when values-based judgements made at all levels of care delivery impact negatively on patient care and become the norm.

Fourth, structures, processes and frameworks generated by the requirements for accountability may, in some circumstances, be counterproductive as individuals in the organisation follow them without questioning the meaning that these procedures may have for their work and roles.

Lastly, managers need to be sensitive to the moral goals of health care, one of which is 'to do no harm and to do good'. Additionally, managers also need to be aware of the diversity that exists among various professional groups, population groups and patients and not to assume that their own values of risk management will be unconsciously shared by the general public or by others with whom they work. This will mean making explicit the values underlying the processes and procedures in which their approach to risk management is embedded.

Clearly, then, following hard and fast rules, frameworks or ethical theories to inform ethical decision making does not necessarily lead one to do that which is morally right. Indeed, Hunt (1994) and Maclean (1994) view the application of philosophical ethical theories to resolve ethical dilemmas as a misconception of the nature of philosophy which, they claim, has very little place, if any, in informing moral thinking or ethical decision making. Similarly,

Managing risk and crisis

others argue that using such theories cannot adequately explain the complexity of moral problems and human interaction. To do so is to reduce morality to a set of absolutes and social goods, which do not reflect the values implicit in the moral or ethical dilemmas experienced within the health care culture.

Values in risk management are driven by both political and economical factors, which are extrinsic in nature because they are instrumental for achieving other things that we value, such as protecting patients from harm. By its very nature, risk management has both a role and a value in serving the interests of society. It has a role because of its value in preventing harm to both service users and service providers. It therefore has a value on account of its role. Thus, it seems that our common-sense distinctions are important ones in health care and it makes very good common sense to *strive* to protect patients from harm as much as is practical.

WHAT ARE OUR MOTIVES AND INTENTIONS FOR IMPLEMENTING RISK MANAGEMENT?

A prescribed risk management system for an effectively run health care service has many benefits but also some tensions. One possible motive for justifying the implementation of risk management in the health care system appears to have both positive and negative connotations. On the positive side, it could be argued that to do 'good' is to recognise that there is a potential for harm, which can be nullified through the risk management process. The negative side to this seems to be based on fear of the public's distrust of professionals. For example, if nothing is done to protect patients from harm and malpractice claims continue to spiral, the backlash from society could be harmful on several different levels, which may include policing of the health care system, with a resultant loss of *so-called* professional autonomy.

Therefore, the end served by the positive and negative aspects of the motive for implementing risk management indicates that risk management does not merely support human interests and neither is it restricted to resolving technical problems of care. It also serves political motives and intentions, as well as politically motivated organisational interests. Clearly, then, the prescription to implement risk management raises important questions about the motives and intentions of all concerned. Broadly speaking, intentions are concerned with choices or aims, whereas motives are what determine the choice or aim (Anscombe 1970, p.147). If the intention of managing risk is to reduce harm to patients, practical reasoning dictates that health care practitioners ought to utilise those strategies or frameworks of care/risk management that will enable that intention to be achieved effectively.

While some actions are freely chosen, other actions may be carried out under compulsion or, as an appeal to different forces at different levels of the hierarchy in the organisation. It is also possible that the primary motive for implementing risk management may not always flow from a *genuine concern* for patient welfare and protection from harm, so far as this is practical; but from an appeal to a higher authority or fear of individual or organisational exposure to tortious liability.

CAN WE ELIMINATE HEALTH CARE RISKS?

Life and, by analogy, health care is not risk free but there is a sense in which, due to some of the harmful outcomes of risky decision taking, risk is perceived as a negative activity that ought to be eliminated. This is an 'is-ought' fallacy in reasoning, in that it does not follow that because risk *is* perceived as negative, it *ought* to be eradicated or that it would even be in our best interests to do so.

Moreover, each time a new drug is given to a patient for the first time, it has the potential to result in harmful outcomes. Fear of these effects does not prevent the drug from being used because its therapeutic effects may be greater than the harmful effects of not taking it. The implication is that, at an organisation level, strategic risk management objectives should be based on effective communication and information management systems to enable informed choices to be made. For example, in North Thames Regional Authority, there are no established systems to help identify adverse events in primary care. While hospitals hold information that may be helpful to the PCTs, there is no 'collaborative venture between them to share such information' (Department of Public Health 1998).

Clearly, then, the real problem is not only about taking risks but also about how the consequences of risks are managed. This may be thought of in two ways. First, the extent to which individuals are empowered by their organisations and professions to take moral responsibility for making available all tangible information about clinical practice and 'good' or 'bad' performance within the organisation, to highlight those areas of practice that fall below their own as well as the public's proper expectations. This approach demands openness and dialogue, rather than a culture of blame and shame, so that there is continuous improvement as a result of learning from experience.

Second, there is a need for those managing and directing NHS organisations to take corporate moral responsibility, promote ideal human values within the organisations and ensure that the strategy for managing risks reflects futuristic thinking in their current decision taking. Models of corporate responsibility, e.g. from Shell UK and the Body Shop, have much to offer managers in NHS organisations regarding a values-based approach to risk management.

The notion of futuristic thinking is consistent with the principle of foreseeability as well as the concept of strategic organisation development. Drucker (1980) states that, from a strategic management perspective, current actions can have a long-term effect but, equally it can take a long time before the effects of some of these actions are known. For example, the NHS currently faces a medical negligence bill of £2.6 billion, double the amount in 1997. Due to the length of time it takes before some claims are received, an additional estimated liability of £1.3 billion has been set aside for negligence that is likely to have happened but has not yet come to light (Ferriman 2001).

Interestingly, it is only when there has been a problem that practitioners get feedback on the effects of their actions. It could be up to 3 or more years before a patient realises that a problem has occurred that is attributable to the health care intervention. However, when this happens, the patient can seek remedy through the Limitation Act 1980, which provides for all actions for personal injury to be brought within 3 years of the particular injury. Sections 11 and 14 provide that if a patient was unaware that he or she had suffered significant injury or did not know that negligence had occurred which could have caused his or her injury, the 3-year period runs only from the time when the patient became aware or should have become aware of what happened.

Implicit in the Limitation Act 1980 is the requirement for the management of risk related to patient-related information. Consequently, the risk management approach should include the process and principles of documentation of patient care to a standard that would satisfy legal requirements and nullify any claims of negligence. These requirements necessitate that the standard of care should be of a good quality, that patient-related information is precise, thorough, truthful, clear and objective, specifically detailing the nature and type of care and treatment given to the patient.

From the foregoing, it can be deduced that there are two broad categories of risk in health care: people risk and organisational risk. At a simplistic level, organisational risks (sometimes called environmental risks) are concerned with the structures, processes and

Managing risk and crisis: legal and ethical implications

systems within the organisation that may restrict the quality of care given to patients. This includes resource-based factors such as staffing levels, skill mix, poor communication and other systems that can negatively affect the environment of care. The preference here is to refer to organisation risk rather than environmental risks. This is because the organisation is responsible for the environment, including the use of dangerous or hazardous equipment and materials in the work and/or care environment.

People risk may also be referred to as clinical risk. The preference is to refer to it as people risk to take account of all people-related activities or clinical interventions that may result in malpractice claims due not only to the side effects of care and treatment but also to the attendant adverse outcomes. This is not to say that side effects do not merit important considerations in the management of risk, because they do. However, an assumption is being made in this chapter that the practitioner will have ensured that, prior to any intervention, he or she has obtained valid consent. To do so would mean disclosing the broad nature, material risks and possible side effects of the intervention to the patient, so far as this is practical. For example, the legal requirements for valid consent dictate that the:

- patient has the capacity to comprehend the information
- practitioner discloses the risks and benefits of the treatment
- patient gives voluntary consent to the procedure.

Where it is not practical to gain valid consent due, e.g. due to the patient's mental status, 'best' practice dictates that practitioners should have uppermost in their minds the will to protect the individual patient's interests and take action which, on the balance of probabilities, would be in accord with the wishes of the individual involved.

These two categories of risks are connected but are not the same and should be treated differently but not dichotomised. Given the complexities that exist in NHS organisations, one problem for managers is the extent to which they can ensure a consistently high standard of care at all times. Three issues flow from this.

First, we have seen that value conflicts can impact on and affect different people at different levels of the organisation. Second, a high standard of care does not always mean getting things right each time with no adverse outcomes of care. It can also mean adopting a timely proactive approach to managing such situations, including accurate explanations of what went wrong rather than for patients being met with a veil of secrecy. Third, ensuring a consistently high standard of care can challenge the manager's ability to:

- build effective working relationships with individuals, teams and groups across the health and social care systems
- empower their staff to take responsibility for the consequences of their actions and the services that they deliver.

WHAT ARE THE CONSEQUENCES OF TAKING RISKS?

There is a sense in which, insofar as medicine, nursing and the allied health professions have a common goal, e.g. health restoration and health promotion, the very ethics of these professions *must* be consequential. That is, if health is an important – and some would say an *ineliminable* – aspect of well-being, it is the one good which health care professionals have a professional, contractual and moral duty to maximise. Therefore, health care professionals have a moral duty to choose that course of action which, on balance, is most likely to provide the greatest benefit to the greatest number.

At a macro level (organisational or government), this is consistent with the idea that:

- if we have an effective risk management approach to care, it may, as a consequence, ensure that scarce financial resources for health care are spent in the pursuit of the broader goals of people's health care rather than on compensation for negligent care
- inclusively calculating outcomes from actions may be interpreted as meaning that we would want to ensure our safety during any future health care interventions that we may experience, so we might as a consequence reduce the cost of compensation with resultant cost-effective but safe care for everyone.

At an individual level, while it is possible to count the financial cost of harm and suffering, it is very difficult to measure the impact of emotional or psychological harms to staff and patients as a result of adverse outcomes of care or environment hazards. Therefore, one difficulty with a consequentialist approach to morality is that, even if everyone who is likely to be affected in this calculation were to be included, uncertainty of the outcomes of decisions as well as individual preferences would militate against anyone reliably predicting outcomes that are of benefit to everyone.

Risk management in health care is therefore a timely and important initiative. The introduction of Crown indemnity, the NHS and Community Care Act 1990 and removal of Crown immunity from the NHS are but three crucially important factors. The introduction

Managing risk and crisis: legal and ethical implications

of Crown indemnity has meant that district health authorities are responsible for negligent claims of malpractice against *all members of the health care professions*. The challenges for managers not only arise from practice and state intervention but also have their roots in the legal system. So, what is the duty of care? And how can this legal principle help?

In tracing the origins of a general principle for risk management, one may draw inferences from the law. Concepts of consequences of actions and risk management are congruent with the legal duty of care and the principle of foreseeability. For example, within the scope of the duty of care, it was Lord Atkin in 1932, in the case of *Donoghue v. Stevenson [1932] AC 562; [1932] 1 All ER 1*, who stated that:

> You must take reasonable care to avoid acts or omissions which you can reasonably foresee would be likely to injure your neighbour. Who, then, in law is my neighbour? The answer seems to be – persons who are closely and directly affected by my act that I ought reasonably to have them in contemplation as being so affected when I am directing my mind to the acts or omissions which are called into question.

Today, in terms of precedent, this principle is still applied in civil law cases and remains the bedrock of the tort of negligence where a breach of duty with resultant harm constitutes liability. Implied in Lord Atkin's statement are the origins of clinical risk management and its interconnectedness with harms as set out within the duty of care, the conditions for a breach of which are that:

- the practitioner (defendant) owes a duty of care to the plaintiff
- there has been a breach of that duty
- the breach caused the plaintiff harm and suffering
- the harm and suffering were foreseeable.

Law, being largely reactive and evidential in nature, serves the interest of justice, but after the harm has been done. The principle of *foreseeability* of harm fits well with managing risks, as well as the outcomes of one's actions and omissions. The four stages of risk management compare well with Lord Atkin's statement on the duty of care that is owed to patients and clients, as outlined in Box 13.1.

Moreover, the neighbour principle and the concept of foreseeability of harms resulting from actions and omissions, established in *Donoghue*, have been developed further in two well-documented cases. In *Caparo Industries plc v. Dickman [1990] 1 ALL ER* the House of Lords considered corporate and professional conduct and the role and responsibilities of professional advisers. In *The Nicholas H [1996] 1 AC 211 (HL) 18, 19*, a cargo was lost after a ship certified by the ship's surveyor as seaworthy sank. These cases are non-medical

> **Box 13.1** Comparison between the statement by Lord Atkin (1932) regarding the principles of the duty of care and the stages of risk management

Stages of risk management	Principles of the duty of care
1. **Identification** – of what can go wrong	1. **Identification** – establishing that a duty of care is owed
2. **Analysis** – of the severity, frequency or likelihood of it going wrong	2. **Analysis** – contemplate the persons who are closely and directly affected by your actions and omissions and *reasonably* foresee the resultant outcomes of these actions/omissions
3. **Control** – the changes that can or should be made to prevent or reduce the effects of it going wrong	3. **Control** – take reasonable care to avoid actions and omissions which . . . would injure your neighbour
4. **Funding** – of losses that are incurred including how this will be paid if it goes wrong	4. **Liability and compensation** – Who pays for compensation. If you are at fault (wrongful breach of duty), then you may be required to pay compensation to the injured party or parties

but the outcomes of such cases may have implications for risk managers who as professional advisers are often called upon to report on the 'seaworthiness' of standards of practice. Indeed, in the draft risk management report from UCLH (1998), one of the nine areas of responsibilities of risk managers was 'provision of advice to all staff' on several key areas of organisational work (UCLH 1998, p.3).

WHAT STANDARD OF CARE OR LEVEL OF RISK SHOULD THE PUBLIC EXPECT?

Legally, an action in negligence may be viewed as a two-pronged activity involving identification of the nature of the negligent act and establishing the amount of compensation to be paid to the plaintiff if negligence is proven. Sources of the principle of negligence are to be found in case law. However, professional issues regarding negligence and competence reflect the principles of the legal duty of care mentioned elsewhere as well as standards of care.

Managing risk and crisis: legal and ethical implications

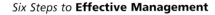

The standard of care delivered to patients has been extensively examined in various legal cases, for example, in *Bolitho v. City and Hackney Health Authority [1997] 4 ALL ER 771 (HL); Wilsher v. Essex Area Health Authority [1986]; Whitehouse v. Jordan (1981) 1 ALL ER; Bolam v. Friern Barnet Hospital Management Committee [1957] 1 WLR.* In *Bolam*, Judge McNair stated that:

> . . . Where you get a situation which involves the use of some special skill or competence, then the test as to whether there has been negligence or not is . . . the standard of the ordinary skilled man exercising and professing to have that special skill.

This means that the legal standard of care expected by practitioners and/or managers is judged according to the skill and expertise that the individual is deemed to have by virtue of being either a learner, manager or qualified practitioner. However, while a high standard of care is the ideal set by practitioners, the law sets the benchmark for the standard of care at a minimum standard.

Being an inexperienced learner is no defence in law to an action for negligence. For example, in *Wilshire v. Essex AHA [1987] QB 730 (1986) 3 ALL ER 801 (CA)*, Lord Justice Musthill commented on the issues facing hospitals, stating that 'wards and departments could not be staffed or junior staff could not learn if such staff' were to be prevented from learning on the job.

The law requires the same standard of the trainee being judged as of his or her more experienced colleague. Therefore, any failure to achieve appropriate standards through ignorance, inexperience, incompetence or lack of knowledge and skill that results in damage or harm to patients may lead to an action of negligence and compensation for the harm caused.

Given the human resource issues facing many NHS trusts, this line of reasoning has some implications for risk managers in relation to the ongoing professional development of all staff and proper supervision of learners in clinical placements. With senior staff moving further away from the bedside to management positions, less experienced practitioners may take on roles and responsibilities that bring additional clinical risks, with resultant legal implications for managers and employers by means of vicarious liability.

SHOULD ORGANISATIONAL GOALS COME BEFORE PROFESSIONAL DUTIES?

Managers and practitioners are individual moral agents and, as such, they are responsible for their actions and are deemed to know

Managing risk and crisis

right from wrong and good from harmful or bad health care practices. They also have vested in them the authority to act to protect patients from harm. This comes from their acceptance of the various domains of their specialised roles as well as the ability and power to take effective, relevant action as and when appropriate.

It is said that experience brings authority but the authority to act does not come from experience alone as this blinds individuals to new ways of working. Indeed, some individuals succumb to situational control in the organisation within which they work to the extent that they allow themselves to be socialised into the often dysfunctional, introspective values that prevail there. This means that they can become so deeply immersed in their roles that they do not take account of the wider consequences of their actions. Therefore, authority comes from the capacity to critically reflect on experience and the duty to take responsibility for the emerging culture of clinical practice. Put another way, authority is like the key that unlocks the door to empower individuals to take responsibility for bringing about reform, overcoming past conventions and harmful outmoded ways of working.

For example, in a study reported by Carmunas (1994), nurse managers identified, amongst others, three issues that most frequently presented ethical conflicts for them when making decisions regarding patient care. These are:

- allocation and rationing of scarce resources
- staffing levels and skill mix decisions
- developing and maintaining standards of care.

It can be deduced from this study that these findings demonstrate a number of important points, for example:

- the tensions between these three items may result in a conflict of role between employee and employer
- a manager with little or no control over the resources available for patient care will employ less well-qualified health carers with poor skill mix, which can result in unintentional risk of harm to patients, employees and the organisation as a whole.

Most importantly, the study demonstrates the connections between individual behaviour, organisational roles and the way in which a manager can succumb to his or her institutional role. This means that in such circumstances, decisions taken regarding the use of resources can mean that the organisation's goals take precedence over professional goals and patient care. While the gap between resources and responsibility can cause pressures of work for health care staff, one cannot assume that scarce resources will automatically mean

Managing risk and crisis: legal and ethical implications

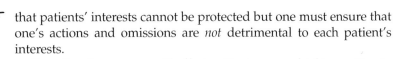

that patients' interests cannot be protected but one must ensure that one's actions and omissions are *not* detrimental to each patient's interests.

Scarcity of resources will affect patient care and taking action to combat this problem demands that individuals have the moral courage to exemplify those values and beliefs that are important to and represented by them. It does not take a crystal ball to realise that reduction of malpractice claims would preserve scarce health care resources. This raises questions about how best to manage health care risks, particularly when prioritising the (often competing) interests of several patients in an entire ward.

The corporate duty of organisations in relation to the rights of individuals has been spelt out by UNESCO (1998) who make explicit the corporate duty owed to individuals. This suggests that the state and public bodies, including NHS trusts, have a duty (negative or positive) to respond appropriately to public concerns about individual rights as well as the universal and special cultural components of managerial and professional conduct, judgement and standards of practice. What is not clear is how this declaration will be enforced, if at all. The policy directives are in place as a means to protect patients from harm, but can they?

Central to these issues is the professional, ethical and legal duty owed to the patient in the health care system. Managing risk is about getting the balance right between a number of conflicting rights and duties. Human interaction, being an important factor within the spectrum of health care, necessitates that NHS institutions recognise their intrinsic obligation and corporate duty to ensure that they respect the rights of managers and practitioners to care for and to protect patients from harm.

CONCLUSION

A number of issues were explored in this chapter, starting with the interrelationship between the intentions of health care, causes of harms and the expectations of society. Harms were addressed in relation to values, motives and intentions, consequences of actions, standards of care and duties and rights, organisationally, individually and professionally. One key question concerned whether it is desirable to eradicate harms.

Throughout the chapter, two themes arose: first, the need for change in the culture of organisational management, to implement effective information management and communication systems. Second, the view that one cannot claim immunity from wrongdoing. Fundamental to determining right from wrong is the ability to draw on one's own moral conscience. As individual moral agents, managers and practitioners each have an individual moral responsibility and duty to ensure that their actions and omissions, for whatever reason, do not harm others. Risk management may be used as a tool to cut the financial cost of suffering but what cannot be counted is the emotional cost of suffering when things go wrong.

References

Anscombe GEM 1970 Intention. In: White A (ed) The philosophy of action. Oxford University Press, Oxford, p 147

Carmunas C 1994 Ethical dilemmas of nurse executives (part 1). Journal of Nursing Administration 24(7/8): 45–51

Department of Health 1998 A first class service. Department of Health, Leeds

Department of Public Health 1998 Clinical governance in North Thames: a paper for discussion and consultation. NHSE North Thames Regional Office, London (www.doh.gov.uk/ntro/summary/htm#top)

Drucker P 1957 The practice of management. Harper and Row, New York

Drucker P 1980 Managing in turbulent times. Butterworth Heinemann, London

Ferriman A 2001 NHS faces medical negligence bill of £2.6bn. British Medical Journal 322: 1081

Hunt G 1994 Book review: The elimination of morality: reflections on utilitarianism and bioethics. Nursing Ethics 1(3): 187–188

Maclean A 1994 The elimination of morality: reflections on utilitarianism and bioethics. Routledge, London

New B 1999 A good-enough service: values, trade-offs and the NHS. Institute for Public Policy Research and the King's Fund, London

Simons R 1999 How risky is your company? Harvard Business Review 77(3): 85–94

Smith BO, Stanley W, Shores J 1957 Fundamentals of curriculum development. Harcourt Brace, New York

UNESCO 1998 Declaration of human duties and responsibilities. UNESCO, New York

University College London Hospitals 1998 Risk Management report (draft) at www.doh.gov.uk/pub/docs/doh/riskuc/h.pdf

World Health Organization 1998 The principles of quality assurance: WHO Working Group Regional Office in Quality Assurance in Health Care. Pergamon Press, Oxford, pp 79–95

Managing risk and crisis: legal and ethical implications

Application **13:1**

Beverley Hunt

Managing risk and crisis

Guidelines and protocols: issues of legal liability

The cases outlined below demonstrate the importance of ensuring not only that guidelines meet certain criteria but that individual practitioners have kept abreast of updated practices in their particular field of practice and that they can legally and professionally justify decisions that they make about client/patient care interventions.

In the case of *Early v. Newham Health Authority [1994] Med LR 214*, the plaintiff, a 13-year-old girl, was being anaesthetised for an appendicectomy. The anaesthetist administered intravenous injection of thiopentone, 100 micrograms of fentanyl and 100 milligrams of suxamethonium, a drug that causes short-term paralysis. The plaintiff came around from the anaesthetic whilst still partly paralysed and was in a state of panic and distress. She claimed that (a) the anaesthetist was negligent in failing to intubate her successfully the first time and (b) the procedure that he adopted when he failed to intubate her was faulty. The claim was dismissed.

Deputy Judge Patrick Bennett QC found the guidelines to be reasonable in that 'a reasonable competent medical authority could have adopted it for their use'. Newham HA laid down the procedure that the anaesthetist used. In this case, the guidelines were developed with consultation with the Division of Anaesthesia and discussions with consultants all of whom decided that the procedures outlined were appropriate.

One point to note is that evidence provided by a key expert witness, Dr McAteer, was founded on medical knowledge drawn from two countries, Sweden and Holland, and two teaching hospitals, the Hammersmith Hospital and the London Hospital. However, beyond this evidence, the judge also placed emphasis on the fact that the 'failed intubation procedure' had been fully discussed within the hospital and the minutes of these discussions were documented. In other words, the consultants had *foreseen* the likelihood of failed intubation occurring and, drawing on the available and responsible body of evidence, had implemented a procedure for managing the risk to bring about the best possible results for the patient.

Issues to consider:

- the legal status of guidelines or protocols
- professional advice and guidelines
- reasonable request.

THE LEGAL STATUS OF GUIDELINES

It is not sufficient for practitioners to accept a practice as standard because everyone else has conformed to it. For example, the standard of practice employed by a 'substantial body of expert medical opinion' was reassessed in the case of *Bolitho v. City and Hackney Health Authority [1997] 4 ALL ER 771 (HL)*. Concerns were expressed regarding whether or not a particular practice described by medical experts as 'accepted by a responsible body of medical opinion' could also be negligent practice. Lord Farquarson stated that:

> It is not enough to call a number of doctors to say that what they had done was in accord with accepted clinical practice. It is necessary for the judge to consider that evidence and decide whether that clinical practice puts the patient unnecessarily at risk. (p. 386)

One conclusion in *Bolitho* is that judges have a prescriptive role to play in determining the standard of care in medical negligence cases. An important point in *Early's* case is that although things did actually go wrong the judge looked at the development process of the guidelines and standards for practice to ensure they were consistent with current approved acceptable standards of practice. It thus seems that:

- clear documentation of the consultation process when developing guidelines can make an important difference when there is alleged negligent care and
- judges set the legal standard of care.

When guidelines are applied in practice with resultant harm to a patient, the potential for a claim of negligence will arise. Many NHS trusts and Primary Care trusts have developed and implemented standards, protocols and guidelines for practice to which practitioners are expected to adhere to avert risk management claims. Simply implementing guidelines cannot ensure safe practices. However, if practitioners are expected to follow standards, protocols and guidelines, there are a number of important lessons that can be learned from the *Early* case. In this regard, managers should ensure that:

- all guidelines for practice are properly ratified; and that individuals responsible for ratifying them are aware of their ethical and legal duties to patients, clients, staff, the organisation and to the public;
- this responsibility also means understanding the contemporary evidence, knowledge, skills and competence available as a benchmark on which to base such standards;

Guidelines and protocols: issues of legal liability

- guidelines are regularly updated to keep abreast with policy, professional and technical developments and research developments, including new knowledge and skills;
- the knowledge-base from which guidelines are developed is supported by a range of appropriate acceptable evidence;
- practitioners do not make decisions solely on the basis of clinical or policy guidelines but must exercise their professional judgement and values base when using guidelines in practice;
- that the organisation learns from its mistakes, analysing the whole complex system of care to identify gaps in the service and to provide the 'organisation with a memory' that is not reliant on any one person (DoH 2000).

Good practice guidelines, for example, *Achieving Effective Practice* (DoH 1998) and the clinical governance reporting structure embraces the general principles of risk management through the call for locally implemented strategies to:

- *inform* the decision making of clinicians, patients and managers
- *change* practice where appropriate and
- *monitor* outcomes.

This calls for a manager who can support the organisation in learning how to learn as well as being a change agent, initiating and adopting change that build on the organisation's capacity to maximise its potential for effective health care.

PROFESSIONAL ADVICE AND GUIDELINES

Health care service providers have adopted various strategies for managing clinical risks. This includes a process of standardisation which calls into question two issues.

- Liability of professional advisers for advice given.
- Enforced use of clinical guidelines for practice.

Firstly, legal deliberations with regard to the liability of professional advisers have some implications for nurse managers who may at times act as professional advisers in the development of standards, guidelines and protocols. There is sufficient proximity in the relationship between the nurse manager, the employing NHS trusts and the practitioner delivering care for a duty of care to be owed to the patient and to each other.

For example, practitioners at the coalface of care often rely on the advice or statements of 'good' practice that are contained within guidelines and protocols for practice. However, professional advisers are legally liable for the advice that they give to others. The question, then, is whether or not it is possible for the deliberations around *proximity*, justness, fairness and reasonableness, by analogy, to be applied to a similar situation where a nurse acts on the professional advice contained in guidelines developed by nurse managers.

The manager will owe a duty of care directly to his or to her employers and indirectly to patients. Therefore, managers ought to take due care when devising such protocols and guidelines for practice. The principle of vicarious liability, in common law, arises out of the legal liability of employers for the negligent acts and omissions of their employees; therefore liability for the negligence of another person will only arise through the doctrine of vicarious liability. While employers may expect nurses to adopt their corporate clinical guidelines in their care interventions, the terms of the employer–employee relationship make the employer liable for the negligent acts of their employees.

ENFORCED USE OF GUIDELINES FOR PRACTICE

In English law, there are implied terms within one's contract of employment that are legally binding between both employer and employee which indicate that each employee must:

- obey all reasonable and lawful instructions of their employers
- exercise reasonable care and skill.

For managers, a decision against using defined corporate guidelines can have equally as contentious outcomes as the decision to adopt them. For example, whilst nurses as employees are expected to obey reasonable and lawful instructions of their employer and exercise reasonable care and skill, an employer cannot 'reasonably' expect a manager to adopt guidelines or procedures that they – the manager/nurse – consider to be at odds with their professional judgement and exercise of that judgement.

The general duties set out in the Health and Safety at Work Act (1974) will be taken into consideration if a member of staff claims that he or she is expected to carry out unreasonable requests in their work environment particularly associated with poor systems and lack of training or instruction. What constitutes a 'reasonable' or an 'unreasonable' request may be interpreted differently by different people. However, the concept of reasonable actions and certain duties were explored. These cases include:

- managing stress at work (*Johnston v. Bloomsbury Area HA [1991] 2 ALL ER 293*)
- the duty to tell employees that they must take breaks and rest pauses (*Pickford v. Imperial Chemical Industries Plc [1997] 8 Med LR*) and
- the statutory duty to ensure a safe system of work (*Health & Safety at Work Act 1974*).

Guidelines and protocols: issues of legal liability

CONCLUSION

The manager's role is not an easy one. However, they must ensure that practitioners are encouraged to exercise sound up-to-date professional judgement and not simply rely on protocols, but this can be difficult to achieve. Protocols or policy development and clinical decisions should include a clearly documented, consultative, patient-centred and partnership approach, rather than a unilateral approach to patient care.

Discussion questions

- What does the clinical guidelines and protocols operated in your sphere of work tell you about the values of your organisation?
- How were they developed and who developed them?
- What will or can you do to ensure that patients and clients remain central to the goals of the organisation?
- Why is it important for your organisation to 'learn how to learn' and to develop a 'memory'?

References

Bolitho v. City and Hackney Health Authority [1997] 4 ALL ER 771 (HL)

Department of Health 2000 An organisation with a memory: Report of an expert group on learning from adverse events in the NHS. Stationery Office, London

Department of Health 1998 Achieving effective practice. Stationery Office, London

Johnston v. Bloomsbury Area HA [1991] 2 ALL ER 293

Health and Safety at Work Act 1974

Pickford v Imperial Chemical Industries Plc [1997] 8 Med LR

Managing risk and crisis

Application 13:2
Lenore Anderson

The importance of documentation in assessing risk

This application looks at an audit document developed by an NHS trust and sets the reader the task of applying this to their own place of work.

BACKGROUND

The importance of documentation has been a long-standing issue in nursing (Gropper 1988). Records provide written evidence of nursing practice and communication about the patient status and their response to care interventions (Tapp 1990). The legal viewpoint is that a nursing document is only what a nurse has done (Cowan 1987, Morrissey-Ross 1988) but it can have wider uses.

The World Health Organization (WHO 1983) published a detailed report on the methods and principles for record keeping. Nurses tend to agree to these in principle but in practice their efforts are poor, many nurses downgrading documentation in favour of patient care (Tapp 1990, Vasey 1979). The WHO (1983) believes that by sharing information through records, nurses would improve the standard and continuity of patient care. Indeed, good record keeping in health care is an issue that will not go away, especially in the current climate of clinical audit and effectiveness for clinical governance and the move to evidence-based research.

LOCAL ACTION

In one particular trust, moves were made to assess the level of good record keeping. Twenty standards were agreed. Nurses were trained in audit techniques and, using the standards, audited 350 sets of nursing notes across the trust. Each auditor used the audit tool shown in Table 13.2.1

Six Steps to **Effective Management**

Table 13.2.1 Clinical audit tool

Standard for nursing documentation audit	1st date	2nd date	3rd date	4th date
1. Patient's full name is on one side of a page				
2. Patient's hospital number is on one side of a page				
3. Patients have a nursing/ midwifery care plan drawn up within 24 hours of admission				
4. Nursing/midwifery care plans are individualised in that they relate to identified problems				
5. Supporting charts relate to plan of care and have been completed 5.A Fluid balance chart 5.B TPR 5.C BP, close observations 5.D Turning chart 5.E Pressure area risk assessment 5.F Wound care assessment 5.G Nutritional status 5.H Manual handling tool 5.I Pain assessment tool 5.J Weight 5.K Height 5.L Other				
6. All entries are clearly dated/timed, ensuring the year is stated 6.A Dated 6.B Timed				
7. All entries are written in chronological order				
8. All entries are signed with usual signature and professional designation				
9. All signatures in nursing notes are in the ward log for that year				

Managing risk and crisis

(continued)

Standard for nursing documentation audit	1st date	2nd date	3rd date	4th date
10. All entries are written in indelible black ink (entries may be underlined in another colour, chart entries may be colour coded)				
11. Any corrections are done with a single line, initialled, dated and timed				
12. Space left at the end of a line is blocked off				
13. Entries made by students are countersigned by a qualified nurse/midwife/ practitioner				
14. Entries made by health care assistants are countersigned by a qualified nurse/ midwife/practitioner				
15. All entries are legible to the auditor				
16. There is a statement in the nursing notes that records all allergies				
17. The next of kin's contact number is recorded				
18. Complex discharge form has been completed				
19. Evidence in nursing notes that patients are receiving information about: 19.A Health promotion 19.B Illness 19.C Treatment				
20. Evidence in the nursing notes about the level of patient's understanding of illness and/or treatment				

(Reproduced with permission from Addenbrooke's NHS Trust.)

The importance of documentation in assessing risk

Six Steps to **Effective Management**

During the audit training, 40 nurses were asked, 'Why should nurses keep records?'; 80% mentioned forming a framework for planning patient care, treatment and evaluation of their progress and meeting legal and UKCC statutory requirements but only 20% indicated the need to provide information for clinical and risk management, quality audits or research (Anderson 1996).

APPLICATION TO OWN AREA OF WORK

If you work in a hospital, use the tool to audit your documentation. Remember to use trained auditors and do not allow self-audit, thereby reducing validity of the findings. The auditing process is only the start; once you have benchmarked the level of adherence to the standards, remember to create a plan of action to address low standard adherence.

If you work in a practice or the community, what modifications to the 20 standards would be needed? Draw up a modified tool for discussion.

'It is inconceivable that in five years' time most clinical process should still be dependent on paper-based manual records' (Dudman 2000). The imminent advent of electronic health records may improve future adherence to the documentation standards and risk strategies will play a big part in any such record.

References

Anderson L 1996 Internal report: nursing documentation audit. Unpublished report. Addenbrooke's NHS Trust, Cambridge

Cowan V 1987 Documentation. Nursing 14: 527–529

Dudman J 2000 Facts at their fingertips. Health Service Journal 110(5728): 9–13

Gropper E 1988 Does charting reflect your worth? Geriatric Nursing Mar/Apr: 99–101

Morrissey-Ross M 1988 Documentation: if you haven't written it, you haven't done it. Nursing Clinics of North America 23(2): 363–371

Tapp RA 1990 Inhibitors and facilitators to documentation of the nursing practice. Western Journal of Nursing Research 12(2): 229–240

Vasey EK 1979 Writing your patient's care plan efficiently. Nursing 9(4): 67–71

World Health Organization 1983 Documentation of the nursing process: report on a working group. WHO Regional Office for Europe, Berne

Chapter **Fourteen**

Assessing and managing risk

Lenore Anderson

- ● Introduction
- ● Risk management programmes
- ● The business case
- ● The role of the risk management team and department
- ● The role of the risk representative
- ● The role of the risk officer
- ● Bringing about change
- ● The role of the employer and employee
- ● Conclusion

OVERVIEW

This chapter will attempt to demystify risk management, enabling the nurse to become proactive in assessing and managing risk in any care setting. The key issues discussed in this chapter are as follows.

- ● What is risk management?
- ● Why do we need risk management?
- ● How does an organisation introduce the concept of risk management?
- ● What is the best framework to achieve effective risk reduction outcomes?
- ● How do people engage with the process?

INTRODUCTION

There is an increasing expectation in all health care sectors that the public require evidence of the level of quality care delivery and service provision. Faugier et al consider that: 'Risk management is a vital component in health service providers' total quality strategies. The future direction may be governed by both patient expectations and the changing nature of the new NHS' (Faugier et al 1997, p. 98). This heightened expectation is reflected in the increasing cost of litigation and complaints that are filed each year (Ham 1995, Stahl 1997). The NHS accounts (April 2000) estimated that its total liability for outstanding claims stood at £2.4 billion. The National Audit Office will be collecting evidence on how the Legal Services Commission evaluates, funds and monitors claims and how well trusts handle and settle them. 'Claims costs is an issue of increasing concern to NHS Trusts, and a comprehensive picture will be useful – Trusts can feel they are working in the dark' (Henderson 2000).

However, Dingwall & Fenn (1991) suggest that litigation is not worth all the attention being lavished on it. The use of litigation as an accurate indicator can be challenged as a rather narrow view. It could be argued that litigation is only the tip of the iceberg as many adverse events are settled out of court or not reported. The government and health care professionals agree that high professional standards from all health care sectors should be the norm and not the exception. Health care workers have a duty of care not to cause harm. Risk management is becoming a necessary and integral part of the working environment in the NHS and private sectors.

The problem is not confined to the UK. A report entitled *To Err is Human: Building a Safer Health System* (Kohn et al 1999) found that in the USA more people die from medical errors than car accidents, making it the fifth leading cause of death. Tingle (2000a) comments that 'healthcare in the USA is 10 years or more behind other high risk industries, both countries need action to improve patient safety'. The USA hopes to introduce wide-ranging strategies to reduce medical errors by 50% over the next 5 years, while in the UK the NHS Executive is working on adverse incident reporting standards and has set out its agenda in *Clinical Governance: Quality in the New NHS* (NHS Executive 1999).

Reason (1995) talks of the human contribution to accidents, in the form of human error. Human error can be described as a failure to adhere to a plan of action, to apply the current knowledge base to the situation or that the plan of action was inadequate and not 'fit for purpose'.

All errors involve some kind of deviation, lapses, slips or trips occur at the level of execution. For mistakes, the actions may go entirely as planned but the plan itself deviates from its path towards its intended goal. (Reason 1995, p. 34)

RISK MANAGEMENT PROGRAMMES

Risk is the possibility of causing harm or loss to patients, visitors or staff or to other assets of the organisation such as information, buildings, equipment and funding or to the reputation of that organisation.

The management of risk is about providing a high-quality and safe service of care by involving the whole health care team in reducing risk and avoiding negligence. Why should an organisation adopt a risk management strategy? A simplistic philosophy would be to claim that everything in our garden is rosy and that all we need to do is to build up sufficient contingency funds to cover any claim. However, the philosophy adopted should include not just consideration of the litigation and legal issues but be broad enough to embrace the moral and ethical dilemma paradigm. It is axiomatic that any health care worker would not ignore any reasonable activity that protects the patient, colleague, visitor or the organisation itself from harm by act of either omission or commission. It is a duty of all health workers to bring risk management into their daily working practice.

> A comprehensive risk management programme needs to address all parts of the service, from clinical services to the management of waste; it is no longer an optional extra. (Nichol 1993)

One of the critical decisions to be faced is how an organisation can introduce the concept of risk management. The danger of introducing departments and/or programmes called 'risk management' is that this can lead to lack of ownership and the development of a mindset that 'It's not my problem, we have a department that deals with that'. The organisation needs to sign up to the continuous commitment of all staff at all levels, to preserve quality of care and protect the public. Gamble & Aires (1994) endorsed the importance of staff working together and using risk management techniques to improve patient care and ensure healthy and safe working conditions.

Risk management should be seen as an essential tool; if it is used in isolation, the results are diminished. There is a need to incorporate risk management into a wider context, so that it can be used in conjunction with other quality initiatives, such as:

- clinical audit and effectiveness
- evidence-based practice
- patient and carer input and advocacy
- complaints
- organisational workload tools
- infection and pressure sore rates
- clinical supervision and reflective practice
- peer review and performance management.

This need was identified in the development and introduction of clinical governance in 1999. This framework, set out in the NHS White Papers *The New NHS: Modern, Dependable* (DoH 1997) and *A First Class Service* (DoH 1998), brings all the above initiatives under one umbrella and the quality of care has an equal footing with fiscal accountability. Health care trusts and authorities have to produce an annual report on clinical governance and failure to provide appropriate standards of care could see trust boards and their chief executives exposed to legal action.

Programmes or strategies must be proactive. For too long the health care sector has been retrospective in nature, taking corrective action after the incident or event. A proactive approach involves the following.

- Engaging all members of staff, visitors and patients.
- Covers all aspects of the organisation's activities.
- Identifies the risk, potential or actual.
- Examines any risk for potential exacerbation.
- Develops strategies that reduce, transfer or eliminate the risks identified.
- Commitment to a continuously evolving programme, fully resourced and accountable to the board of the organisation.

Although the main thrust of risk management is to engage the staff in their place of work and at the customer/professional interface, research by Zeithaml et al (1985) showed the difficulties experienced by service organisations in meeting all customer expectations. They suggest that:

> Quality in a service occurs in the interaction between the customer and the contact personnel and is highly dependent on the performance of the employees. (Zeithaml et al 1985, p. 36)

Management at its highest level needs to be seen to endorse and actively promote the risk reduction concept that will improve that service interaction, by investing in the education of its workforce. It is therefore important to develop a framework that addresses that aspect (Fig. 14.1).

Managing risk and crisis

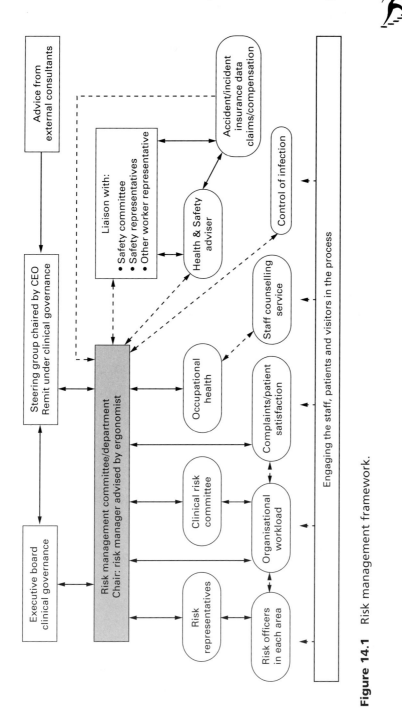

Figure 14.1 Risk management framework.

Assessing and managing risk

Managing risk and crisis

Once an organisation has decided to embrace the concept of risk management, it is important to develop a business case that outlines the cost benefits, options and resources required. This business case must be an integral part of the corporate business plan, thereby ensuring financial support. Nurse managers should include risk management needs in their business plan and look for the following infrastructure within their organisation.

- Preparation for clinical governance, fully developed.
- Organisational, financial and clinical risk strategies.
- Health & Safety framework.
- CoSHH issues discussed and handled appropriately.
- Lifting and handling issues addressed at all levels.
- Security issues highlighted.
- Fire response and prevention procedures.
- Contingency planning for untoward events that have the potential to damage service provision.
- The appointment of a risk management team (RMT), which has the authority to act as and when necessary.
- RMTs are accountable to the organisation's board.
- Access to resources (people, funding and equipment).
- Access to ergonomic advice capable of 'designing out' potential risk problems from the working environment.

Implementation

An implementation framework is essential for engaging the whole organisation in the process. Each part should be clearly defined and reflect the aims of the programme.

1. Creation of risk management steering group chaired by chief executive, to be responsible for the strategic direction, coordination of implementation and decision making.
2. The appointment of a dedicated risk manager and support staff is essential if targets and outcome are to be met.
3. The formation of a risk management group chaired by the risk manager, with membership from across the organisation, each with an overview of operational management. These people would become risk representatives, who would coordinate action across directorates or sectors of care, meeting regularly with the risk manager to formulate approaches, monitor assess-

ment, evaluate the programme and act as a means of communicating changes.

4. At each operational level, the nomination of risk officers would ensure that the risk management message is turned into action.

5. Most health care organisations have had Health & Safety advisors and representatives for many years. These key staff members have been mainly appointed by unions and carry out assessments on Health & Safety issues. It is important to develop a strategy that places this work at the heart of the system envisaged. In small units the role of Health & Safety representative can be merged with the role of a risk officer. This ensures that duplicate assessments and action are not undertaken. In large units, the separate roles can be discussed and where the roles overlap, joint assessments and liaison can make the work less onerous.

6. A clinical risk management committee should be chaired by the risk manager in conjunction with clinical staff and the clinical governance team. It should focus on key areas that are universally deemed as high risk such as:

- obstetric services
- operating theatres
- orthopaedic services
- A&E services
- medical records: all types of documents
- interface between different organisations.

THE ROLE OF THE RISK MANAGEMENT TEAM AND DEPARTMENT

The role of the department and the profile of the people employed are crucial to the success of the whole enterprise. The department needs access to office space, secretarial support and computer databases. The collection and collation of data are of importance but if that is all that happens, the enterprise will not achieve its objectives. The data collected need to be turned into information and then informed action in real time. Many a programme has failed because all the resources have been used to collect data without the same attention given to the implementation of change. Therefore the organisation must have committed funding for activating the change processes that reduce the risk. The nurse will find that such a department will become a partner in the decision-making process.

Assessing and managing risk

329

Information management should cover the areas of communication, trust policies and procedures, reactive accident and incident reporting and monitoring and active monitoring.

Communication

The ability to explore effective ways of communicating with the whole organisation is essential. A risk management framework is an excellent method for cascading information but this should be supported by newsletters, notice boards and reports that detail information and highlight successes and failures. The development of a risk action week enables the RMT to create static displays, host seminars and tours of areas that have made progress in risk reduction. There is nothing like success to raise a profile and encourage further proactive progress.

Trust policies and procedures

The initiation and updating of organisational policies and procedures can be coordinated from this department. The policies should be created by the users and evaluated by the RMT and representatives. Ratification by the board is necessary to ensure continuity and associated accountability and liability. It is important to include the date of ratification and a predicted date for updating.

Reactive accident and incident reporting and monitoring

This mechanism serves two main functions.

1. The collection, collation and analysis of information of loss avoidance, be it fiscal, fabric, personnel, customers or reputation. Using trend analysis, it is possible to indicate if an organisation is improving or deteriorating.
2. Investigation and analysis of individual incidents which have happened to enable the organisation to learn what went wrong and take preventive measures.

The Health & Safety Executive makes a distinction between accidents and incidents.

Accidents are all undesired circumstances which give rise to ill health or injury; damage to property, plant, products or environment; production loss, or increased liabilities. While incidents are:

all undesirable circumstances and near misses which have the potential to cause accidents. (HSE 1991)

Most organisations have not fully utilised incident reporting systems. In December 2000, the government launched an initiative to promote the prevention side of litigation, with a national mandatory reporting system database for errors and near misses.

> The current system of incident reporting and confidential inquiries is a patchwork with no way of picking out current themes. Some information is not systematically available, for example NHS Litigation Authority database has not been looked at but is a rich seam of information. (Donaldson 2000)

When an organisation implements a risk management programme, there is usually an increase in reporting but most authors agree that there are still many incidents that never reach the light of day. The organisation needs to promote a 'no blame' culture and support staff in reporting incidents.

> Completing an incident report when an unexpected 'event' occurs is the first step in identifying practice issues and potential problems. (Stern 1997)

Clements (1995) has advocated this more positive approach. An investigation of incident reports and/or analysis of case notes can identify common triggers that lead to adverse events. The triggers can then be avoided, transferred or the risk reduced by the creation of protocols to guide staff through the potential problem. Each protocol is drawn up by the team and ratified as appropriate practice, communicated and audited.

In the clinical risk management field, Clements (1995) comments that 'without doctors such programmes are not effective'. Medical, nursing and professions allied to medicine (PAMs) should all be involved in the creation of a clinical trigger incident proforma, its usage and subsequent changes in clinical practice, so that it is based on the best evidence available. Figure 14.2 lists the trigger incidents in an obstetric domain.

Clinical guidelines or protocols can be dangerous if not fully documented and covering all the process of care. Tingle (1997) comments that such documents are used in cases that have gone to court and therefore the style and content are of paramount importance to staff and their patients, while Dukes & Stewart (1993) describe protocols as 'in potential conflict with holistic individualised patient care'.

The Human Rights Act 1998, fully implemented in October 2000, implements the European Convention on Human Rights and

Assessing and managing risk

Six Steps to **Effective Management**

Use this form to record critical incidents occurring in Maternity Care. The events listed below are considered high risk and therefore must be reported. However, this list is not exhaustive so for this reason a box labelled 'other' has been provided. Use this to notify any other situation that you believe constitutes either a potential or actual risk to an individual. Death or serious injury must be reported to the Risk Management Coordinator immediately. All other incidents are to be recorded on the main Incident Report Form.

Section A: Details of person affected by the incident
Surname: Forename(s):   Title:
Home address:
                                         Postcode:
Phone No:
Status: Patient ID:
Date of incident: Time: Location:

Section B: Critical event (please tick the relevant event)

Tick	Maternal Events	Tick	Neonatal Events
	3rd degree tear		Birth trauma: Erb's palsy, scalpel blade trauma, fractures, severe bruising
	Bladder injury during LSCS		Cord pH of 7.1 or below
	Cord prolapse		Delay in paediatrician's attendance at delivery (more than 5 min from time of request by phone)
	Delayed delivery (doctor busy in theatre)		Infant of 36 weeks, gestation or above requiring intubation
	Eclampsia		Postnatal admission to hospital
	Failed induction		Undiagnosed congenital abnormality: spina bifida, abnormal wall defects, Down's syndrome, other
	Hb of less than 9 g/dl in labour		Unexpected admission to NICU
	Maternal death		Unexpected difficult resuscitation, equipment failure or absence, difficult intubation, structural abnormality, other
	Postpartum haemorrhage >700 ml		Other event
	Prolonged 2nd stage of labour (>3 hours)		
	Readmission to postnatal ward		
	Retained swab/instrument		
	Return to theatre following LSCS		
	Rupture of the uterus		
	Shoulder dystocia requiring medical help		
	Transfer to ITU		
	Two unsuccessful attempts at instrumental delivery		

Con't

Figure 14.2a Maternity services critical incidence report form (reproduced with permission from Addenbrooke's NHS Trust).

has the potential to make enormous impact on the NHS. Patients and their lawyers will be considering how to use the act to advance their cases. Similarly, defendant NHS law firms will be considering how the act could be used to ensure their clients comply with the

Section C: Add any other information (fact, not opinion)

Section D: Other important information
Was a device or equipment involved YES/NO. If Yes, complete an Equipment/
Consumable Report and attach it to this report. Place a "Withdrawn from Service"
label on the item concerned. Labels for this purpose are found at the back of the main
incident books.

Section E: Details of person completing form
Name: Directorate/Speciality/Ward/Department:
Title:
Post   Box No.   Phone:
                              Signature:

For use by risk management coordinator only
Date of receipt: Time of receipt:
Significance score: 0   1   2   3   4   5
Incident class:
Initial action taken:

Signature:
Notes and references (initial each entry, continue on separate sheet)

Synopsis

Figure 14.2b

act. Tingle (2000a) doubts whether the average risk manager or health care professional is fully prepared for the potential problems the new act may provoke. Under English law, the dissemination of medical data anonymised, even for commercial gain, is lawful. However, the European Convention on Human Rights takes the dissemination of personal data extremely seriously. For example, it is common practice at present to give any member of the patient's family a large amount of confidential information without the patient's express consent. This will have to stop in the light of European Convention on Human Rights Article 8, advisory confidential protocols, and professionals will have to change their practice.

Analysis of the causes of accidents lends itself to the domino theory, which states that a lack of control may produce the basic cause for a potential incident. This potential incident leads to a substandard condition and an actual incident occurring where a loss is sustained. One deficit leads to another; hence the analogy of the fall of dominoes. If attention is directed towards identifying substandard conditions, the domino sequence of events is broken.

Active monitoring

Reactive monitoring on its own is an insufficient measure of safety performance.

> A low accident rate, even over a period of years, is no guarantee that the risks are being effectively controlled. This is particularly so in organisations where there is a low probability of accidents but where major hazards are present. (HSE 1992a)

Active monitoring involves all staff in the following activities.

- Quarterly Health & Safety assessments, with reporting and appropriate action plans to address any problem found. These fit within the framework of RIDDOR (see p.341), enabling the HSE to identify where and how risks arise and to investigate serious accidents, while providing advice on prevention and reduction of injury.
- Quarterly risk assessment that identifies potential hazards and ranks them according to likely occurrence and enables an action plan to be created to address the problem.
- Yearly CoSHH assessments as per CoSHH Regulations (HSE 1994a) that investigate the type of substances in use, their transportation, storage, handling and waste disposal.
- Display screen assessment at each workstation for staff who use the station. This is likely to be an increasing problem with the introduction of hot desking in which a workstation has multiple users of all shapes and sizes.
- Security at work assessments that address the internal security of the workplace, including personal belongings, equipment, access to the building, the use of phones, email, Inter- and Intranets, storage of confidential data (Caldicote Report 1997) and personal safety when working alone.
- Dissemination of hazard warnings to all staff.
- Yearly audits of each working area to ensure that the above assessments are documented and that action has taken place to reduce the risk.

When both reactive and active monitoring data are available for the same incident event, it is possible to establish what effect, if any, a particular safety activity is having on key incident events.

THE ROLE OF THE RISK REPRESENTATIVE

The role flourishes when incumbents are enthusiastic; a volunteer is worth three conscripts. The role is about coordination, communication and continuity. They give operational advice and feedback to the risk manager and facilitate the work of the risk officers during regular meetings. Their inclusion in an officers' workshop can become a powerhouse for improvement. The representative and officers take time out to review their assessments, actions and plans. This enables the new officers to learn from the old hands and encourages a standardisation of approach. Each officer is charged with researching one or two problems common to all and that information is pooled, each officer adapting the findings to their own environment.

THE ROLE OF THE RISK OFFICER

This role is very much 'hands-on', day-to-day assessment of the working environment to ensure that risk reduction is working, the emphasis being on the changing work environment, practice and behaviour. Once the initial assessment and action plans are implemented, the main problem encountered is a changing status quo. When the working environment changes temporarily or permanently, this usually increases the risk. The previous assessments and action to reduce, transfer or eliminate risk are thrown back into the melting pot.

BRINGING ABOUT CHANGE

Training strategies

The launch of a risk management strategy should coincide with a training programme, to ensure maximum benefits and satisfactory outcomes are achieved. The organisation should give consideration to the use of outside consultants if there is limited expertise internally. The programme is most effective if it follows a 'big bang' process, as a programme spread over months leads to a patchy creation and implementation of risk management and the mutual support between staff being trained is diluted. The training should embrace the theory, legal, statutory and practical matters, at all

Assessing and managing risk

levels of the framework. A balance between theory and practice is paramount. On many courses the trainee returns with a large folder full of theory and assessment pro formas but little practical knowledge of how to complete the assessments and what to do with the results. The support of other risk officers and representatives will do much to ameliorate such problems.

Changing the culture

The development and implementation of risk management strategies will only be truly consolidated into the staff culture of an organisation if behaviour changes. It is therefore useful to identify change strategies that will encourage a shift in current behaviour and practice. Wright (1989) defines change as 'an attempt to alter or replace existing knowledge, skills, attitudes and norms of individuals or groups'. However, change is difficult to sustain if it does not take into account beliefs, attitudes and values that may block our path to change. Lancaster & Lancaster (1982) comment that 'people tend to be comfortable with change as long as it does not affect strongly held values, beliefs and ideals'. Lewin's (1951) and Rogers' (in Lancaster & Lancaster 1982) theories of change (Table 14.1) throw light on the process in relation to risk management.

Central to Lewin's change theory is the concept of force field analysis in which the individual is at the centre of several forces that

Table 14.1 Change theory comparison between the phases of change and the implementation of risk management

Lewin	Rogers	Risk management
Unfreezing	Awareness	Organisation's realisation that something needs to be done
	Interest	Participation in development of a risk strategy
Moving to a new level	Evaluation	Development of risk management framework and process to find best solutions
Refreezing	Adoption	Consolidation of that framework and process into the organisation's culture Assessment of appropriate action being undertaken across the organisation

336

are either driving or resisting change. Knowledge and identification of those forces can enable the change agent to move the organisation and/or individual along the change continuum (see Table 14.2).

Induction at ground level

The risk officer is usually responsible for introducing all new staff members into the risk reduction programme and the maintenance

Table 14.2 Force field analysis

Resisting forces	Driving forces
• We are already providing quality care (head in the sand behaviour)	• The desire to improve the standard of care delivered
• The problem lies in another department/community/government/management	• Moral ethical duty to do no harm
• It has never happened/will not happen to us	• Improvement in working conditions
• We do not have the money for that kind of thing	• Alternative funding for changes to the environment/new equipment
• Why do you need to assess such insignificant activities?	• Enhanced job satisfaction
• I/we do not have time, I/we are too busy doing the job	• Improved communication between areas, leading to a platform to discuss overlapping problems in care and service delivery
• It has always been done that way	• Reduction in injury to staff
• I do not like doing it this way, it takes too long to do it that way	• Less sick leave, more staff available to work
• Another management two-minute wonder, I have seen it all before	• No-blame culture promoted
• What we say is not what we do	• Organisation's reputation as a caring place enhanced

Assessing and managing risk

of evidence that staff have attended annual refresher programmes. It is advisable to integrate fire, risk management, manual handling, confidentiality and security into one refresher session. Bank and agency staff can miss out in the induction programmes and there is a need to have basic information available in each area in which they work. To ensure that they and their work areas comply, it is effective to have an induction checklist on the back of time sheets. An agreement of non-payment unless the form is signed off certainly increases compliance and protects not just the employee but the patient and employer.

THE ROLE OF THE EMPLOYER AND EMPLOYEE

The Health & Safety at Work Act (1974) confers responsibilities on employers to:

- ensure safety of all employees, patients, visitors and contractors
- provide and maintain safe plant and equipment
- provide safe systems of work
- provide safe storage, transport and handling
- provide adequate instruction, information, training and supervision
- provide and maintain safe access and egress.

Employees' responsibilities are threefold:

- to cause no harm by act of omission or action
- to cooperate with the employer
- no employee shall intentionally or recklessly interfere with or misuse anything provided in the interest of health, safety or welfare at work.

The staff have a duty to conform and cooperate with the risk reduction programme but this may prove difficult. For example, a risk officer carried out a display screen equipment (DSE) assessment as described in the HSE DSE Regulations (HSE 1992b) across a department and advised changes to the workstations to reduce the potential risk. One member of staff repeatedly changed the workstation back to how they previously worked and refused to use an adjustable chair. The officer referred the problem to the risk representative, who endorsed the advice and spoke with the staff member. The occupational health department undertook a formal DSE review and confirmed the original findings. The staff member was informed that they were required to conform to the changes and they continued to defy the order. The person was employed on the bank scheme so the bank was asked to withdraw them from the organisation, until such time as they conformed to the DSE action plan.

The employer is responsible for carrying out a general assessment of risk. Most assessment pro formas involve a score system that promotes action when certain agreed scores are reached and a time frame for remedial action is calculated (see Fig. 14.3).

When the assessment has been carried out and a hazard rating number (HRN) obtained, discussion should centre on what the recommended action to reduce the risk should be. Advice may be

GENERAL RISK ASSESSMENT RECORD

Workplace: wards Location: Dirty linen storage, sluices
Task: manual handling of linen bags into linen chutes Hazard: Back injury

Probability of exposure to/contact with hazard		Frequency of exposure to hazard		Maximum probable loss		No. persons at risk	
Exposure/Contact	PE	Frequency	FE	Loss	MPL	Number	NP
Impossible	0	Infrequent	0.1	Fatality	15	(1–2)	1
Unlikely	1	Annually	0.2	Perm. major illness/injury	8	(3–7)	2
Possible	2	Monthly	1.0	Temp. major illness/injury	4	(8–15)	4
Even chance	5	Weekly	1.5	Major injury/illness	2	(16–50)	8
Probably	8	Daily	2.5	Minor illness/injury	1	(>50)	12
Likely	10	Hourly	4.0	Puncture wound	0.5		
Certain	15	Constantly	5.0	Scratch/bruise	0.1		

1. Please circle level at which risk is assessed in each of the four values for each task. 2. Please calculate hazard rating number (HRN) using the following equation:

PE	x	FE	x	MPL	x	NP	=	HRN
2	x	2.5	x	1	x	2	=	10 HRN

HRN	RISK	AGREED ACTION REQUIRED
(0–1)	ACCEPTABLE	ACCEPT RISK
(1–5)	VERY LOW	WITHIN 1 YEAR
(5–10)	LOW	WITHIN 3 MONTHS
(10–50)	SIGNIFICANT	WITHIN 1 MONTH
(50–100)	HIGH	WITHIN 1 WEEK
(100–500)	VERY HIGH	WITHIN 1 DAY
(500–1000)	EXTREME	IMMEDIATELY
(>1000)	UNACCEPTABLE	STOP THE ACTIVITY

Signed _____ Designation _____

Date _____ If HRN is 100 or above send to Risk Management

con't

Figure 14.3a Example of an assessment form (reproduced with permisson from Addenbrooke's NHS Trust).

Recommended action to reduce risk	Action to be taken by whom/date	Completed signed/dated
1. Instruct staff to half-fill linen bags	Chief nurse/risk manager/immediately	
2. Place notices in every ward sluice re filling of linen bags	Ward managers/ immediately	
3. Investigate manual handling techniques of staff handling linen bags	Manual handling trainer/within 1 week	
4. Enhance training in manual handling techniques of staff	Manual handling trainer and link nurses/within 1 month	
5. Identify bags that have the potential to be a manual handling risk, i.e. wet linen do not move until help is obtained	Staff handling bags/ immediately	
6. Monitor and evaluate action taken	Risk and ward managers/within 1 month	

NB: To be periodically reviewed until all action is completed and assessment/ remedial action is formally 'signed off' (column 3).

Year	Action	Signed/Designation/Dated

NB: Each yearly assessment can be signed off if no change has occurred.If the result of this assessment is different, a new assessment form must be used to quantify that change.

Figure 14.3b

sought from the manufacturers or outside consultants or research undertaken to obtain a consensus on best practice. It is important to remember that there are various options available when managing risk.

- Risk avoidance: is it possible to stop doing the activity altogether?
- Risk reduction: change practice, enhance training.
- Risk spreading: break down the task into smaller parts, that reduce the risk.
- Risk transfer: move the task to another, more appropriate environment or person.
- Risk acceptance: accept that the activity cannot be modified by the above strategies and that the activity is a core task for the organisation.

Managing risk and crisis

The nurse may have to weigh up the relative merits of the HRN and possible options, before making a decision on the appropriate action. The language and content of assessments, policies, procedures, protocols and plans for action are of great importance to their adoption by the staff into their everyday working practices.

Physiotherapists, occupational therapists and nurses have commented that 'no lifting policies' are difficult to defend in practice. They find that when they need to start mobilising and/or rehabilitating patients, it is at times impossible not to contravene Health & Safety manual handling advice, if that advice is a no lifting policy. Many professionals feel that this order can place them in an untenable position, because if the policy is fully adhered to, that action prevents or prolongs the rehabilitation process, whereas a minimal lifting policy enables the professional to act appropriately within the guidelines.

The guidance for any risk acceptance discussion should be well researched and communicated in unambiguous language. If the organisation's policy is seen to be unworkable, the staff may circumvent that policy. Green's (1996) exploratory study of moving and handling practices suggested that risk assessment of the task, load and environment was often incomplete. The study highlighted insufficient equipment, lack of space, unsuitable uniforms and negative attitudes towards changing practice as the main causes of non-compliance with risk management policy. Certainly the purchase of manual handling equipment without assessment of the space available in which to use the equipment can cause problems. Most hoists are of necessity rather large and if the nurse has difficulty in placing the equipment next to the patient due to lack of space, or the toilet or bathroom is too small, the temptation to return to old practices will be great.

The distribution of the incident pro forma does not in itself cause a change in practice. Some risk management measures assume that staff recognise and report hazards and risks. Elinsky et al (1997), after a survey of nurses working in the acute sector, advised nurse managers not to use the level of incident reporting as a quality measure. A proactive risk officer who promotes and manages staff towards changes in practice is the most effective resource in risk reduction and control.

RIDDOR

Every employer has a duty to have knowledge of or act in accordance with the Health and Safety Executive (1995) *Reporting of Injuries, Diseases and Dangerous Occurrences Regulations* which applies to all work activities and came into force in April 1996. The information enables the HSE to identify where and how risks arise

341

and to investigate serious accidents, while providing advice on prevention and reduction of injury.

CONCLUSION

The findings of all assessments and incidents identified are worthless unless action takes place. Only the individual's knowledge and enthusiasm limit the range of action available. Even a decision to take no action is valid as long as it is not the result of apathy. Reduction in risk or the potential risk to staff, patients and the organisation will depend on the ability to change culture, attitudes and beliefs and also upon an advocate in high places to champion the cause.

The adoption of a risk reduction culture in the workplace has the potential to change the face of care and care provision and it is people who will make it work. However, the mental health of staff has not received the same attention as the prevention, reduction and elimination of physical injuries. In many organisations there is an acceptance of the immediate role of counselling following exposure to stressful incidents, rather than scrutiny of organisational issues that may be the real cause of mental stress. The 1994 HSE guidance *OH Series for NHS Staff* argues that 'plain good management that enables people to receive feedback and support on their performance will help to reduce stress' (HSE 1994b).

Management should monitor its staff workload and introduce action plans to ameliorate it if it becomes burdensome, by increasing staff, reengineering the way activities are undertaken or the closure of beds. This aspect of risk management will need greater recognition in the coming decade, as staff are faced with an ever-increasing workload and as a knowledgeable public demands quality health care for all.

References

Caldicote Report 1997 Report on the management audit of patient identifiable information. Stationery Office, London

Clements RV 1995 Essentials of clinical risk management. In: Vincent C (ed) Clinical risk management. BMJ Books, London, pp. 335–349

Department of Health 1997 The new NHS: modern, dependable. Stationery Office, London

Department of Health 1998 A first class service. Stationery Office, London

Dingwall R, Fenn P 1991 Is risk management necessary? International Journal of Risk and Safety in Medicine 2: 91–106

Donaldson L 2000 National new-miss reporting system. Health Care Risk Report 6(8): 5

Dukes J, Stewart D 1993 Be prepared. Health Service Journal 103: 24–25

Elinsky C, Nichols B, Palmer K 1997 Are hospital incidents being reported? Journal of Nursing Administration 27(11): 40–46

Faugier J, Ashworth G, Lancaster J, Ward D 1997 An exploration of clinical risk management from a nursing perspective. Nursing Research 2(2): 97–107

Gamble P, Aires P 1994 Caring for health and safety counts. British Journal of Theatre Nursing 4(9): 5–9

Green C 1996 Study of moving and handling practices on two medical wards. British Journal of Nursing 5(5): 303–304

Ham C (ed) 1995 NHS handbook. JMH Publishing, Tunbridge Wells

Health and Safety Executive 1991 Successful health and safety management. HMSO, London

Health and Safety Executive 1992a Five steps to successful health and safety management. HMSO, London

Health and Safety Executive 1992b Display Screen Equipment Regulations. HSE Books, London

Health and Safety Executive 1994a Control of Substances Hazardous to Health Regulations. HSE Books, London

Health and Safety Executive 1994b Occupational Health Series for NHS Staff. HSE Books, London

Health and Safety Executive 1995 Reporting of Injuries, Diseases and Dangerous Occurrences Regulations. HSE Books, London

Henderson A 2000 Audit Office investigates negligence claims. Health Care Risk Report 6(8): 4

Kohn IT, Corrigan JM, Donaldson MS (eds) 1999 To err is human: building a safer health system. Committee on Quality of Health Care in America, Institute of Medicine, Washington DC

Lancaster J, Lancaster J 1982 The nurse as a change agent. Mosby, London

Lewin K 1951 The nurse as a change agent. In: Lancaster J, Lancaster J (eds) Change management. Mosby, London, ch 5

NHS Executive 1999 Clinical governance: quality in the new NHS. Department of Health, London

Nichol D 1993 Foreword: Risk management in the NHS. NHS Management Executive, Department of Health, London

Reason J 1995 Understanding adverse events: human factors. In: Vincent C (ed) Clinical risk management. BMJ Books, London, pp. 31–54

Stahl DA 1997 Subacute care: creating alternatives. Managing risks in subacute care. Nursing Management 28(10): 26–27

Stern DF 1997 Handling clinical incidents. Nursing Management 28: 9–48

Tingle J 1997 Ethical and legal. Healthcare litigation: working towards a culture change. British Journal of Nursing 6(1): 56–57

Tingle J 2000a The report that rocked a nation. Health Care Risk Report 6(8): 20–21

Tingle J 2000b (ed) The new, new millennium bug? Health Care Risk Report 6(8): 1

Wright S 1989 Changing nursing practice. Edward Arnold, London

Zeithaml V, Berry L, Pasasuraman A 1985 Communication and control processes in the delivery of a quality service. Journal of Marketing 52: 35–48

Assessing and managing risk

343

Application 14:1

Lenore Anderson

Implementing risk management strategies

This application should be used to compare the content of Chapter Fourteen with your own practice. Working through the three exercises below should give you a clear understanding of the issues in implementing risk management strategies.

Exercise 1: Practice checklist

- Use the force field analysis format (Table 14.2) to create a list of resisting and driving forces within your own workplace.
- Compose an action plan that would reduce those resisting forces and capitalise on the driving forces you have identified.
- Compare and contrast the organisational risk management framework shown in Figure 14.1 with your own.
- Have you changed practice as a result of the risk assessment? If so, review your action; if not, use the risk assessment pro forma at the end of this chapter.
- Have you checked your incident report book to see if there are any common problems or causes? If there is a common thread emerging, for example falls occurring at a specific time or to a specific group of patients, draw up a plan of action to reduce the incidence. Read Trummer et al (1996) for inspiration; they developed an algorithm for managing confused patients who fall.

References

GRASP © Systems, Nurse Consultants International Ltd, 82 Deepwell Avenue, Halfway, Sheffield S20 5ST, UK. Workload tool (2000).
Trummer KH, Foster BB, Hartmann L, Lewis-Vais C, Sullivan H 1996 Managing falls. American Journal of Nursing 7: 16

Exercise 2: Your attitude

Evaluate your approach to risk management; is it proactive? Use an attitudinal scale to decide. Base your decision on Table 14.1.1 as follows.

Is there evidence that each risk management activity is in place and has been acted upon?

4 More than satisfactory (complete compliance)
3 Satisfactory (more than 75% compliance)
2 Barely satisfactory (less than 50% compliance)
1 Unsatisfactory (minimal compliance)

Please circle the most appropriate score, based on the evidence for either your organisation as a whole or your area of responsibility, using the above ranking.

Add up your total score to find this year's results. If you score 10 or below, your risk management is not proactive. A score between 10 and 14 indicates some awareness, while 15–18 indicates a proactive stance; above 18 indicates you have risk management cracked (for now). Remember your environment, staff, case mix and practice will change over time so repeat this exercise yearly to ensure you are on track.

Table 14.1.1

Engaging all members of staff, visitors and patients 1	2	3	4
Covers all aspects of the organisation's activities	1 2	3	4
Identifies the risks, potential or actual	1 2	3	4
Examines any risk for potential exacerbation	1 2	3	4
Develops strategies that reduce, transfer or eliminate the risks identified	1 2	3	4
Commitment to a continuous evolving programme, resourced and accountable to the board of the organisation	1 2	3	4

Implementing risk management strategies

345

Managing risk and crisis

Exercise 3: Comparative analysis of a 24-bedded ward (indicates the high workload is causing higher incidences of the items below)

Period	Complaints	Incidents	Accidents	GRASP © workload average	Audit of care delivered	Hospital-acquired infection rate	Sick leave	Staff turnover
Quarter	7	48	14	145%	71%	12.8%	6%	7%
Norm	0	23	3	100–130%	90%	9%	2%	4%

GRASP© Systems Workload Average Utilisation % (the balance between nursing care required and that provided) indicates:

below 90% utilisation – not cost effective but may be required for safety reasons

90–110% utilisation – creates a quality climate for patients and staff but does not guarantee quality care

111–130% utilisation – staff working to maximum capacity

130–150% – staff prioritising care, creating a quality gap

151% and above – staff on course for 'burnout'; possible increased incidents, errors, complaints, sick leave and staff turnover

Your Ward

Period	Complaints	Incidents	Accidents	% Workload	Audit of care	Infection rate	Sick leave	Staff turnover

Application **14:2**

Mike Flynn

Managing children's services: a risky business

This application shows that, while risk can never be eliminated, a proactive approach to managing risk can be implemented.

'Murder on Ward 4' and 'Doctor Death' are emotive media headlines that were used to describe events surrounding Beverley Allitt and Harold Shipman. In a similar vein, the detrimental effects of being treated at certain paediatric cardiac units have lead to alarm and almost disbelief.

When learning of the tragedies that befell not only the patients but their families and local communities many of us, if honest, probably took the opinionated stance 'it couldn't happen here'. Yet to someone, somewhere, it did happen and it is only now, when the full reality of what took place has become clear, that we have all had to come to terms with the fact that, sadly, yes it could.

All these incidents are undoubtedly at the extreme end of a spectrum relating to risk. But if robust systems of benchmarking, audit and action are not in place, history may repeat itself. The purpose of this exercise is not, however, to go back over what did or didn't happen; the inclusion of these events is intended to illustrate why we need to take risk management seriously.

WHAT EXACTLY IS MEANT BY RISK MANAGEMENT?

A risk can be defined as a decision to exert influence (by action or inaction) on a particular event or set of circumstances to try to achieve a predetermined, desired outcome. The risk can be undertaken by an individual (personal), a number of people (group) or an organisation (corporate).

In its simplest form, every waking moment of our own lives involves an element of risk and how we manage it. For example, when we leave the house and cross the road to catch the bus, whether or not we reach our destination will be self-determined. If we exclude the variables that are outside our control, e.g. it doesn't turn up or it is full and drives past, we instinctively manage a series of risks so that we get where we want to go.

- We look at the clock so we leave the house in time.
- We check to make sure we have everything with us so we don't have to go back.
- We make sure we have money to pay the fare.
- We take care with crossing the road to avoid sustaining personal injury from other traffic.

If we can accept these principles it is easy to translate them into a clinical context. By doing so, we can see that the degree to which we successfully deliver care (or not, as the case may be) is significantly influenced by a series of risk management strategies that are set at key stages along the care pathway.

CHILD CARE AND RISK MANAGEMENT

The best way of illustrating this is to use a practical example. The one we will use is unique to children but the principles identified can be applied across the wider spectrum of health care.

We will cite and then critically appraise an established trust procedure for an incident involving a child going missing. Before considering this we need to recognise that all children and young people up to the age of 16 years should be regarded as being a potential risk to themselves and that a trust must assume *in loco parentis* responsibility in the absence of a parent.

Every stage of the protocol (Fig. 14.2.1) must be able to be justified within the context of risk management. If such a validation cannot be made, any inclusion and likely effective contribution to the process must be questioned.

- *Stage 1* is having a protocol in place to anticipate a child going missing. This proactive approach can considerably influence a positive outcome, especially when the critical incident itself may be a relatively rare event.
- *Stage 2* is a means of ensuring that the risk is more effectively managed by passing control to one designated person. This adds clarity to the exercise of the local search.
- *Stage 3* is a measured response to achieve a widening of the search. It ensures a rapid response and, if the child is still on the premises, means that they will be found.
- *Stage 4* is primarily to ensure that the parents are aware of the situation but it may also provide clues to possible destinations that the child may be making for.

A child appears to have gone missing.

↓

Senior person on shift alerts colleagues and institutes a local search.

↓

If child not found, switchboard must be contacted and procedure for checking site instituted.

↓

If parents are not present they must be contacted and informed. (If care proceedings are involved, social services must be informed.)

↓

The local police must be involved and they should be fully briefed regarding any special circumstances, e.g. child protection issues.

↓

Situational review must be undertaken and the possibility of abduction should always be considered.

Figure 14.2.1   Trust protocol for when a child goes missing.

- *Stage 5* will allow the rolling out of the search across the wider community by involving professionals who can lend considerable expertise and networking.
- *Stage 6* will hopefully be a winding-down operation once the child is found. This stage is just as important as the others, especially if lessons need to be learned.

This example demonstrates that focus and explicitness of approach can greatly increase the chance of success, in this case of ensuring the safety and well-being of the child.

By thinking through the issues and anticipating the possible outcomes, the degree of risk is significantly lowered. But what should also be manifest is that the methodology used in this approach can be used to consider risks associated with other aspects of children's services.

Managing children's services: a risky business

MANAGING RISK SUCCESSFULLY

Successful risk management does not just happen. It has to be facilitated by an organisation and its managers to ensure that:

- there is a pervasive culture which values all staff
- there is openness and participation
- research and development are active components of management and clinical practice
- there is explicit support from the management board.

But are these ideals achievable? How can risk management avoid being consigned to the management filing cabinet until something goes badly wrong?

There is not one single answer to this but the following model identifies some potential barriers which can be turned into tools for success.

Table 14.2.1 Constraints and how to overcome them

Barrier	Corrective action
Misunderstanding	Provide clear information
Misgivings	Offer personal support
Lack of people skills	Educate and empower
No established benchmarking	Develop pathways
Poor data collection	Enhance software
Add-on job	Allocate time and resources

In conclusion, the ideal of delivering an optimal standard of service by itself is rarely achievable, but a measured approach using risk management as a proactive tool has a much greater chance of success.

Chapter **Fifteen**

Crisis management: creating order out of chaos

Trevor Dolan and Nigel Northcott

Life can only be understood backwards; but it must be lived forwards. (Kierkegaard 1955)

- ● **The 'new' NHS**
- ● **Reflective practice**
- ● **Thriving on the edge of chaos**
- ● **Culture**
- ● **Stephen Covey's first habit**
- ● **Leadership issues**
- ● **Time management**
- ● **Taking risks**
- ● **Conclusion**

O V E R V I E W

Crisis management seems to have become an inevitable part of decision making in the NHS. Although crises will occur in any health care setting, they can never be completely avoided. Reported cases where care has been jeopardised, whether in the A&E department, the maternity ward or the child health department, are depressingly familiar and seemingly increasingly frequent. Clinical staff shortages, exhausted and burnt-out professionals, cost cutting of support and middle managerial posts, a system that is functioning at higher capacity levels and a greater public awareness all work together to lead to a vicious circle.

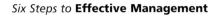

Staff become caught up in a 'band aid' approach to crises where organisational first aid leaves little time and energy for organisational health promotion. Unfortunately, being on a crisis problem-solving treadmill means that today's solutions are often tomorrow's problems, a situation in which quick fixes may potentially be doing more harm than good. A culture of short-term remedial management develops that plays down the importance of longer term generative management.

It is the argument of this chapter that, even in adverse conditions, some more proactive approaches can be taken. The chapter sets out to explore a series of practical solutions to the ways in which clinical team leaders can develop a culture within their teams where generative working predominates. It starts with a general discussion of the context in which these problems arise. It goes on to explore how metaphors and models of organisations tend to support disabling rather than enabling ways of tackling issues which then become habitual and continue to 'boomerang' around to the detriment of longer term problem solving.

Two key themes are introduced in this chapter and make up the main body of discussion: reflecting before action and welcoming chaos and uncertainty as integral to changing practice. In conclusion, suggestions are made on ways to develop the decision maker's own thinking around these areas of complexity and chaos theory. These involve critical reflection on management practice in a way that moves from habitual ways of working towards new and innovative approaches, thereby enabling the practitioner to build on good practice.

THE 'NEW' NHS

Within a customer and market-oriented health care system, many changes have had a profound impact upon professionals working in the NHS. These include restructuring the way in which health care is being delivered as a result of trust mergers and the move towards health care delivery by primary care groups and trusts. Changes in health care technology such as innovative treatments, new drugs, minimally invasive surgical procedures, demographic changes, life expectancy and changing expectations of consumer involvement all impact upon practice. More recent modifications of the purchaser/provider split with innovative forms of health care delivery rely more on collaborative interagency and interprofes-

Managing risk and crisis

sional partnerships than adversarial tribalism (Isles 1997, NHS Executive 1997).

Along with these changes, government policies aim to focus services towards health inequalities rather than purely offering health care (Secretary of State for Health 2000). This bid to provide a seamless acute/community-based care system aims to meet the health needs of patients and families, rather than overemphasising the need to deliver health care efficiently, economically and effectively. It will provide a matrix of services across health, social services, education and the voluntary sector that is committed to meeting the needs of local health economies.

These changes mean increases in nursing and midwifery activity and changes in the ways in which nurses and midwives relate to patients. Not surprisingly, there are physical and emotional consequences to increased workloads and changing relationships (Seedhouse 1994). The challenge for leaders of health care is therefore to develop cultures that balance caring for staff with effective promotion of good health and health care delivery. The question is posed as to how to develop clinical leaders with the skills and capabilities that these types of innovation and rapid changes require.

The author's experience with a wide range of clinical leadership development initiatives supports the belief that these changes need to be underpinned by a critical approach to leadership practice through reflective practice and critical thinking. Developing critical models of leadership and management that match the complexities of our practice situations will move professionals away from simple mechanistic models towards collaborative and transformational models that are based on the new sciences of complexity and chaos.

REFLECTIVE PRACTICE

It is suggested that nurses, teachers and managers take a broad personal and professional interest in contemporary theories and ideas. This in part is an attempt to 'make sense' or learn from experiences, exposures and situations. Apps (1985) and Mezirow (1990) suggested learning from experiences in order to leave behind the old and develop new ways of thinking and acting. Most nurses recognise the term 'reflection' or 'reflective practice' but how many actually acknowledge what this means to them? The process of reflective practice has been identified by Ecclestone (1995) as

Crisis management: creating order out of chaos

becoming little more than a mantra, with little impact on professionals' practice or lives.

Mezirow (1991) recognised that an understanding of reflection should include the notion of 'mindfulness'. This forms a neat connection that is probably unintentional; the use of a mantra is as central to Buddhism as is a concept of mindfulness. Buddhists use the term to indicate the need to be constantly aware of the world and the individual's place and actions in it. This accords with Benner's (1984) 'on-the-spot experimentation' and 'reflection-in-action'. This is a process of considering the effect and impact of actions in order to then act 'mindfully' according to personal skills and abilities. Each day infuses us with knowledge that we carry into tomorrow.

The process of reflection-in-action is complemented by reflection-on-action, which was alluded to as far back as 1954 when Flanagan described the process of collecting observations of human behaviour to guide future problem solving: the 'critical incident technique'. The analysis of behaviour and experiences as a foundation for learning offers a useful process for understanding life 'backwards'. The challenge, however, is to live it forwards; to learn from experiences and become truly a lifelong learner who learns continuously and who acts today as a result of all that has gone before. However, the analysis of experiences to bring about change and learning may not be enough. Reflection-on-action can enable professionals to revisit and learn from the past, reflection-in-action can make them mindful of the present but how can individuals be best prepared for the future?

Reflection-before-action

The following sayings come from nursing staff working on development projects (probably bastardised from other sources and with apologies for the lack of individual acknowledgements!).

> Some people watch things happen. Some make things happen. Some don't realise things are happening.

> Some see themselves as they are and think, why? Some see themselves as they could be and think, why not?

> Too many do things 'because'. Too few do things 'in order to'.

These three sayings confirm the additional need to reflect *before* action; the manager, in particular, should plan and prepare for the future.

We now turn to examine some of the theories that either support or militate against a proactive approach.

THRIVING ON THE EDGE OF CHAOS

The concept of organisations as mechanistic creations flourished in the age of bureaucracies. Organisations worked in linear ways and followed clearly laid-down procedures and policies and were resistant to change. Admittedly many of these organisations lasted many years but, like dinosaurs, their age has passed. They have been and are being replaced by organisations that possess almost living qualities; they learn, adapt, change and see chaos not as something to fear but as reality that has to be worked with rather than against. They emphasise making things happen rather than thinking about how they were.

Margaret Wheatley (1992) confirmed this organic quality of many new and successful organisations that have given up despairing about the ever-changing world, a world where linear thinking has been replaced by quantum thinking and acting. The linear approach is entrenched in rules and 'because' and following clearly laid-down pathways and patterns. The quantum organisation prefers reasons and 'in order to' and seeing the future only as something that will be different from today and to be welcomed. The linear organisation examines its activity and tries to understand why things happen, constantly looking back. The quantum approach is framed in the future and in 'why not?' and seeks to use the past as a learning opportunity or, as Kierkegaard (1955) suggests, 'understood backwards but lived forwards'. It expects and welcomes change, chaos and confusion as opportunities and not impediments.

Chaos and complexity theory

The terms 'chaos' and 'complexity' introduce uncomfortable and jarring connotations in many minds. Chaos and complexity are what people tend to move away from, rather than move towards. So how might a way of working based on these ideas help individuals to cope with today's chaotic and complex environment?

The term 'chaos' is misleading. It actually aims to help understand the behaviours of individuals and teams that do not work in a purely linear way. It helps recognition and appreciation of the patterns in individual and team behaviour and responses. It

Crisis management: creating order out of chaos

encourages people to work with, rather than against the chaotic situations. It is the antithesis of the strict scientific and medical model that influenced managerial thinking for much of the 20th century. It is creative and imaginative and despite the impression of the term as pejorative, its impact is highly positive but unconventional.

Chaos theory has its own principles and terminology that need more than simple explanations. Its key principles are outlined below.

Non-linearity

The size or quality of interventions in a situation may produce a change larger, smaller or more complex than the initial intervention. Being stuck on the M6 in a 5-mile tailback that disappears with no sign of an obstruction is an example of this. Often seemingly small problems create diverse and complex responses. Think of the effect of the ward clerk going sick!

Ability to change

The unstable character of chaotic systems means that they have a tendency towards change and looking to the future, rather than stability and being embedded in the past and present. This is both exciting and anxiety provoking. Anyone who has experienced or is going through a trust merger or moving into a primary care trust will appreciate this.

Common principles

Although situations appear chaotic and unpredictable, they have sets of organising principles such as the shared values and beliefs of the team that make up the culture of the workplace and influence the way staff behave towards each other, patients and families.

Scoping

In complex situations, it is often difficult to 'see the wood for the trees' because situations are viewed from one point in time, rather than through time. Individuals can be too close to situations and this does not allow them to take the broad view of things. Chaos theory is an invitation to take a 'helicopter view' of situations, before, during and after they happen. It also asks individuals to respond rather than react. The day after a dilemma or crisis, the intensity is less, the panic reduced and more solutions arise if professionals stand back to take an overview.

Self-organisation and self-renewal

Organisations have an innate ability to generate their own sets of rules and guidelines to work from. They are able to reorganise themselves without external involvement. However, despite policies, procedures, guidelines and memos, there is always one section or team that 'does its own thing'.

In a sense, therefore, chaos theory is emancipatory but the price for this open-endedness may be extreme uncertainty and loss of self-control.

So far, this chapter has focused on two agendas for health care professionals: the importance of reflection-before-action and the inevitability of change and chaos and living 'forwards'. Five management ideas and concepts are now explored that assist in the practical application of these agendas:

- culture
- Stephen Covey's first habit
- leadership
- time management
- risk taking.

CULTURE

Culture can be defined as '. . . how things are done around here' (Johnson & Scholes 1999) along with what is called the psychological contract to establish the environment within which staff work. Positive links have been established between a constructive culture and the morale, staff retention, service enhancement and even decreased mortality of patients (McDaniel & Stumpf 1993). Hawkins & Shohet (1989) identify five distinct cultures that may operate and these play a major role in creating the attitudes, style of working and effectiveness of the workplace. Three of these cultures are relevant to health care: the bureaucratic, the reactive/crisis and the learning/development cultures.

In the *bureaucratic* culture, the clearly laid down rules, regulations and lists of procedures will determine that actions are based upon what has happened before. This can strip patients and staff of their individuality, undermine the ability and potential of professionals and create a cumbersome and unresponsive organisation, one that operates 'because' and not 'in order to'. This is not to say that protocols and principles should not be set out but they should be framed as guidelines that allow and encourage professionals to ensure they meet the exact needs of individuals. The introduction of primary nursing (Manthey 1980) challenges bureaucratic work patterns by enhancing the autonomy of individual practitioners to care for unique individual patients. The move towards patient-centred nursing has created a more flattened hierarchy that allows a much more therapeutic relationship with the patients where outcomes and 'reasons' are more valued than 'rules' and conformity.

The *reactive/crisis* culture is a problem-solving culture where attention is only focused on immediate problems with no concern for development or visionary activities. This culture operates in many busy departments especially if the leadership is short-sighted and tentative. Plans are not laid down and some staff in such cultures even pride themselves on their ability to cope in a crisis. Indeed, in an emergency situation problem solving and crisis management may be attractive and important. However, in everyday working such a mode is unnecessarily authoritarian and has little regard for individuals. It is also the culture that is typical of the health service as it puts its head in the sand and waits for all the confusion and chaos to go away.

By contrast, the *learning/development* culture is one where growth, development and learning are all central to the organisation. The notion of the 'learning company' (Pedlar et al 1991) is a clear example of this culture, which has the following features.

- Learning is seen as a life-long activity for all staff.
- All work situations may potentially create learning opportunities.
- Problems are learning opportunities.
- Good practices arise from exploring learning cycles.
- Feedback exists at all levels and is ongoing.
- Time is an expected dimension of change.
- Regular review and evaluation are part of the individual and organisational activity.

This concept is advanced further by Peter Senge (1990) who advocates a new role of manager as 'researcher and designer', a manager who is seeking improvement and who is future thinking. Senge recognises that as the world becomes more interconnected and complex it must also become more 'learningful' and that learning should exist at all levels and not rely upon the 'boss' to have all the good ideas. Within this culture, work and life use the past and present to prepare for an inevitably different future by reflecting and learning.

These three cultures will impact significantly upon individuals and organisations. The bureaucratic and reactive cultures are firmly set in the past and present. They are cultures of 'because' and 'watching things happen', whereas the learning culture is about the future, 'in order to' and 'making things happen'. The challenge for the manager is in attempting to shift the organisation towards the third culture.

Consider the following case study.

> Adam is a reliable and committed nurse who has been in the ward team for the past 6 months. Yesterday he offered a patient extensive dietary advice. The patient's wife telephones the hospital dietician who realises the wrong advice has been given which has serious implications for the patient's health. The dietician advises you that this has happened and that the mistake has been corrected.
> What action would you take?

Comment

You should see the nurse as soon as possible to ensure he understands that an error has been made and to check why you feel it happened. You have to decide if the action was a mistake, which we all make, or was the result of 'recklessness'. Recklessness implies a degree of intention or carelessness and should be dealt with within the established disciplinary procedure and perhaps the professional body.

If it was a mistake, by taking a positive and non-punitive approach you encourage staff to feel able to accept that mistakes can happen and when they do, to ensure a solution is created. Taking a punitive approach can lead to staff covering up errors and failing to accept the need to learn lifelong. A punitive approach to a human error may result in fewer errors being reported and corrected. A learning approach may actually help reduce the number of incidents. It is also a culture that nurtures; it develops and enhances the skills and practice of its staff. It dynamically seeks to improve constantly.

STEPHEN COVEY'S FIRST HABIT

Stephen Covey (1992) suggested that highly effective people were characterised by seven habits: be proactive; begin with the end in mind; prioritise; think win/win; seek to understand then be understood; synergise and sharpen the saw.

Crisis management: creating order out of chaos

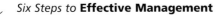

The notion of 'making things happen' can be summarised by the term 'proactive', the first of the seven habits. Habit 1 emphasises that between stimulus and response, there is choice: 'response-ability!'. Individuals should be encouraged to think about their response to situations rather than reacting automatically to them and should seek to create, choose and initiate. This habit is about thinking and initiating which again should use reflection-before-action to analyse and consider the possible outcomes.

Stephen Covey describes living and working at three levels: dependence is the lowest, moving through independence to inter-dependence. Each level indicates a difference in people's effectiveness at managing themselves, their work and their colleagues. Habits 1–3 are about moving from dependence to interdependence; the first habit makes things happen.

LEADERSHIP ISSUES

Organisations that are forward thinking and that seek to make the future happen have moved away from traditional styles of leadership. The three styles of leadership most readily recognised are those established by Lewin in 1939:

- autocratic
- democratic
- laissez-faire.

Autocratic leaders are often reactive or bureaucratic and tend to promote 'person pathology'. The autocratic leader typically uses orders to achieve results, showing little regard for the skills and abilities of individuals unless they have failed to achieve. Mistakes and lack of success will often be seen by the autocratic leader as the signal to punish those who have failed. Autocratic leaders are not renowned for their imagination or for being forward thinking. They apply rules and regulations to situations. They rarely have a long-term outlook or vision and concentrate on the here and now.

The *democratic* leader is much more people centred and if anything is slow to react and to plan for the future for fear of not gaining consensus. They are so busy worrying about everyone having a fair say that often the moment is lost.

The *laissez-faire* leader doesn't care much for anything. Whether success or failure arises is not important nor, for that matter, is leading. They abrogate or abdicate their responsibilities.

Arising from these three styles has been the concept of a leader who uses democratic processes but who has distinct vision, energy and direction. This leader values team members and seeks to use and combine their skills. Terms applied to this type of leader vary but include the benevolent dictator, the charismatic leader or the transformational leader.

Transformational leaders:

- develop a shared vision
- inspire and communicate
- value others
- challenge and stimulate
- develop trust
- enable.

Senge (1990) takes this stand on leaders further. He challenges the assumptions in many of the interpretations of leaders that people are powerless, lack the ability to effect change and have few good ideas. He sees leaders as designers, stewards and teachers who are responsible for building organisations. Senge's leaders promote creative tension between what is and what could be. They energise organisations to learn, adapt and move towards their vision.

The following case study illustrates a less than useful leadership style.

Philippa has been the senior member of the team of health visitors for the past 2 years and has been asked to identify a training needs analysis for the team for the next year. Personnel ring her 2 days after it is due in and ask for it at the latest that evening at 1700. At a regular team meeting that lunchtime she tells her colleagues, 'I'm being hassled for a training needs analysis by 5 o'clock. Any ideas anyone?'. 'I've got a free 10 minutes this afternoon; I know what we need so I'll write it,' says Rebecca. 'Thanks, that'll save any arguing,' says Philippa.

What style of leadership does Philippa show?

Comment

This approach is typical of the laissez-faire leader who operates with a reactive/crisis culture. The training needs analysis is a crucial feature for the success of the team in the future and is an area in which Philippa should have demonstrated a more effective leadership style. Further, had she managed her time, this problem would not have been handled by her allowing a colleague to quickly put

361

something together. How would a transformational leader have handled this issue?

This leads on to a consideration of one of the most pervasive arguments against breaking out of a crisis approach to managing care: lack of time.

TIME MANAGEMENT

Time is the only irreplaceable resource that individuals and organisations have to manage. Primarily time management requires a key question to be answered: 'What am I here for?'.

This question can be broken down into a number of additional questions.

- What are the essentials of my job/business?
- What will my boss and customers expect me to achieve?
- What should I *not* spend my time doing?
- What should I delegate to someone else?
- What are my role outcomes?

Time management allows the focus of energy to be on the expected outcomes of the business. This may be influenced by what has happened before but, more importantly, is directed towards the future. Effective time management allows all tasks to be considered in two ways. First, the simple 4Ds.

Do → Now
Delay → Do later
Ditch → Do much later or never
Delegate → Someone else does!

Or in a more complex form all work can be considered with regard to its importance and urgency as shown in Figure 15.1.

Using such an approach ensures tasks are allocated time that reflects their significance to the goals of the individual or organisation and time is set aside for additional and unexpected work.

TAKING RISKS

The final consideration in this chapter that explores reflection-before-action and proactivity is the need to embrace risk taking. It is not enough to accept an ever-changing future; it is more important to 'make things happen' and this will often involve taking risks.

Drucker (1989) emphasised the importance of maximising opportunities rather than minimising risks. He indicated the

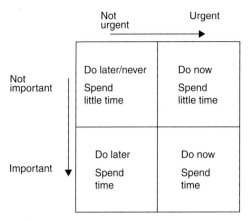

Figure 15.1 Effective time management of tasks.

importance of considering the organisation as a whole when assessing risk, rather than in parts. Risks need to be carefully evaluated and again this emphasises the need for a proactive approach. Risks assessment should seek to eliminate them by anticipating them. However, if mistakes occur they should become the focus for learning and not a trigger for reaction or crisis management. Mistakes, as mentioned earlier, should not be pathologised towards individuals but, as part of a 'no-blame culture', be a part of learning.

CONCLUSION

We live in a dynamic, creative and ever-changing world and must accept that or suffer the consequences. Sitting like King Canute, willing the tide of change to turn, will lead to disaster. If health care professionals are not, as individuals, making the future happen then someone else will and nurses will have to accept it. Nursing will be delivered tomorrow differently from today and exactly how this happens is a major professional responsibility. Health care staff are good at 'blame culture' and almost seem to prefer to blame anyone else, for their education, salaries, status and position in health care. However, Eleanor Roosevelt suggested, 'No one can devalue you without your consent'.

This chapter is a wake-up call for those working in health care. Chaos is the paradigm of the new millennium and being proactive in the face of it is preferable to 'watching things happen' or, worse still, not realising they are happening.

Crisis management: creating order out of chaos

References

Apps J 1985 Improving practice in continuing education: modern approaches for understanding the field and determining priorities. Jossey-Bass, San Francisco

Benner P 1984 From novice to expert. Addison-Wesley, California

Covey S 1992 The seven habits of highly effective people. Simon and Schuster, London

Drucker P 1989 Managing for results. Heinemann Professional, London

Ecclestone K 1995 The reflective practitioner: mantra or model for emancipation? Unpublished paper. University of Central Lancashire

Flanagan J 1954 The critical incident technique. Psychological Bulletin 51: 327–358

Hawkins P, Shohet R 1989 Supervision in the helping professions. Open University Press, Milton Keynes

Iles V 1997 Really managing health care. Open University Press, Buckingham

Johnson G, Scholes J 1999 Exploring corporate strategy, 5th edn. Prentice Hall, London

Kierkegaard S 1955 Kierkegaard: selected and edited by WH Auden. Cassell, London

Lewin K 1939 Patterns of aggressive behaviour in experimentally created social climates. Journal of Social Psychology 10: 271–299

Manthey M 1980 The practice of primary nursing. Blackwell, London

McDaniel C, Stumpf L 1993 The organisational culture. Journal of Nursing Administration 4: 54–60

Mezirow J 1990 Fostering critical reflection in adulthood. Jossey-Bass, San Francisco

Mezirow J 1991 Transformation dimensions of adult learning, Jossey-Bass, San Francisco

NHS Executive 1997 The new NHS: modern, dependable. DoH, London

Pedlar M, Burgoyne J, Boydell T 1991 The learning company. McGraw Hill, New York

Secretary of State for Health 2000 The NHS Plan. The Stationery Office, Norwich

Seedhouse D 1994 Fortress NHS: a philosophical review of the NHS. Wiley, Chichester

Senge P 1990 The fifth discipline. Doubleday, New York

Wheatley M 1992 Leadership and the new science. Berrett-Koehler, San Francisco

Application **15:1**

Mary Cooke

Interview with a clinical manager in A&E

The interviewee, an experienced member of the A&E team, sees her role as very much being in the centre of crisis management. However, she differentiates between levels of crisis and comments on how she uses her experience and learning to manage in this environment. She accepts that other individuals may have different styles of dealing with crisis management but emphasises the importance of reflection whatever process is used.

Manager: Managers in health care; there are, I suppose, two groups of managers now. Managers like me who worked clinically. Most of my career has been in A&E and that's been about, for the most part, crisis management in terms of not knowing what's coming through the door next and then being able to react to that. I guess that some of what we do is proactive because we have already thought through what we are going to do with a particular patient with a particular diagnosis, taking into account that there are other factors that need to be considered.

Then there are the group of managers who come up via a management training scheme or come from a different setting where they have really been brought up to be much more proactive. They plan and aim to get it right first or trust that what they put in place will actually work. I think that there are those two types and we probably end up with the same thing but the way that we actually get to the outcome is possibly different, particularly our thinking processes.

For example, maybe we think more quickly and miss out some of the steps that another type of manager would go through. I suppose in A&E you don't have an awful lot of time really, so you dismiss those steps quickly instead of working through them.

Interviewer: And the safety features of those steps are built into your planning?

Manager: Yes and I guess that what a manager like me will do is to use that experience and put it into management of other things that you do. But projects may sometimes fall down because you do actually then need to revert to that step-by-step process, much more methodical and probably taking much more visible steps.

Interviewer: So when you are making your managerial decisions from an A&E clinical historical perspective, is it intuition that you are using to move through those stages or is it knowing that you can from experience?

Manager: I am sure a lot of it is experience. It's actually saying I've been there before, this is what I did and this is what the outcome was. It feels as though it's the same and I can use that process, that very quick process that gets me to where I want to be. Or, if it didn't work before but it feels the same, then what was it that I could have done that would have made a difference? So I would say that a lot of it is experience.

However, I am sure that the formal management training that I have had along the way has helped. I guess the one that has the biggest impact was probably the managing health services course because I use some of the tools that I learnt, some of the theory when I'm in practice. I see that more in reflection than perhaps when I'm doing it.

Interviewer: So you reflect while you're doing it or you reflect on what's happened, using the theoretical background. Where do you bring that into your personal learning?

Manager: I suppose I bring that in when I think about the way I'm going to do something. Sometimes the theory will sit there and seem quite real, sometimes it will not. But then I begin to think of what options I am going to use this time, which one is most appropriate for what I've got to do.

Interviewer: And do you do that with a specific outcome in mind?

Manager: When I'm dealing with people then generally I do. With people I tend to have a strategy and I've learnt that strategy in a formal sense but I've also learnt it from other people who've acted as role models. There are some things that role modelling can help you with no end.

Interviewer: Do you see yourself as a role model for other people?

Manager: I would like to think that I was a role model. There are some things that I would like to rub out and have another go at. I like to think that I'm a role model, particularly for fairness, because I think that one of the things that makes you a reasonable manager is fairness. If you are unfair, things can go completely wrong. Being fair enables you to manage the biggest thing which is managing people.

Interviewer: Do you have any resources that you draw upon in order to use your strategies?

Manager: Yes and that resource is different depending on what I'm doing. I can go out into the department to find some of the resources that I need but I use other people quite a lot, people around the trust because it's their speciality.

Interviewer: Getting back to how you learn from the strategies that you have used and then disseminate that as best practice to other people. Apart from those things that you would rather forget about, what about things that you have learned from? Are there best ways of doing things in this particular trust because of the culture of the trust that wouldn't necessarily be helpful elsewhere?

Manager: It's difficult to make that sort of comparison because I have been with this trust a long time and because things have changed such a lot. But I suppose that if I feel that something has worked well, if it's something that's consistent, then I will use that in teaching people shadowing me. I don't say, this is the only way to do it, but this is the way that I have found has worked for me in a particular situation.

Interviewer: What about the use of scenario building and planning? I know that comes into training specifically for A&E staff. Do you see it as a good way of building up resources as a manager and for your staff?

Manager: It is a good way of doing it but it's probably not the easiest. Generally, somebody wants something done, they want it now and they haven't got time to do it themselves. There is the temptation, and I fell into that trap, of doing it yourself as opposed to showing somebody the way to go and supporting them in doing it themselves. I will try and do that but sometimes I will have to sort of remind myself or somebody might remind me to do that. There is the temptation to help the situation along by doing it yourself because more and more I can see how stressed staff are and I feel that I'm distanced from it.

Interviewer: You have explained about developing strategies for dealing with crises where there are some certainties and you are able to plan to some extent. But what tools do you call on to deal with situations of increasing uncertainty? How can you cut down this uncertainty?

Manager: I guess there are some fundamental things, interpersonal skills, communication, not being afraid to ask, having confidence and looking at somebody who manages uncertainty well with good outcomes and following that. We tend to have this very narrow path that we tread because our experience is fairly narrow but, as we tread the path, it hopefully stretches out so that there are more and more options. Often there is not one particular way of doing something to get a good outcome. It's about trying to choose the one that fits best with the information that you have got, the task that you have to complete. It is experience and not being afraid to use what you have got around you, to help you to actually learn. It is making sure that you have considered all of these things.

I suppose all of us start off with this fairly rigid frame . . . you know, just do this, if it's not like this, then do that. But managing uncertainty is about taking risks. I wouldn't have said that I was a person that takes risks. However, there are times when I consciously calculate the balance between two options. Neither of them is particularly what I want to do but this one I can justify probably more than that one. It has to be about stopping and thinking it through. It's all too easy where you are being pressurised either by the service because there are lots of other things to do or by the person that you are working with who wants things to be done and dusted quite quickly, you can be pressurised into missing things. But if I have this plan that addresses all these issues, then whatever happens at the end, I will have done the best that I can do and I can justify my actions.

One thing that helps in this whole process, and I enjoyed, was having a trainee with me for 3 days. That's quite good fun because you end up hearing yourself talking about what you do and the way that you do things and that's quite good in confirming things that you put into practice but you don't think about. But every now and again you do need to sort it out in your mind. I think, as a manager, one of things that I should do more often is that, if somebody comes along to me and they are interested and I can feel that interest, I should think through and explain the processes I have used.

Interviewer: It's a kind of partnership.

Manager: Yes, but you need to feel that somebody wants something from you and the benefit of the experiences that you have is one way of being able to give something back into the system.

Index

Indexer's note: Pagination prefixed by (A) refers to Applications

A&E manager
    interview with, (A) 365–8
Accidents
    distinction from incidents, 330–1
    monitoring, 334
Accountability, 301
    measures, 16–18
    user participation, 159–61
ACN see Associate Charge Nurse
Action for Sick Children, 191
Action on Smoking in Health, 186
Acts of Parliament, 8
    Community Care (Direct Payments)
        Act 1996, 190
    Data Protection Act 1998, 214
    Disability Discrimination Act 1999, 190
    European Rights Act 1998, 159
    Health & Safety at Work Act 1974, 338
    Human Rights Act 1998, 186, 218, 331;
        2000, 191
    Limitation Act 1980, 305
    Local Government Act 2000, 217
    NHS and Community Care Act 1990,
        31, 194, 307
Acupuncture, 169
Addenbrooke's NHS Trust, Cambridge,
    UK, 281
    maternity services critical incidence
        report, 332, 333
    nursing strategic direction document,
        244–5, 246
    standard for nursing documentation
        audit, 320–1
Advanced practice roles
    development of, (A) 39–45
Aggressive character type, 267, 268
Aims and outcomes of decisions
    matching, 7
Alzheimer's Disease Society
    website, 200
Annual patient surveys, 217
Arnstein's ladder of citizen participation,
    188–9
Arthritis and Rheumatism Council
    website, 200
Arthritis Association, 193
Assertiveness
    exercises, (A) 276–7
Associate Charge Nurse (ACN), 115

Association for Improvement in Maternity
    Services, 191
Association for Improvement in
    Midwifery Services, 186
Asthma and Allergy Research
    website, 200
Audits, 241
    care outcomes, 164
    documentation, (A) 319–22
    working areas, 334
Australia
    patients' rights, 208
    recruitment from, 23
Autocratic leadership, 360
Autonomy
    in implementing strategic decisions,
        256–71

Behavioural disorder unit manager
    interview with, (A) 72–5
Belbin's team roles, 264–5; (A)
    148–50
Biotechnology, 225
BMA see British Medical Association
Bounded rationality, 97
British Diabetic Association, 191
British Digestive Foundation
    website, 201
British Heart Foundation, 191, 281
British Medical Association (BMA), 159,
    223
Bureaucratic culture/structure, 56–7, 357–8

Cambridge Cancer Help Centre, 173
Campaign against Health Fraud see
    Healthwatch
Cancer Bacup, 186, 193
    website, 201
Cancer-Help, 191
Cancer Research Campaign, 281
Cancer support groups, (A) 173–4
Career development of nurses, 122–3
Carers, 168, 190
Caring, diminution of, 226
Case studies
    complaints and complainants, (A)
        180–1
    development of specialist and
        advanced practice roles, (A) 39–45

Case studies (*Contd.*)
    evaluating decisions in a rural practice,
      (A) 108–12
    influencing decisions through group
      processes, 140
    reengineering, (A) 251–5
Centre for Health Information Quality,
    202
Change in health care structures
    history of, 15–16
Change theory, 336–7
Chaos and complexity theory, 355–6
Character types, 267–8
Charters
    Charter of the United Nations (1945),
      211
    Citizen's Charter, 203
    Mental Health Charter, 204
    Patient's Charter, 17, 204, 215–16, 220
    Primary Care Charter, 204, 221
CHCs *see* Community Health Councils
Chemical pathology unit
    strategic information planning, (A)
      247–50
'Cherry-picking' solutions, 253
CHCs *see* Community Health Councils
CHI *see* Commission for Health
    Improvement
Chief Nursing Officers (CNOs), 31
Children's services
    risk management, (A) 347–50
CI *see* Consumers International
Citizens
    distinction from consumers, 194
Citizens' Advice Bureaux, 162, 168
Citizen's Charter, 203
Citizens' juries, 196
Civil service, 8–9
Claims against NHS, 305, 324
Classical management, 60
Clinical audit committees, 136–7
Clinical governance, 166–7, 241, 326
*Clinical Governance: Quality in the New
    NHS* (NHS Executive, 1999), 324
Clinical Negligence Scheme for Trusts
    (CNST), 298
Clinical practice development (CPD)
    research studies, 281–9, 291–2
Clinical supervision, 109
Clinical trials management, 49
'Closed-mind' decision making system,
    95, 96
Cluster structure, 58
CNOs *see* Chief Nursing Officers
CNST *see* Clinical Negligence Scheme for
    Trusts
College of Health, 202
Commission for Health Improvement
    (CHI), 110, 193, 218, 297
Commissioning for health care, 241
Committees
    access to information, 135

emergency meetings, 134
expert advice, 134
forward planning, 135
meeting dates, 134
reasons for using, 136–7
record keeping, 134–5
selection of members, 133–4
statement of purpose, 135–6
see also Groups, organisational
Community Care (Direct Payments) Act
    1996, 190
Community development, 163–9
Community Health Councils (CHCs), 159,
    160, 161, 181, 220
Community-oriented primary care
    (COPC), 163
Competitive forces external to
    organisations, 93
Complaints, (A) 180–1
    as part of user involvement, 163–5
    right to make, 214
Complaints procedures
    and patients' rights, 205
    and regulatory bodies, 300
Complementary therapies, 169
Completer team role, 149, 264
Compliant character type, 267, 268
Confidentiality
    and patient's family, 333
    and patients' rights, 205
Consent
    and patients' rights, 205
    legal requirements for validity, 306
Conservatism, 10
Conservative governments/policies, 19,
    203, 235
Consultant nurses, 43–4
Consultations, doctor/patient, 158
Consumer groups, 182–99
Consumerism, 204, 210–11
Consumers
    distinction from citizens, 194
Consumers International (CI)
    framework for patients' rights, 211–12
    surveys, 208
Contacts, professional, 138–9
Contingency approach to management,
    116
Control
    financial, 13
    judicial, 9
    political, 7–9
    professional knowledge, 14
    psychological, 266–9
Control techniques, organisational, 259–62
Coordinator team role, 148, 264
COPC *see* Community-oriented primary
    care
Coronary Prevention Group, 191
CoSHH Regulations, 334
Covey's seven habits, 359
CPD *see* Clinical practice development

Creative decision making in groups, 137–8
Crisis management, 351–64
  legal and ethical implications, 295–313
Crown immunity
  removal from NHS, 307
Crown indemnity, 307, 308
Culture, organisational, 50
  and performance, 51
  and risk management, 298–300
  and structure, 55–8
  changing of , 19, 336–7
  control techniques, 262
  management of, 4–5, 59–63
  reflection in job descriptions, (A) 65–71
  subcultures, 54
  transmission and maintenance of, 52–3
  types of, 357–9
Customers
  definition of, 94

Daily decision making, typical, (A) 100–7
Data Protection Act 1998, 214
Deaf and hard of hearing website, 201
Decision making
  and Belbin's team roles, (A) 148–50
  and clinical research, 280–90
  and organisational culture, 50–64
  daily, (A) 100–7
  in groups, 128–38
  individual/organisational parallels, 80–3
  influence of professional and statutory
    bodies, 27–38
  political context of, 3–21
  strategic, 233–46
  user participation in, 151–229
Decision making, conflicts in
  nursing home management, (A) 125–7
  urgency of, 120–2
Decisions
  categories of, 81–2, 83–7
  delayed, 82–3
  non-rationality, 82
Decisions, local
  role of RCN interest groups, (A) 46–9
Defence mechanisms, psychoanalytic,
  267–8
Delegation, 118–19
Democracy
  decision making in, 4–5
  health service provision in, 194–5
Democratic leadership, 360
Denmark
  patients' rights, 209
Dental phobics information website, 201
Department of Health publications
  A First Class Service (1998), 297, 326
  Local Voices (1992), 193
  Making a Difference (1999), 43
  The New NHS: Modern, Dependable
    (1997), 32, 326; (1999) 158, 160
  The NHS Plan (2000), 158–9, 161, 170,
    186, 223, 224–8, 241

websites, (A) 25–6
Detached character type, 267, 268
Devolution, 225
Diabetes website, 201
Disability Discrimination Act 1999, 190
Disabled Living Foundation
  website, 201
Discussion questions
  complaints and complainants, 181
  internet use, 26
  legal liability of guidelines and
    protocols, (A) 314–18
  user empowerment, 179
Disease, shifts in burden of, 226
Diverse Minds programme, 175
Doctor, right to choose a, 214
Doctors
  incentives for professional
    development, 219
Documentation
  risk assessment, (A) 319–22
  see also Patients' records
Double-loop learning, 96
Duty of care principle, 308, 309

Efficiency tests
  measurement of outcomes, 226–8
Electronic health records, 322
ELS *see* Existing Liabilities Scheme
Employees/Employers
  responsibilities for risk management,
    338–42
Empowerment of patients, 155–72; (A)
  173–6, 177–9
Environments, organisational, 92–4
Epilepsy website, 201
Ethical conflicts
  in nursing homes, (A) 125–6, 127
  in patient care decisions, 310–12
Ethical considerations
  and decision/policy making, 191–2, 302–3
  and patients' rights, 205
  clinical trials, 49
  networking, 147
Ethnic minority users, 168–9, 175
Europe
  patients' rights, 204–8
European Community, 8
European Convention on Human Rights
  (1950), 211, 331, 333
European Rights Act 1998, 159
Evaluation of decisions/strategy, 95
  in rural practice, (A) 108–12
  see also Audits
Exercises
  assertiveness, (A) 276–7
  leadership skills, (A) 278–9
  risk management implementation
    strategy, (A) 344–6
Existing Liabilities Scheme (ELS), 298
Experimentation on human beings
  right to refuse, 211

Index

Fairness, 366
Feedback, learning from, 95–6
Financial control, organisational, 13
    A First Class Service (DoH, 1998), 297, 326
Force field analysis, 336–7, 344
Foreseeability of harm, 308
Freud's developmental theory, 266–7

Gelling, Leslie, 46
Gendering of professions, 121
General Medical Council (GMC), 223
General Nursing Councils (GNCs), 29
Geographical inequality of health care,
    157, 158, 223
Global health targets, 240
GMC *see* General Medical Council
GNCs *see* General Nursing Councils
GP fundholding, 237
GRASP © Systems, 254, 255, 344
Groups, organisational
    brainstorming, 137–8
    conflicts between members, 132
    development of meetings, 129–30
    leadership and management, 131
    membership, 130
    networking, 138–42
    pressures to conform to norm, 265
    reasons for joining, 131
    role distribution, 131–2; *see also* Belbin's
        team roles
    team building, 133
    work environment, 130–1
    see also Committees *and* Interest groups
Groups, patient *see* Consumer groups *and*
    User support groups/ organisations
Guidelines, 331
    legal liability, (A) 314–18

Hakesley-Brown, Roswyn, 49
Hazard warnings, 334
Health & Safety Assessments, 334
Health & Safety at Work Act 1974, 338
Health action zones, 236
Health care, right to, 213
Health for All programme, 240
Health indices, 236
Health insurance systems, 207
Health Select Committee, 164, 300
Health Service Commissioner (HSC), 300
Health Service Ombudsman, 164, 181
Health services
    local authority scrutiny, 217–18
Health surveys, 236
Health systems
    world ranking, 184–5
Health visitors, 31
Health workers
    role in developing strategy, 243–4
Healthwatch (*formerly* Campaign against
    Health Fraud), 191
Help for Health Trust, 202
Hepatitis Network website, 201

Higher level practice, 42–3
History of change in health care
    structures, 15–16
Homoeopathy, 169
Hong Kong
    patients' rights, 208–9
Hot desking, 334
HSC *see* Health Service Commissioner
Human relations management, 60–1
Human Rights Act 1998, 186, 218, 331;
    2000, 191

Implementation, strategic, 18–19, 95
    assertiveness and leadership skills, 276–9
    autonomy and initiative, 256–71;
        (A) 272–5
    in clinical research, 280–90
    practitioner role in, 233–46
    reengineering, (A) 251–5
    risk management, (A) 344–6
    user involvement in, (A) 247–50
Implementer team role, 149, 264
Incidents
    distinction from accidents, 330–1
Incremental decision making, 97–8
Indonesia
    patients' rights, 209
Inequalities of health care, 242–3
    geographical areas, 157, 158, 223
Infant mortality, 223
Information, Patient *see* Confidentiality
    and Patients' records
Information gathering
    chemical pathology unit, (A) 247–50
    for strategic analysis, 92–4
Information services for users, 193
Information technology, 215
Initiative
    in implementing strategic decisions,
        256–71
    managerial perceptions of, (A) 272–5
Institute of Psychiatry website, 201
Interest groups, 28, 139
    role in local decisions, (A) 46–9
Internet, 215, 227
    use for networking, 139
    see also Websites
Interviewing/interviews, 23, 24
    behavioural disorder unit manager, (A)
        72–5
    clinical A&E manager, (A) 365–8
    middle managers (initiative in the
        workplace), (A) 272–5
Involvement in decision making
    and organisational culture, 61–3
Ireland
    patients' rights, 209
Irreversible decisions
    avoidance of, 97
Isolation, professional
    in big organisations, 144
    in rural practice, 108–9

Index

Job descriptions, managerial
  reflection of organisational culture, (A) 65–71
Job fairs, 23–4
Judge Institute of Management Studies, 281, 282
Judiciary, 9

Keen, Ann, 34
King's Fund, 35, 146, 163, 202
Knowledge, control of, 14

Labour governments/policies, 19, 20, 34, 160, 186, 187, 216, 237
Laissez-faire leadership, 360
Language communication problems, 168
Le Grand's theory of social behaviour, 189–90
Leadership, 56
  exercises, (A) 278–9
  practice development, 292
  styles, 360–2
League tables, 215, 237
Learning/development culture, 358
Legal cases
  duty of care, 308
  foreseeability of harms concept, 308
  liability for guidelines and protocols, (A) 314–18
  neighbour principle, 308
  standard of care, 310
Legal implications
  risk and crisis management, 295–313
Life expectancy, 223
Lifespan Trust, Cambridgeshire, 33
Lifting policies, 341
Limitation Act 1980, 305
Live studies, 253–5
Local advisory forums, 217
Local Government Act 2000, 217
Local strategy
  influence of national policy, 234–40
  see also Implementation, strategic
Local Voices (DoH, 1992), 193

Maastricht Treaty, Social Chapter of, 8
Making a Difference (DoH, 1999), 43
Management science/theories, 115–16
  and organisational culture, 59–63
Managers
  interviews with, (A) 72–5, 365–8
  job descriptions, (A) 65–71
  networking, (A) 144–7
  perceptions of initiative, (A) 272–5
  teams, (A) 149–50
  transition from practitioners, 113–24
  typical days (A) 100–6
Marie Stopes Institute
  website, 201
Market model, 17
  see also Private health care
Maternity services critical incidence report, 332, 333

Matrix structure, 57–8
Measles, mumps, rubella (MMR) vaccine, 240
Media, 225
  raising awareness of patients' rights, 185, 206, 214–15
Medical errors, 324
Medical Research Council (MRC), 281
Mental health
  empowerment, (A) 177–9
  support groups, (A) 175–6
Mental Health Charter, 204
Mental Health Foundation
  website, 201
Mentors, 139
Midgeley's system boundaries, 192
Midwives, 31
MIND, 175, 186, 191
Mindfulness, 354
MINDLINK, 175
Mission, organisational, 89–90
Mission statements, 234
'Mixed scanning', 98
MMR *see* Measles, mumps, rubella vaccine
Moffat, Laura, 34
Monitor-evaluator team role, 149, 264
Monitoring, accident, 334
Motivation studies, 115
MRC *see* Medical Research Council
Multiple sclerosis website, 201
Muslim patients, 168–9

NAMRU *see* Nursing and Midwifery Research Unit
National Childbirth Trust, 191
National Health Service (NHS), 30–2
  claims against, 305, 324
  league tables, 215, 237
  managerial job descriptions, 66–7
  'new' NHS, 352–3
  provider/purchaser policy, 235–7
  removal of Crown Immunity, 307
  see also under NHS
National Health Service Litigation Authority (NHSLA), 298
National Institute of Clinical Excellence (NICE), 297
National policy
  influence on local strategy, 234–40
National Schizophrenia Society, 186
National Service Frameworks (NSFs), 157, 297
National Statistical Office
  website, 237
National Vocational Qualifications (NVQs), 14
Negligence claims *see* Claims against NHS
Neighbour principle, 308
Netherlands
  health care structures, 15
  patients' rights, 209

Index

Networking, 109, 138–42; (A) 144–7
Networks, 72–3
  patients' rights, 207
  The New NHS: Modern, Dependable
    (DoH, 1997), 32, 326; (1999) 158, 160
New Zealand
  patients' rights, 209
  recruitment from, 23
NGOs *see* Non-governmental
  organisations
NHS and Community Care Act 1990, 31,
  194, 307
NHS Centre for Reviews and
  Dissemination (CRD), 202
NHS Direct, 165, 187, 227
  The NHS Plan (DoH, 2000), 158–9, 161,
    170, 186, 241
  and patients' rights and
    responsibilities, 216–18; (A) 223–9
NHS *see also under* National Health
  Service
NHS Trust Nursing and Midwifery
  Advisory Committee, 23
NHSLA *see* National Health Service
  Litigation Authority
NICE *see* National Institute of Clinical
  Excellence
NMC *see* Nursing and Midwifery Council
Non-governmental organisations (NGOs),
  206
Non-maleficience, principle of, 295
Non-programmed decisions, 83, 84
Nordic School of Public Health, 207
Norway
  health care structures, 15
NSFs *see* National Service Frameworks
Nurse consultants, 43–4
Nurse researchers, 46–7, 48–9
Nurses/nursing, 31
  and changes in health care system, 33
  and political decision making, 33–7
  career specialisation, 40, 122–3
  negligence, 300
  professional development, 35–6
  professional status, 32
  subordination of, 32, 36
  training, 32, 41
  see also Clinical practice development;
    Practice roles *and* Practitioners
Nursing and Midwifery Council (NMC),
  29–30, 32, 167
Nursing and Midwifery Research Unit
  (NAMRU), 48
Nursing home management
  conflicts in decision making, (A) 125–7
NVQs *see* National Vocational
  Qualifications

Objectives, organisational, 90–2
Operational decisions, 83, 84–5, 106
Organisational approach to management,
  116

Organisational level change, 18–19
OSCs *see* Overview and Scrutiny
  Committees
Outcomes, strategic
  visibility of, 258
  see also Aims and outcomes of
    decisions
Outpatient department manager
  typical day, (A) 100–3
Overview and Scrutiny Committees
  (OSCs), 217–18

PAF *see* Performance Assessment
  Framework
PALS *see* Patient Advocacy and Liaison
  Service
Parkinson's Disease Society, 169, 186, 191
  website, 201
Participation of users in decision making,
  151–229
Patient Advocacy and Liaison Service
  (PALS), 159, 161–2, 166, 217
Patients
  empowerment, 155–72; (A) 173–6, 177–9
  representation on boards, 216
Patient's Charter, 17, 204, 215–16, 220
Patients' councils, 217
Patients' forums, 166, 216–17
Patient's Pictures, 201–2
Patients' records
  access to, 167, 205
  fragmentation, 140
Patients' rights
  and health care consumerism, 210–11
  and *The NHS Plan*, 216–18; (A) 223–9
  European, 204–8
  implications for professionals, 218–19
  international review, 208–10
  media role in, 214–15
  principles of statutory involvement,
    211–13
  see also Charters
PCGs *see* Primary care groups
PCTs *see* Primary care trusts
Peach, Sir Len 32
People First, 191
Performance Assessment Framework
  (PAF), 297
Periodic control decisions, 83, 85–6
Person culture, 58
PEST factors, 93
Philippines
  recruitment from, 23
Pilot studies, 253
Planning process, 87–9
Plant team role, 149, 264
Policies, national
  influence on local strategy, 234–40
Policy directives
  risk management, 296–8
Policy making
  and ethics, 191–2

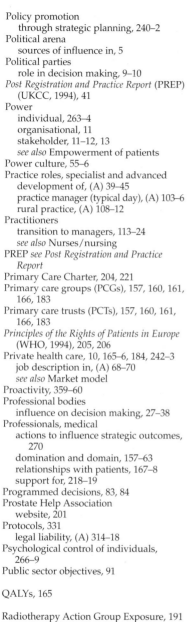

Policy promotion
   through strategic planning, 240–2
Political arena
   sources of influence in, 5
Political parties
   role in decision making, 9–10
Post Registration and Practice Report (PREP)
   (UKCC, 1994), 41
Power
   individual, 263–4
   organisational, 11
   stakeholder, 11–12, 13
   see also Empowerment of patients
Power culture, 55–6
Practice roles, specialist and advanced
   development of, (A) 39–45
   practice manager (typical day), (A) 103–6
   rural practice, (A) 108–12
Practitioners
   transition to managers, 113–24
   see also Nurses/nursing
PREP *see Post Registration and Practice Report*
Primary Care Charter, 204, 221
Primary care groups (PCGs), 157, 160, 161, 166, 183
Primary care trusts (PCTs), 157, 160, 161, 166, 183
Principles of the Rights of Patients in Europe (WHO, 1994), 205, 206
Private health care, 10, 165–6, 184, 242–3
   job description in, (A) 68–70
   see also Market model
Proactivity, 359–60
Professional bodies
   influence on decision making, 27–38
Professionals, medical
   actions to influence strategic outcomes, 270
   domination and domain, 157–63
   relationships with patients, 167–8
   support for, 218–19
Programmed decisions, 83, 84
Prostate Help Association
   website, 201
Protocols, 331
   legal liability, (A) 314–18
Psychological control of individuals, 266–9
Public sector objectives, 91

QALYs, 165

Radiotherapy Action Group Exposure, 191
Rational decision making, 97
RCN *see* Royal College of Nursing
Reactive/crisis culture, 358
Records *see* Patients' records *and* Risk assessment records
Recruitment, (A) 22–5
Reengineering, (A) 251–5
Reflective practice, 353–5

Reporting, accident/incident, 330–4
Reporting of Injuries, Diseases and Dangerous Occurrences Regulations (RIDDOR) (HSE, 1995), 334, 341–2
Research
   and patients' rights, 205
   to underpin decision making, 280–90
Research nurses, 46–7, 48–9
Research Society, RCN, 47, 48
Resource-investigator team role, 149, 264
Resource scarcity, 312
Restructuring of health care system, 15–16
RIDDOR *see Reporting of Injuries, Diseases and Dangerous Occurrences Regulations*
Rights *see* Patients' rights
Risk assessment records, 339–40
   importance of, (A) 319–22
Risk management
   business case for, 328
   children's services, (A) 347–50
   defined, 347–8
   framework, 327
   legal and ethical implications, 295–313
   motives, 303–4
   programmes, 325–7
   role of department/team, 329–34
   strategy implementation, (A) 344–6
Risk officers/representatives, role of, 335
Risk reduction
   induction programmes, 337–8
Risks
   categories, 305–6
   consequences, 307–9
   elimination, 304–7
   public expectations, 309–10
   taking, 362–3
Role culture, 56–7
Role transition
   from practitioner to manager, 114–15
Royal College of Nursing (RCN), 30, 34–5
   role of interest groups in local decisions, (A) 46–9
Rules
   as organisational control techniques, 259–61
Rural practice
   decision evaluation, (A) 108–12

Sainsbury Centre for Mental Health, 176, 193
Salvage, Jane, 35
San Marino
   patients' rights, 209
Schizophrenia Society, 193
Scope of Professional Practice (UKCC, 1992), 35–6, 40
Scottish Association of Health Councils, 202
Seacroft Hospital, Leeds, 140
Security at work assessments, 334
Self-help groups, 191
Self-regulation, professional, 28–30

Index

Shaper team role, 148, 264
Single-loop learning, 96
SMART acronym, 90
Socialism, 10
Specialist roles
  development of, (A) 39–45
  specialist nursing roles, 122–3
  specialist team role, 149, 264
Spina bifida and hydrocephalus website, 201
Staff intimidation, 181
Stakeholder analysis, 11–12
Stakeholders
  health care professionals as, 12–13
Standard of care, 310
State institutions
  role in decision making, 7–9
Status quo
  challenges to, 302
  pressures to maintain, 259
Statutory bodies
  influence on decision making, 27–38
Statutory rights *see* Patients' rights
Stephen Covey's first habit, 359–60
Strategic analysis
  information gathering 92–4; (A) 247–50
Strategic choice, 94–5
Strategic review and evaluation, 95
Strategies, local
  influence of national policy, 234–40
Strategy *see* Decision making *and*
  Implementation, strategic
Structure, organisational
  and culture, 55–8
Success factors, organisational, 91
Survivors Speak Out, 175, 191
Sweden
  health care structures, 15
  patients' rights, 209
SWOT analysis, 94
Systems approach to management, 116

Targets
  as control techniques, 261–2
  for global health, 240
Task culture, 57–8
Team roles *see* Belbin's team roles *and*
  Groups, organisational: role
  distribution
Team worker team role, 149, 264
Teenage pregnancy reduction policies, 238–40, 243–4
Terrence Higgins Trust, 191
  website, 200
Theories
  change, 336–7
  chaos and complexity, 355–6
  management, 59–63
  psychoanalysis, 266–7
  user involvement, 187–91
Time management, 362, 363
Total quality management (TQM), 16

Trainees
  expected standard of care, 310
Training
  nurses, 32, 41
  risk management, 335–6
Trust within organisations, 96
Twins and Multiple Births Association
  website, 201

UK Advocacy Network, 175
UKCC, 29, 41, 42, 167, 300
UKCC publications
  Post Registration and Practice Report
    (PREP) (1994), 41
  Scope of Professional Practice (1992),
    35–6, 40
UNESCO, 312
UNISON, 22, 23, 35
United States of America
  health care system, 16
  medical errors, 324
  patients' rights, 209
Universal Declaration of Human Rights
  (1948), 211
University of Cambridge, UK, 207, 281
University of Canterbury, UK, 207
Urgent decisions, conflicts in, 120–2
User support groups/organisations, (A)
  173–6
  websites, (A) 200–2
Users *see* Carers; Consumers *and* Patients

'Value chain analysis', 93
Values
  in risk management, 300–3
Voluntary charitable associations, 185–6, 190
Voluntary Organisations Internet Server, 201

Web structure, 55–6
Websites
  Department of Health, 241; (A) 25–6
  National Statistical Office, 237
  recruitment, 24
  user support organisations, (A) 200–1
  see also Internet
Wellcome Trust, 281
WHO *see* World Health Organization
Withdrawal of Guidance on the Extended Role
  of the Nurse, 40
Women's infertility website, 201
Work colleagues, previous, 139
Working area audits, 334
Working relationships
  and subcultures, 54
Workload measurement
  research methodologies, 255
World Health Assembly, 36, 240
World Health Organization (WHO), 182,
  184, 240, 297, 319
World Health Organization publications
  Principles of the Rights of Patients in
    Europe (1994), 205, 206

05194475

Index